CLINICAL PATHWAYS IN NURSING

A Guide to Managing Care from Hospital to Home

CLINICAL PATHWAYS IN NURSING

A Guide to Managing Care from Hospital to Home

Gail P. Poirrier, RN, DNS
Acting Dean and Associate Professor
College of Nursing
University of Southwestern Louisiana
Lafayette

Melinda G. Oberleitner, RN, DNS, OCN
Acting Department Head and Associate Professor
Department of Nursing
College of Nursing
University of Southwestern Louisiana
Lafayette

SPRINGHOUSE CORPORATION • SPRINGHOUSE, PENNSYLVANIA

Staff

Vice President
Matthew Cahill

Clinical Director
Judith Schilling McCann, RN, MSN

Art Director
John Hubbard

Managing Editor
David Moreau

Clinical Consultants
Clare Brabson, RN, BSN; Patricia Kardish Fischer, RN, BSN

Editors
Karen Diamond, Margaret MacKay Eckman,
Carol Munson

Copy Editors
Cynthia C. Breuninger (manager), Mary T. Durkin,
Brenna H. Mayer, Pamela Wingrod

Designers
Arlene Putterman (associate art director), Cindy
Marczuk (designer), StellarVisions (project manager)

Manufacturing
Deborah Meiris (director), Patricia K. Dorshaw
(manager), Otto Mezei (book production manager)

Editorial Assistants
Beverly Lane, Liz Schaeffer

Indexer
Gerry Lynn Messner

Printed in the United States of America.

CPIN-011198

Ɍ A member of the Reed Elsevier plc group

Library of Congress Cataloging-in-Publication Data
Poirrier, Gail P.
   Clinical pathways in nursing: a guide to managing care from hospital to home/Gail P. Poirrier, Melinda G. Oberleitner.
      p.   cm.
   Includes bibliographical references and index.
   1. Nursing care plans. 2. Critical path analysis. I. Oberleitner, Melinda G. II. Title.
RT49.P65 1999
610.73—ddc21   98-38636
ISBN 0-87434-930-3 (alk. paper)   CIP

Contents

Contributors, consultants, and reviewers

Contributors

Regina L. Payne, RN, EdD, CETN
Professor
Department of Nursing
Florida Gulf Coast University
Fort Meyers

Martha L. Kuhns, RN, PhD
Associate Professor
Department of Nursing
University of Southwestern Louisiana
Lafayette

Consultants and reviewers

Eugene Anderson, RN, MSN, CCRN
Patient Care Specialist: MICU/SICU/SCU
Lehigh Valley Hospital, Allentown, Pa.

Elizabeth A. Ayello, RN,CS, PhD, CETN
Clinical Assistant Professor, School of Education, Div. of Nursing
Clinical Associate Nurse, Enterostomal Therapy Service, Dept. of Nursing
New York University

Linda Carman Copel, RN,CS, PhD, CGP
Associate Professor
Villanova (Pa.) University

Diane M. Ellis, RN,CS, MSN, CCRN
Clinical Educator–Critical Care Neuro Clinical Specialist
Allegheny University Hospitals: Graduate, Philadelphia

Eileen Erskine, RN, MSN
Clinical Instructor, Howard Community College, Columbia, Md.
Staff Nurse, St. Joseph Medical Center, Towson, Md.

Mary Kay Flynn, RN, DNSc, CCRN
Professor of Nursing
Mesa Community College, Sun City, Ariz.

Latrell P. Fowler, RN, PhD
Assistant Professor
Medical University of South Carolina, Florence, S.C.

Ellie Z. Franges, RN, MSN, CNRN, CCRN
Director of Neuroscience Services
Sacred Heart Hospital, Allentown, Pa.

Bonita K. Handerhan, RN, MSN, CCRN
Critical Care Educator
North Penn Hospital, Lansdale, Pa.

Donna Iszler, RN,C, MA, MSN
Associate Professor, Psychiatric Nursing Education
University of North Dakota, Jamestown

Lisa Kosciolek, RN, BSN, CCRN
Staff Nurse, Neurosurgical–Trauma ICU
Hospital of the University of Pennsylvania, Philadelphia

Pat S. Kupina, RN, MSN
Nursing Educator
Joliet (Ill.) Junior College

Tamara Luedtke, RN, MSN, CCRN
Nurse Manager, Critical Care Unit
Hendrick Medical Center, Abilene, Tex.

Dawna Martich, RN, MSN
Clinical Manager
University Family Practice Associates, Inc
Moon Township, Pa.

Carol Lynn Maxwell-Thompson, RN, MSN, CCRN
University of Virginia School of Nursing Faculty, Charlottesville

Lora McGuire, RN, MS
Nursing Faculty and Pain Consultant
Joliet (Ill.) Junior College

Donna B. Schaffer, RN, BSN, CETN
Enterostomal Therapy Nurse–Education and Development
St. Joseph Medical Center, Joliet, Ill.

Brenda K. Shelton, RN, MS, CCRN, AOCN
Critical Care Clinical Nurse Specialist
The Johns Hopkins Oncology Center, Baltimore

Larry Simmons, RN, MSN
Clinical Instructor
UMKC School of Nursing, Kansas City, Mo.

Naomi Walpert, RN, MS, CDE
Clinical Nurse Specialist: Endocrinology
Sinai Hospital, Baltimore, Md.

Pamela A. Wendt, RN, BSN
Vice President of Clinical Services
Nursefinders, Inc., Arlington, Tex.

Preface

As managed care continues to drive health care delivery systems in our country, the role of the professional nurse will undergo profound change. To practice in today's health care environment, nurses must weave outcomes, cost, resources, and process within multiple or integrated care systems to expedite effective patient care.

Nursing education and practice must keep abreast of the rapid changes in care planning methods to prepare nurses to provide quality care and collaborative health care to consumers. Clinical pathways are tools that help the health care provider refocus roles to include accountability for outcomes throughout a patient's illness and take responsibility for length of stay and effective use of resources. These tools offer new alternatives to traditional care planning methods in a variety of health care settings.

The clinical pathways presented in this book generally cover a predictable course of illness, surgery, recovery, or event. They are designed for acute care hospital and home settings as opposed to critical care settings. This book provides a comprehensive approach to critically examining delivery of collaborative, outcome-driven health care across a timeline. The care settings represent the latest in health care trends, from preadmission to home care.

Other outstanding features of this book include:
- an emphasis on the nursing process as a conceptual and operational basis for clinical pathways
- an educational perspective in addition to a clinical perspective
- home care interventions and hospital care
- patient outcomes for home and hospital settings
- inclusion of multidisciplinary health team providers
- implications for nursing research
- patient education guides
- a listing of community resources to assist in discharge planning.

This book is an educational guide for nurses to use clinical pathways — within the context of the nursing process — to plan multidisciplinary health care delivery in the hospital and home settings. In the practice arena, this book will help nurses and health care providers to plan and deliver outcome-driven care.

This text will also help students and faculty in the teaching and learning process of providing care incrementally, day-by-day.

PART 1

Overview

Introduction to clinical pathways

Clinical pathways in nursing

Introduction to clinical pathways

The challenge of managed care

Managed care was originally intended to enhance health care delivery by setting and following primary care objectives, thereby decreasing the complications of disorders and effectively preventing an increase in disease. In the 1990s, its role has expanded dramatically in response to escalating health care costs, growing populations of elderly and uninsured patients, and decreasing government reimbursements.

The American Nurses Association (ANA) defines managed care as a health care system that integrates the financing and delivery of health care services to covered individuals, most often by arrangement with selected providers such as health maintenance organizations (HMOs) and preferred provider organizations (PPOs). Managed care is financed by prospective payments. A dollar amount is paid to the health care provider, who is then responsible for arranging the delivery of all health care services required by the covered individual under the terms of the contract.

Managed care today has several overall goals. It is expected to lower the costs for consumers of health care, improve their access to that care, improve communication among health care providers, maintain satisfactory levels of service and quality of care, improve consumer satisfaction with care delivery, and improve job satisfaction for health care providers.

In a managed care environment nurses are part of an interdisciplinary team that follows patients from preadmission through postdischarge care at home in an effort to help patients achieve optimal outcomes. As crucial members of managed care teams, nurses have increased responsibility for decision making, with more autonomy and expanded roles in disease prevention and health promotion.

Case management is an integral part of managed care. It involves balancing the use of personnel and material resources to provide optimal outcomes of care. Case management is used from preadmission care through postdischarge home care. The nursing case manager coordinates care and assists the patient and family in the decision-making process. Case managers assume most of the responsibility for patient outcomes and often assume the leadership role in a collaborative model of health care delivery that is based on interdisciplinary teams.

The promise of clinical pathways

Within this restructured system of case management, nurses must consider the costs, process, and expected outcomes within a collaborative model of delivery. One of the most effective tools a nurse can use is the clinical pathway developed by the collaborative health care team. Simply stated, a clinical pathway is a guideline for the nurses and other members of the healthcare team. It functions as a documentation tool that describes an expected sequence of events and processes that moves the patient to a desired goal and can help nurses achieve better control, quality care, and cost outcomes.

Clinical pathways direct the health care team in achieving daily patient care goals for specific health care problems. These pathways are multidisciplinary plans of care designed to reduce patient discharge delays and use resources efficiently, while providing optimal quality patient care. As monitoring tools, pathways help identify activities that require improvement. They can be useful in identifying quality assurance issues, and assisting in setting quality assurance goals. Pathways also foster continuity of patient care by allowing the healthcare team to pinpoint exactly which goals the patient has achieved during his stay.

A pathway follows the patient wherever he may be transferred in the healthcare environment, and can be easily identified throughout the health care organization. Clinical pathway tools can be used by multidisciplinary teams in hospital, ambulatory, community-based, and home-care settings.

Designed properly, clinical pathways control operations in a health care system, allowing more provider-based internal control of processes and systems. Clinical pathways must include the following to control operations:

- processes, tasks, and interventions, which are the projected resources in an anticipated timed relationship
- outcome progressions, results, and projected responses to those resources.

Clinical pathways are an important part of — but do not supplant — the nursing process, which still serves as the basis for nursing practice in all health care settings. The standard of care for clinical nursing practice is described by the ANA as a competent level of nursing care as demonstrated by the nursing process, which (1) encompasses all interventions and actions that nurses perform to provide care to all patients and (2) forms the basis for clinical decision making. Thus, clinical pathways must be incorporated *within* the context of the nursing process. Used in this way, the clinical pathway is a tool that nurses can use to recognize human responses to actual or potential health problems. Finally, clinical pathways should include nursing diagnoses that direct dependent, independent, and interdependent patient care. The clinical pathways in this book reflect the nursing process and the use of nursing diagnoses within that process.

Origins of clinical pathways

Clinical pathways are derived in part from project management techniques long used in nonmedical spheres such as manufacturing and construction. These techniques include the critical path method (CPM) and Program Evaluation and Review Technique. These basic planning tools outline and determine the timing of work on a project. They consist of visual or mathematical models that convey what is to be done and when it is to be done and then communicate this information to those involved in the work. In today's health care delivery systems, clinical pathways are variously referred to as clinical paths, critical paths or pathways, care maps, care paths, collaborative plans of care, multidisciplinary action plans, and anticipated recovery paths.

CPM is the most common network method used in planning complex projects. It identifies the activities critical to finishing the project on time.

At the same time, the use of CMP presents the following problems:
- difficulties in communication
- difficulties in monitoring and controlling progress
- difficulties that may arise in time management.

Today's critical pathways are formulated to overcome these problems. They foster improved communication and enhance abilities to monitor patient progress, and, in many settings, they are used as an operational plan. The CPM network is clearly useful for project planning, because it forces project staff to identify carefully the tasks that need to be undertaken and to determine precisely the relationships of those tasks to each other.

The CPM network is also useful in planning because it allows planners to develop "what if" scenarios within the clinical paths to explore the impact on overall project scheduling of slippages and speed-ups (variances) of individual tasks. Because activities off the pathway have some slack associated with them, the CPM network can tolerate some slippage in schedule. Nurse case managers, along with other members of the interdisciplinary team, continually review and revise plans of care as variances occur.

Components of clinical pathways

Although clinical pathway formats vary among institutions, the core components should include comprehensive aspects of care within the framework of the nursing process, time references, multidisciplinary interventions, and expected patient outcomes.

Comprehensive aspects of care include subjective and objective assessment data, including functional health patterns and physical findings in biological systems; the plan of care, which presents laboratory and diagnostic tests; relevant medical and nursing diagnoses; and medications, treatments, diet, activity level, elimination and hygiene needs, teaching needs, discharge planning, appropriate consults, and various other aspects of care.

Time references provide realistic information relevant to the sequencing of interventions. These time references vary among health care settings. For example, inpatient care utilizes day-by-day time references; intensive care units, hour-by-hour; and home care, week-by-week or visit-by-visit.

Multidisciplinary interventions are presented within the relevant time references and represent collaborative efforts by several health care professionals in developing and implementing the pathway.

Expected patient outcomes generally include daily as well as discharge outcomes. These outcomes should reflect the expected patient outcomes at the time of discharge from the health care setting.

Variances

Certain complex health care problems require deviations from the core clinical pathway format for patients with special needs. These situations are documented on a variance form, which may be attached to the core clinical pathway. (See Using a variance form.) This is a related document to be used concurrently with a clinical pathway, usually as an attachment. For example, if the patient could not tolerate clear liquids on postoperative day 2, the nurse would note this on a variance form as a deviation from the expected outcome documented on the clinical pathway. The nurse would also include an assessment as to why the patient experienced the variance.

Variances require detailed documentation and analysis and form a separate subject beyond the scope of this book.

Quality control

Clinical pathways that incorporate quality improvement indices are valuable to the clinician and the health care organization. The quality improvement process is a structured series of steps designed to plan, evaluate, and propose changes for

Using a variance form

When a patient with a complicated health care problem deviates from the path, a variance form is required for documentation. Below is an example of a variance form used for a patient who has had an appendectomy and is unable to tolerate clear liquids on postoperative day 2.

Code		Discipline specific codes			
C = Comment	NSG Nursing	ST Speech therapy		ET Enterostomal therapy	
E = Evaluation	RT Respiratory therapy	NT Nutritional therapy		OM Outcomes manager	
V = Variation	PT Physical therapy	PC Pastoral care		PAC Patient activity coordinator	
I = Intervention	OT Occupational therapy	SS Social services		CR Cardiac rehabilitation	
O = Outcome	TR Recreational therapy	DE Diabetes education		RAD Radiology	

Date	Time	Code	Discipline Code	Notes	Initials
9/2/98	1030	V	NSG	C/O nausea. Bowel sounds absent in all quadrants on auscultation at 0915.	
		I	NSG	Dr. Harper called. I.M. neostigmine ordered and given at 0930. Hypoactive bowel sounds heard in RUQ.	J.C.
9/2/98	1430	E	NSG	Bowel sounds distant but present in all quadrants. Tolerating ice chips.	J.C.
9/2/98	2200	E	NSG	Continues with hypoactive bowel sounds. Denies nausea, but refusing all p.o. except ice chips and sips of water.	G.A.

Print name and title: Janet Cohen, RN
J.C.

Print name and title: Gloria Altman, RN
G.A.

Print name and title:

health care activities. Quality improvement goals to measure patient care outcomes or certain indicators can be established based on standards such as those set by the state nurse practice act, Joint Commission on Accreditation of Healthcare Organizations, Community Health Accrediting Program, Medicare, Health Care Financing Administration (HCFA), and other sources such as nursing research, as well as by internal policies and procedures. For example, improvement in health care activities would be necessary when: (1) multiple variances occur; (2) patients do not achieve expected outcomes; (3) referrals are not seen within a specified time period; (4) length of stay is extended; (5) patient/family education in progress is not documented within a specified time period; and (6) specified diagnosis-related group (DRG) indicators are not met. (See Using a DRG indicator form for quality control for a DRG indicator form for cerebral vascular accident [CVA].) Indicators are generally used by the institution quality control team and are not a permanent part of the chart, but may be attached to the pathway to ensure assessment by the health care team.

Presentation of clinical pathways

The clinical pathways in this book include the medical diagnoses with their DRG codes and the geometric mean length of stay (GMLOS). The GMLOS is a statistical tool used to compute reimbursement for a given DRG and represents an adjusted value of all cases, making allowances for the outliers, transfer cases, and negative outlier cases that would normally skew the data. The GMLOS is calculated by HCFA and is published in the *Federal Register*.

The specific health care problems identified by the collaborative health care team represent potential physiologic complications; they mainly require monitoring the patient's condition and preventing development of the potential complication. These problems require both medical and nursing interventions for definitive treatment of the condition. Several current nursing diagnoses as specified by the North American Nursing Diagnosis Association (NANDA) are included with each pathway. Inclusion of nursing diagnoses and collaborative problems helps nurses, who are in most situations the case managers, to focus on the problems associated with specific medical diagnoses. Nursing diagnoses and collaborative problems form the basis for the plan of care and expected patient outcomes.

Expected outcomes reflect the evaluation phase of the nursing process and relate directly to the nursing diagnoses. The effectiveness of interventions and the plan of care are measured by the patient's achievement of the expected outcomes. Progress toward achievement of the expected outcomes is evaluated daily for acute problems, during which time the plan of care may be modified, continued, revised, or discontinued. Home care agencies and long-term care facilities may need to modify the plan according to the patient's particular situation and frequency of care.

The assessment phase of the nursing process is reflected by the pertinent assessment data. All listed assessment data for each clinical pathway validate the stated nursing diagnoses. Subjective assessment findings and data include the past health history, medication history, and functional health patterns. Objective assessment findings and data include physical findings and associated pertinent laboratory and diagnostic tests. A plan of care is only as good as the assessment data collected. Pertinent assessment data must be routinely collected on all patients by nurses and all other members of the health care team. A daily baseline assessment should be performed. Baseline assessment data include the patient's general appearance, including posture and hygiene; motor activity; skin condition; orientation and men-

Using a DRG indicator form for quality control

Diagnosis-related group (DRG) indicator forms are used to gather care information about patients with the same condition to help manage the care of future patients with similar conditions. Below is a sample DRG indicator form for cerebrovascular accident (CVA) risk factors.

CVA risk factors (please check all that apply)

☒ Black/Hispanic	☐ Previous CVA/transient ischemic attack	☒ Hypertension	☐ Heart surgery
☒ Age 55+	☐ Cholesterol > 200	☐ Smoker _____ packs per day	
☒ Diabetes	☐ Coronary artery disease	☐ Former smoker	

Indicators	ICU/4 North				Med/Surg			
	Yes	No	NA	Comments	Yes	No	NA	Comments
1. PATIENT (PT) ASSESSMENT/MEDS								
Correct CVA pathway placed on chart	X							
Physical medicine and rehabilitation (PM&R) consulted on Day 1	X							
Pt prophylaxed for deep vein thrombosis (DVT)	X							
If so, with what method?				heparin protocol				
Heparin gtt	X							
Heparin S.C.					X			started day 4
Antiembolic (TED) stockings/Pneumatic compression boots (PCBs)					X			TEDS
Indwelling urinary catheter inserted	X							
2. PATIENT EDUCATION								
Stroke education packet reviewed with patient/family	X				X			
Documentation of education in progress notes/24 hr record	X				X			
3. VARIANCES								
Pt developed urinary tract infection		X			X			Catheter D/C'd day 3; Amoxil given
Pt developed DVT		X						
Pt developed infection		X						
Other variance			X				X	
4. UTILIZATION MANAGEMENT								
Length of stay (LOS)	5 days							
Place of discharge	7th floor rehab							

tal status; vital signs; pulmonary and cardiovascular function; urinary and bowel function; signs of distress; and presence of odors.

The plan of care, or planning phase of the nursing process, includes the following nine categories that characterize the comprehensive aspects of care:
- diagnostic tests
- medications
- procedures
- diet
- activity level
- elimination needs
- hygiene needs
- patient teaching needs
- discharge planning.

Timelines represent sequencing of interventions related to each comprehensive aspect of care category. Timelines appear to the right of the plan of care column, and include the preadmit phase, days of stay for inpatient care, and numbers of visits for home care. Interventions make reference to a multidisciplinary approach, directing nurses to consult other health team providers. Most interventions listed represent dependent, independent, and interdependent nursing actions. Agency protocols, standards of care, and nursing and doctor orders are frequently listed as interventions.

References

Bates, B., et al. *A Guide to Physical Examination and History Taking*, 6th ed. Philadelphia: Lippincott-Raven, Pubs., 1991.

Corbett, C.F., and Androwich, I.M. "Critical Paths: Implications for Improving Practice," *Homehealth Nurse* 12(6):27-84, 1994.

Ignatavicius, D.D., and Hausman, K.A. *Clinical Pathways for Collaborative Practice.* Philadelphia: W.B. Saunders Co., 1995.

Kozier, B., et al. *Fundamentals of Nursing: Concepts, Process, and Practice,* 5th ed. Menlo Park, Calif.: Addison-Wesley-Longman Publishing Co., 1995.

Lewis, S.M., et al. *Medical-Surgical Nursing Assessment and Management of Clinical Problems.* St. Louis: Mosby–Year Book, Inc., 1996.

Marquis, B.L., and Huston, C.J. *Leadership Roles and Management, Functions in Nursing: Theory and Application.* Philadelphia: Lippincott-Raven, Pubs., 1992.

Moder, J.J., et al. *Project Management with CPM, PERT, and Precedence Diagramming,* 3rd ed. New York: Van Nostrand Reinhold, 1983.

Nursing Facts: Managed Care: Challenges and Opportunities for Nursing. Kansas City, Mo.: American Nurses Association, 1995.

Schull, D., et al. "Clinical Nurse Specialists as Collaborative Care Managers," *Nursing Management* 12(3):30-33, 1992.

St. Anthony's DRG Guidebook 1997. Reston, Va.: St. Anthony Publishing, 1996.

Standards of Clinical Nursing Practice. Kansas City, Mo.: American Nurses Association, 1993.

Yoder Wise, P.S. *Leading and Managing in Nursing.* St. Louis: Mosby–Year Book, Inc., 1995.

Zander, K. "Evolving Mapping and Case Management for Capitation: Part III: Getting Control of Value." In *The New Definition* (Vol.11,2). South Natick, Mass.: The Center for Case Management, Inc., 1996.

Clinical pathways in nursing

In the last chapter we briefly examined what clinical pathways are, how they were developed, and why they are becoming so important in today's managed care environment. Also, we reviewed the presentation of clinical pathway tools in this book, including the use of variance forms and diagnosis-related group (DRG) indicators. In this chapter, we will examine more thoroughly the issues that are bringing clinical pathway tools to the forefront of nursing practice.

Current social and economic realities make it necessary to optimize access to care and the quality of care, as well as control its costs. Changes must be made in the areas of health care delivery, professional practice, nursing and medical education, health care financing, and public policy. Although access, quality, and cost of care are relatively simple concepts, there is no "quick fix" available.

Professional schools of nursing can foster gradual change within health care provider organizations by preparing their students in innovative ways. New skills and knowledge, greater focus on attitudes and values that health care workers can bring to the delivery arenas, and fundamental curriculum changes are needed. As an important step, clinical pathways should be introduced as a major focus in teaching the application of the nursing process to students in professional schools of nursing.

Clinical pathways, care plans, and the nursing process

Traditionally, nurses have been taught how to assist patients and families to resolve actual and potential problems by using the nursing process as documented in care plans. However, the format for documenting the nursing process has changed from the traditional care plan to the clinical pathway.

Both of these documentation formats rely on the nursing process. To review briefly, the nursing process is a method of organizing thought processes for clinical decision making and problem solving. It allows nurses to focus on patients' individual responses to actual and potential health care problems, and to think and reason critically and perform psychomotor and affective skills to plan care for an individual patient. The nursing process provides the framework for nursing practice in five major areas: assessment, diagnosis, planning, implementation, and evaluation.

The clinical pathway may replace care plans previously used, but it does not replace the nursing process; rather, it provides an innovative method of documenting assessment, diagnosis, planning, implementation, and evaluation specific for each day of care. Traditional care plans often focused on completion of nursing tasks without addressing the impact of other disciplines on cost issues in the care of patients. In contrast to traditional care plans, the clinical pathway is often based on the DRG services that are to be provided by all disciplines for the patient's particular DRG classification. This unique cost monitoring aspect makes the clinical pathway a tool that can decrease patient length of stay and improve insurance reimbursement when used correctly by care managers or coordinators of patient care.

The clinical pathway tools in this book include the relevant DRG numbers to assist in this purpose. This method of documenting the care plan actualizes competencies required for training health care practitioners in 2005 as defined by the Pew Health Profession Commission Report issued in 1991.

The Pew Health Profession Commission is an interdisciplinary charitable trust group representing both the private and public sectors. The Pew Commission aims at analyzing forces that will shape health care in the future. Some examples of the competencies defined by the 1991 Pew Report include emphasizing primary care, participating in coordinated care, ensuring cost-effective and appropriate care, involving patients and families in the decision-making process, promoting healthy lifestyles, accommodating expanded accountability, participating in a racially and culturally diverse society, and continuing to learn.

As viewed by the Commission, clinical pathways represent a model that permits new ways of organizing the work of health care providers, decision making, and patient care. Professional schools of nursing should begin to incorporate this new model to help prepare future health care providers to respond to pressing issues of access, quality, and cost.

Benefits for nursing practice and education

Multidisciplinary clinical pathways ensure expected patient outcomes and collaborative care in a quality, cost-efficient manner.

Practice

Benefits of utilization of clinical pathways by health care providers include (but are not limited to) the following:

- Clinical pathways enhance the nursing process, especially in the area of evaluation of expected outcomes based on pertinent assessment data and a timely plan of care.
- Clinical pathways as a form of documentation are important for institutional accreditation and licensing, financial reimbursement, quality improvement, and contracting for managed care systems.
- Clinical pathways provide a visual record of the practitioner's or multidisciplinary team's efforts to incorporate and balance cost and quality in the decision-making process. They ensure a plan of care that encourages decreased length of stay in hospitals, thereby reducing hospitalization costs.
- Institutions that utilize clinical pathways may attract more third-party payers who provide incentives and discounts.
- Use of clinical pathways provides a better means of communication among multidisciplinary health care providers. Provider expectations and patient outcomes are clearly presented, thereby helping individuals, families, and communities maintain and promote beneficial health behaviors.
- Patient and family education related to illness is achieved and documented in a structured fashion.
- Clinical pathways facilitate identification of areas for clinical research, such as quality improvement, management strategies, innovative intervention applications, multidisciplinary approaches to care, risk management, trends in health care, patient and staff satisfaction, cultural value identification, professional competencies, and cost-effective care.

Education

Clinical pathways can assist professional schools of nursing to address curricular issues that will shape future graduates, who must possess skills necessary to meet the evolving health care needs of the public. According to the Pew Report, schools should redefine their educational core and examine specific curricular issues as follows:

- Offer educational opportunities that provide expanded skills, knowledge, and attitudes necessary to ensure competencies that will be required to meet health care needs in the year 2005.
- Shift from hospitals to community-based settings that emphasize prevention.
- Focus on teaching-learning processes that promote inquiry skills with the ability to manage large amounts of information for decision making.
- Provide clinical learning opportunities that enhance health care teamwork.
- Focus on assessment of curricular effectiveness utilizing process and outcome evaluations.
- Offer greater flexibility to allow easier access to professional training, crosstraining, and exploration of professional career options.

Clinical pathways can be used to teach the application of the nursing process in multiple educational settings such as hospitals and community-based centers, including school health clinics, ambulatory clinics, home health settings, gerontology centers, mental health centers, child and elder day care facilities, and shelters.

Professional students learn inquiry and communication skills, as well as cost-efficient and timely care planning skills, by using clinical pathways. What's more, because clinical pathways can be multidisciplinary, students are introduced to integrated health care and can function as team members with other providers and managers in a variety of health care settings.

Clinical pathways are comprehensive and effective teaching tools that address access, quality, and cost of care issues in a multicultural society. These teaching tools will assist nursing education leaders to better prepare future practitioners.

Research and patient teaching

More nursing and multidisciplinary clinical research is needed to advance the science of nursing. Clinical pathways can play an integral role in the development of such research studies and projects. The clinical pathways provided in this book include a quick nursing research focus that cues health care providers to think critically about potential clinical nursing research areas.

In addition, the clinical pathways in this book are designed to present a continuum for continuity of care from an inpatient to a home care setting. To further enhance continuity of care and collaborative care, these pathways provide patient-teaching guidelines and a national resource list for each clinical pathway. This feature helps focus on the shifting trends from hospital to home and community-based care, the new frontier of nursing practice.

Policy issues and new directions

Naturally, where there are advantages to using clinical pathways, there are also problems and concerns. Questions continually arise as to whether or not these pathways are truly multidisciplinary or collaborative in nature and concerns exist that some agencies allow a particular discipline, such as doctors, to dominate or direct the pathways.

Doctors and other medical staff may perceive the clinical pathway as yet another restriction imposed on them in this era of managed care. Compliance with clinical path tools can be improved by involving medical staff directly in their design and development, and by emphasizing that these tools are guidelines for care and are not intended to supplant individualized clinical judgments and decisions. For their part, nurses must insist that collaboration is essential in developing clinical pathways for patient care.

To ensure quality patient care in a timely manner, all members of the multidisciplinary team must adhere to and accept the pathway. Noncompliance by any member of the team will cause the clinical pathway to be ineffective, resulting in poor quality of care and increased length of stay.

Because multidisciplinary teams are now involved in activities and documentation practices that were previously confined to specific departments, another potential source of concern is the issue of confidentiality. More people will have access to patient information when creating or reviewing pathways. However, as more health care systems convert to computerized documentation systems, a password will be needed to access documents such as the clinical pathway.

There is general skepticism as to the true value of clinical pathways. Can pathways generate meaningful care, cost, and quality reports? The overuse of variance forms makes analyzing the value of clinical pathways difficult. Clinical pathway tools have been developed only for the most common illnesses that occur in hospital and home settings. Diseases may be grouped according to commonalities and pathways may be developed based on the common features. For example, a pathway may be developed for patients with diarrhea, instead of creating a separate plan for each type of *Escherichia coli* as the causative agent.

As with other documentation tools, clinical pathways could hold one accountable in a court of law. Health care providers could become easy targets for attorneys in malpractice suits if a pathway is not followed correctly, if a patient develops a variance that is not carefully identified, or if the patient suffers an injury because a team member failed to follow the pathway or followed the pathway incorrectly. For this reason, it is wise to involve appropriate legal counsel at the outset when creating pathways. Some experts recommend giving legal counsel the task of determining what legal pitfalls to avoid prior to implementation. Agencies need to carefully examine the terminology used in their pathways and to carefully consider when and how to use each pathway. The pathway must also be accessible to all members of the multidisciplinary team to facilitate adherence and accomplishments in a timely manner. The team must determine where the pathway will be stored so the patient receives quality care within an efficient time period, as evidenced by appropriate documentation.

Clinical pathways need to be computerized, as does variance analysis. Costing-out issues can be determined via computer tracking and coding systems. This could assist with third-party payments to nurses for nursing services identified in the clinical pathway. In addition, the data provided via computer systems could support research related to the efficiency and accuracy of clinical pathways.

What are the next steps in terms of utilization of clinical pathways? As the trend in health care moves from hospital settings to home and community-based settings, the agencies involved need to collaborate. There is a need for all parties to come together to develop comprehensive clinical pathways that address care needs from preadmission to surgery to home care and alternative care settings. Now is the time for partnerships to emerge among nursing practice arenas and between nursing practice and nursing education.

References

Carpenito, L.J. *Nursing Diagnosis: Application to Clinical Practice,* 6th ed. Philadelphia: Lippincott-Raven, Pubs., 1995.

Graybeal, K., et al. "Clinical Pathway Development. The Overlake Model," *Nursing Management* 24(4):42-45, 1993.

Lewis, S.M., et al. *Medical-Surgical Nursing Assessment and Management of Clinical Problems.* St. Louis: Mosby–Year Book, Inc., 1996.

Sugars, D.A., et al. *Healthy America: Practitioners for 2005, An Agenda for Action for U.S. Health Professional Schools.* Durham, N.C.: The Pew Health Professions Commission, 1991.

PART 2

Respiratory problems

Asthma

Chronic obstructive pulmonary disease

Pneumonia

Tuberculosis

Asthma

DRG: 97 Mean LOS: 3.6 days

Asthma is a reversible chronic lung disorder characterized by airway obstruction, wheezing, and coughing. The pathophysiology of asthma includes inflammation and hyperresponsiveness (bronchoconstriction), which may be antigen-mediated (allergic), to physical, chemical, or pharmacologic stimuli. Because asthma's symptoms and causes vary, therapeutic intervention can follow numerous avenues. The clinical course of the disorder is unpredictable and may range from mild coughing, wheezing, and paroxysms of dyspnea to severe status asthmaticus symptoms with drastically altered activities of daily living (ADLs) and even death.

Worldwide, the prevalence of asthma is increasing. The reason is unknown but may be linked to the spread of urban living conditions and greater exposure to environmental and occupational pollutants. Also, passive exposure to cigarette smoke in childhood (that is, parental smoking) likely plays a role in the development of asthma.

This disorder has a high mortality especially among blacks. Socioeconomic factors, such as limited access to health care, inadequate medical treatment, and noncompliance with prescribed therapy, are closely associated with high rates.

Subjective assessment findings

Health history
Allergic rhinitis, exposure to environmental and chemical irritants (pollen, dander, mold, dust, smoke, weather changes, feathers, inhaled irritants), sinus infection, exercise, gastroesophageal reflux

Medication history
Corticosteroid use, sympathomimetics, methylxanthines, bronchodilators, cromolyn sodium, drugs that precipitate asthma attacks (aspirin, cholinergics, antibiotics, nonsteroidal anti-inflammatory drugs, beta blockers)

Functional health patterns
Health perception–health maintenance: recent upper respiratory infection (URI) or sinus infection, fatigue, family history of allergies or asthma
Activity-exercise: chest tightness, decreased tolerance to exercise, cough, dyspnea, sputum production, difficulty breathing, shortness of breath, feelings of suffocation
Sleep-rest: interrupted sleep, insomnia
Coping–stress tolerance: fear, anxiety, emotional distress

Objective assessment findings

Physical findings
Cardiovascular: tachycardia, jugular vein distention, hypertension or hypotension, premature ventricular contraction, pulsus paradoxus

General: signs of anxiety, restlessness, body position that facilitates breathing, fatigue to exhaustion, confusion

Integumentary: diaphoresis, cyanosis (circumoral and nail bed)

Respiratory: adventitious breath sounds (wheezing, crackles, rhonchi), decreased or absent breath sounds, white and tenacious sputum, use of accessory muscles for breathing, labored breathing, thorax retractions (intercostal and supraclavicular), tachypnea with hyperventilation, prolonged expiration

Diagnostic tests

Arterial blood gases (ABGs), pulmonary function tests (PFTs), allergen skin tests, chest X-ray, theophylline level, serum immunoglobulin E, complete blood count, serum electrolytes, white blood cell count (eosinophils), pulse oximetry

Related nursing diagnoses

1 Ineffective breathing pattern
2 Ineffective airway clearance
3 Impaired gas exchange
4 Activity intolerance
5 Anxiety
6 Ineffective individual coping
7 Sleep pattern disturbance
8 Ineffective management of therapeutic regimen: individual

Expected outcomes

The following expected outcomes pertain to the patient or family. Numbers in parentheses refer to related nursing diagnoses above.

- Exhibit absence of wheezing and chest tightness (1,2,3).
- Have normal breath sounds with respiratory rate of 12 to 18 breaths per minute (1,2,3).
- Have ABGs, pulse oximetry, and PFTs within normal limits (1,2,3).
- Demonstrate increased energy to do ADLs (4).
- Demonstrate less anxiety (5).
- Use coping mechanisms to control anxiety to stimuli (6).
- Seek appropriate support groups and referrals to maintain well-being (6).
- Experience feelings of being rested (7).
- List general knowledge of disease process and factors that trigger attacks (8).
- Agree to adherence to medical management plan, including drug therapy (8).
- Recognize signs and symptoms (S/S) to report to doctor or to seek emergency room care (8).
- Control environment to prevent asthma attack (8).
- Do not smoke (8).
- Monitor uncontrollable environmental factors to prevent attacks (air quality index) (8).
- Comply with the medical health management plan and drug therapy (8).

Other possible nursing diagnoses

Risk for infection; risk for fluid volume deficit

Potential complications

Hypoxemia

(Text continues on page 19.)

Asthma

PLAN OF CARE	PREADMIT PHASE	INPATIENT CARE Day 1	Day 2
DIAGNOSTIC TESTS	• Immunoglobulin (IgM) • Complete blood count (CBC), serum electrolytes (lytes) • Arterial blood gases (ABGs) • Pulmonary function tests (PFTs) • Sputum culture (if indicated) • Electrocardiogram if age 40 or older • Chest X-ray (CXR)	• Theophylline level • IgM analysis • CBC • Pulse oximetry or ABGs	• Theophylline level • Lytes • CBC • ABGs • Sputum analysis (if indicated) • Pulse oximetry • CXR
MEDICATIONS	• Methylxanthines • Sympathomimetics • Cromolyn sodium • Antibiotics • Corticosteroids • Anticholinergics • Bronchodilators	• I.V./P.O. methylxanthines • I.V./P.O. corticosteroids • I.V./P.O. antibiotics (if indicated) • Bronchodilators • Sympathomimetics • Maintain I.V. with 5% dextrose in water (D_5W) or 5% dextrose in 0.45% sodium chloride (D_5 ½ NS).	• I.V./P.O. methylxanthines • I.V./P.O. corticosteroids • I.V./P.O. antibiotics (if indicated) • Bronchodilators • Sympathomimetics • Maintain I.V. (D_5W or D_5 ½ NS).
PROCEDURES	• Check baseline vital signs (VS). • Establish I.V access. • Obtain respiratory therapy (RT) consult.	• Check VS q 4 hr. • Maintain oxygen saturation (O_2 sat) > 94% inhalation. • Check nebulizer. • Perform chest physiotherapy (CPT). • Monitor I.V. site.	• Check VS q 4 hr. • Maintain O_2 sat > 94%, inhalation. • Check nebulizer. • Perform CPT. • Monitor I.V. site.
DIET	• Assess current diet.	• Give diet as tolerated (DAT). *Dietary consult:* • Avoid food allergens if indicated. • Give low-sodium diet if steroid-dependent.	• Give DAT.
ACTIVITY	• Institute energy conservation measures.	• Encourage bed rest with bathroom privileges.	• Gets up in chair b.i.d. • Assess tolerance for activity.
ELIMINATION	• Assess for diaphoresis.	• Measure intake and output (I & O). • Have patient force fluids. • Provide bedside commode if needed.	• Measure I & O. • Have patient force fluids.
HYGIENE		• Oral hygiene before and after meals and before and after RT	• Same as Day 1
PATIENT TEACHING	• Explain need for inpatient care.	• Teach deep-breathing (DB) exercises and postural drainage.	• Explain dynamics of disease process. • Discuss environmental control measures to prevent future attacks. • Explain importance of therapeutic management.
DISCHARGE PLANNING	*Social services:* • Determine needs for home care, support groups.	*Psychological consult:* • Determine need for counseling (self-image and coping). *RT consult:* • Pulmonary rehabilitation *Social services consult:* • Assess needs.	*Social services:* • Arrange for home health, RT equipment.

Day 3

- Theophylline level
- CBC
- Lytes
- PFTs
- Pulse oximetry

- Convert I.V. to P.O.
- Methylxanthines
- Corticosteroids
- Antibiotics (if indicated)
- Bronchodilators
- Sympathomimetics
- Discontinue (D/C) I.V. to heparin or saline lock.

- Check VS q 4 hr.
- Maintain O_2 sat > 94%, inhalation.
- Check nebulizer.
- Perform CPT.

- Same as previous day

- Walks in room.
- Assess tolerance to activities and self-care.

- Same as previous day

- Same as Day 1

- Evaluate patient performance of DB and postural drainage.
- Reinforce previous teaching.

Social services:
- Support group visit patient while inpatient.
Home health:
- Visit patient and family while inpatient.

Day 4

- Theophylline level
- Pulse oximetry
- CXR

- Methylxanthines
- Corticosteroids
- Antibiotics (if indicated)
- Bronchodilators
- Sympathomimetics

- Check VS q 4 hr.
- Maintain O_2 sat > 94%, inhalation.

- Same as previous day

- Walks in hall.
- Assess tolerance to activities and self-care.

- Same as previous day

- Same as Day 1

- Discuss home drug therapy.
- Reinforce previous teaching.

- Assess patient's and family's knowledge of home health and support group contacts.

(continued)

PLAN OF CARE	HOME CARE Visit 1	Visit 2	Visit 3
DIAGNOSTIC TESTS	• Complete blood count • Serum electrolytes • Theophylline level	• Refer to doctor for arterial blood gases (ABGs) and pulmonary function tests (PFTs) if indicated.	• Same as previous visit
MEDICATIONS	• Evaluate effectiveness of medications. • Evaluate compliance with drug regimen.	• Evaluate compliance with drug regimen. • Assess for positive and adverse effects of drug therapy.	• Reassess same as previous visit.
PROCEDURES	• Refer to respiratory therapy (RT) if indicated. • Observe patient performing postural drainage and deep breathing (DB) exercises. • Assess proper use of O_2 and other respiratory equipment (if ordered). • Assess VS, breath sounds, sputum production (amount and color), use of accessory muscles for breathing, presence of cyanosis.	• Reassess same as previous visit. • Refer to RT if indicated.	• Same as previous visit
DIET	• Assess nutritional intake. • Assess medication interactions with food. • Encourage to force fluids 2 to 3 L/day.	• Reinforce previous visit. • Refer to dietary consult if indicated.	• Same as previous visit
ACTIVITY	• Assess sleep activity. • Assess response to activity.	• Reinforce previous visit.	• Same as previous visit
ELIMINATION	• Assess urine output.	• Reinforce previous visit.	• Same as previous visit
HYGIENE	• Evaluate home environment for allergens. • Encourage oral hygiene before and after RT.	• Reinforce previous visit.	• Same as previous visit
PATIENT TEACHING	• Discuss signs and symptoms to report to doctor and seek medical care • Reinforce postural drainage and DB exercises. • Discuss medication (name, dosage, purpose, time and route of administration, side effects, food interaction). • Teach safe use of RT equipment necessary for drug administration. • Explain need to control the environment for allergies and cigarette smoke. • Teach patient to avoid outdoors on high-humidity days and to check the air quality index (if poor, stay inside). • Teach relaxation measures (imagery, DB) to decrease anxiety to stimuli.	• Define factors that trigger asthma attacks. • Discuss lifestyle modification and environmental control measures, smoking cessation, and need for regular follow-up care.	• Reinforce and evaluate teaching sessions from previous home visits.
DISCHARGE PLANNING	• Assess home support and resource needs (for example, economic status to purchase medication and equipment). • Refer to appropriate agency or social services as indicated.	• Assess home support and resource needs. • Refer to RT/counselor if indicated.	• Assess home support and resource needs.

Patient teaching

Preventing recurrence
- Maintain natural resistance to illness (adequate nutrition, rest, exercise, clean living environment).
- Avoid persons with infections, especially URIs.
- Avoid fatigue and stressful situations.
- Do not use tobacco, and avoid persons who smoke; seek local smoking cessation group to stop smoking if necessary.
- Express anxieties and fears.
- Avoid known irritants and allergens, especially in bedroom (dust, feather pillows, wool blankets, any dust-collecting articles, house pet's dander, house plants).
- Humidify indoor air by using humidifiers (instruct as to care and cleaning).
- Develop a clear understanding of the disease process; know what to expect and how to manage self-care during attacks.
- Reinforce knowledge of asthma by reading appropriate materials, watching videos, and attending question and answer sessions with appropriate health care providers.
- Report evidence of respiratory infection promptly to the doctor.
- Adhere to prescribed medication regimen.
- Participate in regular follow-up care.

Signs and symptoms
- URIs
- S/S of influenza
- Elevated temperature
- Increased wheezing
- Sore throat
- Chest tightness
- Prolonged expirations
- Increased difficulty breathing

Activity
- Avoid activities that produce shortness of breath, and limit activities during extreme hot or cold temperatures.
- Stay indoors if local air quality index indicates high air pollution.
- Plan rest periods between activities.
- Avoid fatigue, and adjust activities according to individual fatigue patterns.

Medications
- Know the dosage, time of administration, purpose, and side effects.
- Avoid overuse of nebulizers to prevent toxic effects.
- Wear a medical alert band with asthma identification.

Health care equipment
- Know how to use and clean home humidifier.
- Use inhalers, nebulizers, and aerosols properly, and perform oral hygiene after each treatment.

Reducing bronchial secretions
- Use humidifier in room.
- Increase fluid intake (2 to 3 L/day).
- Sleep with head of bed elevated 30° to 60°.
- Explain importance of postural drainage and deep breathing (DB) exercises after each postural position.
- Demonstrate postural drainage and DB exercises.

Nutrition
- Explain importance of maintaining a well-balanced diet.
- Drink at least 3 L/day unless contraindicated.
- Weigh daily and keep weight log; avoid unnecessary weight gain.

Critical thinking activities
1. List coping strategies that help asthma patients deal with feelings of depression.
2. List psychosocial variables that influence perception, self-care, treatment, and emotional reactions to an asthmatic attack.
3. Describe how a nurse identifies the asthma patient at greatest risk.
4. Explain the correlation between restored sleep patterns and predicted life satisfaction among chronic asthma patients.
5. Explain why chronic asthma patients who use support groups do or do not experience fewer asthma attacks over time.
6. List the interventions that a patient's significant others could engage in to help the patient during an asthma attack.
7. Identify myths and misinformation about asthma that are found in the general public.
8. Identify how the patient with asthma can avoid the common triggers of asthma attacks.
9. Relate the clinical manifestations of asthma to the pathophysiologic processes that occur.
10. Identify the expected assessment findings that result from hypoxemia and forced exhalation with the use of abdominal muscles.

Suggested research topics
- Coping strategies for asthma
- Emotional reactions to asthma
- Effectiveness of support groups
- Sleep patterns

Chronic obstructive pulmonary disease

DRG: 89 Mean LOS: 4.9 days

Chronic obstructive pulmonary disease (COPD) refers to a group of lung conditions (chronic bronchitis, emphysema, and asthma) that may lead to chronic obstruction of airflow. Usually, more than one of these underlying conditions, such as chronic bronchitis and emphysema, coexist. Chronic bronchitis and emphysema can occur without an airway obstruction. When an airway obstruction is present, remission is not the usual response to treatment as with an asthmatic airway obstruction, which may be partially reversible.

Prevalence, incidence, and mortality for COPD increase with age and are higher in males than females and in whites than nonwhites. Incidence and mortality are generally higher in blue-collar workers and in those with fewer years of formal education. Tobacco smoking and age are the most predominant risk factors for developing COPD in the United States, and exposure to environmental and occupational pollutants ranks next. COPD mortality rates are relatively insensitive to smoking cessation.

Subjective assessment findings

Health history
Chronic bronchitis; emphysema; bronchiectasis; asthma; smoking; long-term exposure to air and chemical pollutants, respiratory irritants, occupational fumes, dust; previous hospitalizations

Medication history
Oxygen (O_2), bronchodilators, steroids, antibiotics, over-the-counter (OTC) drugs, anticholinergics

Functional health patterns
Health perception–health management: recurrent upper respiratory infection (URI), fatigue, family history of respiratory disease
Nutritional-metabolic: anorexia, weight loss or gain
Activity-exercise: decreased ability to perform activities of daily living (ADLs), pedal edema, palpitations, dyspnea, recurrent cough, orthopnea, sputum production
Sleep-rest: insomnia, paroxysmal nocturnal dyspnea, sleeping in an upright position
Cognitive-perceptual: chest and abdominal soreness, headache

Objective assessment findings

Physical findings
General: anxiety, debilitation, body position that facilitates breathing, restlessness to confusion and somnolence
Cardiovascular: hypotension, tachycardia, arrhythmia, pulsus paradoxus, edema of lower extremities, right-sided S_3 heart sound, jugular vein distention
Integumentary: bruising, poor skin turgor, cyanosis, pallor or ruddy color
Musculoskeletal: increased anteroposterior diameter (barrel-chest), muscle atrophy

(Text continues on page 25.)

PLAN OF CARE	PREADMIT PHASE	INPATIENT CARE Day 1	Day 2
DIAGNOSTIC TESTS	• Arterial blood gases (ABGs) • Complete blood count (CBC) • Chest X-ray (CXR) • Electrocardiogram • Serum electrolytes (lytes) • Albumin	• ABGs • Pulse oximetry q4hr • Sputum analysis • CBC, lytes, theophylline level • Pulmonary function tests (PFTs) • CXR	• ABGs • Pulse oximetry q 8 hr • CBC, lytes, theophylline level • Sputum analysis
MEDICATIONS	• Assess current medication (pre-scriptions and over-the-counter). • Bronchodilators • Antibiotics • Corticosteroids • Diuretics • Cardiotonics	• Bronchodilators • Antibiotics • Corticosteroids • Diuretics • Cardiotonics	• Same as Day 1
PROCEDURES	• Oxygen (O_2) • Aerosol nebulization • Vital signs (VS) • Establish I.V. access.	• Check VS q 4 hr. *Respiratory therapy (RT) consult:* • Give O_2 therapy to maintain O_2 saturation (O_2 sat) at 92%. Provide nebulizer. Provide chest physiotherapy (CPT). Assess breath/heart sounds. • Maintain I.V. and monitor site.	• Check VS q 4 hr. • Give O_2 therapy to maintain O_2 sat at 92%. Provide nebulizer. Provide CPT. Assess breath/heart sounds. • Maintain I.V. and monitor site.
DIET	• Weigh patient. • Give high-protein, moderate fat, low-carbohydrate diet. • Give low-sodium diet if steroid-dependent.	• Weigh patient. *Dietary consult:* • Dietary management by nutritionist to plan and prepare for dietary needs. • Increase fluid intake as tolerated.	• Weigh patient. • Increase fluid intake as tolerated.
ACTIVITY	• Institute energy conservation measures.	• Turn, position frequently. • Bed rest (BR) with bathroom privileges (BRP). Elevate head of bed (HOB) 30° to 60°. Provide overbed table with pillow for leaning.	• Turn, position frequently. • Encourage BR with BRP. Elevate HOB. Provide overbed table with pillow for leaning. Have patient get up in chair as tolerated. • Assist with activities of daily living (ADLs).
ELIMINATION	• Assess presence of GI tract disturbance and fluid retention.	• Measure intake and output (I & O). • Assess presence of edema. • Assess bowel function.	• Same as Day 1
HYGIENE	• Assess skin integrity.	• Moisturize skin and assess skin integrity. • Provide frequent oral hygiene. • Assess mucous membrane for moisture.	• Same as Day 1
PATIENT TEACHING	• Discuss need for inpatient care.	• Teach alternative cough and breathing techniques.	• Reinforce previous teaching. *RT consult:* • Instruct in proper use of home O_2.
DISCHARGE PLANNING	*Social services consult:* • Determine home care and smoking cessation support group needs. *Dietary consult:* • Provide dietary counseling. *Psychosocial consult:* • Determine need for counseling.	*Social services:* • Assess needs.	*Social services:* • Prepare for home health O_2, other health care devices. • Refer for psychosocial counseling if indicated.

Day 3	Day 4	Day 5
• ABGs or pulse oximetry every day and as needed • CBC • Albumin • Theophylline level	• Repeat ABGs or pulse oximetry and CBC if indicated. • Theophylline level • PFTs	• Same as previous day
• Same as Day 1	• As ordered by doctor	• As ordered by doctor
• Check VS q 4 hr. • Give O_2 therapy to maintain O_2 sat at 92%. • Provide nebulizer. Provide CPT. • Assess breath/heart sounds and teach controlled breathing • Discontinue (D/C) I.V. to heparin lock. • Monitor I.V. site.	• Reinforce RT.	• Observe patient demonstration of postural drainage and controlled breathing.
• Weigh patient. *Dietary consult:* • Maintain high-protein, low-carbohydrate diet. Give low-sodium diet if steroid-dependent. Increase fluid intake as tolerated.	• Weigh patient. • Evaluate nutritional intake. • Reinforce importance of dietary management.	• Same as previous day
• Have patient get out of bed as tolerated. • Assess ability to perform ADLs. • Assess response to activity. *Consult physical therapy:* • Instruct about appropriate exercise. *Consult occupational therapy:* • Discuss devices to assist with activity.	• Have patient perform self-care with assistance as necessary. • Have patient walk in hall q.i.d.	• Patient performs self-care with assistance as necessary. • Patient walks in hall q.i.d.
• Same as Day 1	• Same as Day 1	• Same as Day 1
• Same as Day 1	• Same as Day 1	• Same as Day 1
• Reinforce previous teaching.	• Reinforce previous teaching. • Discuss home medications and RT equipment.	• Reinforce previous teaching.
Home health and support group (for example, smoking cessation): • Visit patient and family while inpatient.	• Assess patient's and family's knowledge of home health, support groups, and counseling contacts.	• Same as previous day

(continued)

PLAN OF CARE	HOME CARE Visit 1	Visit 2	Visit 3
DIAGNOSTIC TESTS	• Complete blood count • Serum electrolytes	• Refer to doctor for arterial blood gases (ABGs) if indicated. • Refer for chest X-ray (CXR) if indicated. • Review lab work with patient and family.	• Refer to doctor for ABGs if indicated. • Refer to CXR if indicated.
MEDICATIONS	• Evaluate effectiveness of medications. • Evaluate compliance with drug regimen. • Explain need to avoid over- the-counter medication without doctor approval.	• Evaluate compliance with drug regimen. • Assess for positive and adverse effects of drug therapy.	• Reassess same as previous visit.
PROCEDURES	• Assess vital signs, breath/heart sounds, and thorax. • Observe patient performing pursed-lip, abdominal, and deep breathing (DB) techniques. • Assess proper and safe use of oxygen (O_2) and other respiratory equipment. • Assess proper sitting techniques. • Refer to respiratory therapy (RT) if indicated.	• Reassess same as previous visit. • Refer to RT if indicated.	• Reassess same as previous visit. • Refer to RT if indicated.
DIET	• Have patient force fluids to 2 to 3 L/day if tolerated. • Assess weight. • Assess nutritional intake. • Encourage high-protein, low-carbohydrate foods. • Assess sodium intake if steroid dependent. • Refer to dietitian if indicated.	• Reinforce previous visit. • Explain importance of diet maintenance. • Refer to dietitian if indicated.	• Reinforce previous visit.
ACTIVITY	• Assess response to activity. • Assess exercise tolerance. • Assess O_2 needs. • Assess ability to perform activities of daily living.	• Reassess same as previous visit.	• Reassess same as previous visit.
ELIMINATION	• Assess presence of edema. • Instruct to keep daily weight log.	• Assess presence of edema. • Evaluate daily weight log.	• Reinforce previous visit.
HYGIENE	• Assess home environment for recurrence factors (adequate heating/cooling, absence of persons with infections, fresh air, lack of dust and other irritants). • Encourage frequent oral hygiene. • Assess skin integrity.	• Reinforce previous visit.	• Reinforce previous visit.
PATIENT TEACHING	• Discuss signs and symptoms to report to doctor • Reinforce pursed-lip, abdominal, and DB techniques. • Explain need to slow down disease process. • Teach to continue O_2 during meals. • Instruct to eat a balanced diet in frequent and small portions. • Teach O_2 safety and use. • Discuss medication (name, dosage, purpose, time and route of administration, side effects).	• Discuss definition and causes of COPD, lifestyle modification, and risk factor reduction (for example, smoking cessation). • Refer to physical therapy, occupational therapy, and psychosocial counselor, if indicated, need for regular follow-up care.	• Reinforce and evaluate teaching sessions from previous home visits.
DISCHARGE PLANNING	• Assess home support and resource needs (for example, economic status for ability to purchase medications and equipment). • Refer to appropriate agency or social services as indicated.	• Assess home support and resource needs.	• Assess home support and resource needs.

Respiratory: difficulty speaking, audible expiratory wheeze, prolonged expirations with forced effort, pursed-lip breathing, use of accessory muscles of respiration, diminished breath sounds, crackles, rhonchi, hyperresonance or dullness on percussion, bronchospasm, cough (productive/nonproductive) or hacking (ineffective)

Diagnostic tests
Arterial blood gases, complete blood count, pulmonary function tests, chest X-ray, electrocardiogram, theophylline level

Related nursing diagnoses
1 Ineffective airway clearance
2 Ineffective breathing pattern
3 Impaired gas exchange
4 Self-care deficit
5 Anxiety
6 Altered nutrition: less than body requirements
7 Sleep pattern disturbance
8 Self-esteem disturbance
9 Fatigue
10 Activity intolerance
11 Ineffective management of therapeutic regimen: individual

Expected outcomes
The following expected outcomes pertain to the patient or family. Numbers in parentheses refer to related nursing diagnoses above.
- Maintain a patent airway (1,2,3).
- Exhibit a normal respiratory rate, rhythm, and depth (1,2,3).
- Demonstrate improved mental status and skin color (3).
- Increase independence in ADLs (4).
- Demonstrate less anxiety (5).
- Maintain body weight (6).
- Adhere to prescribed diet therapy (6).
- Maintain adequate nutritional and fluid intake (6).
- Verbalize feelings of being rested (7).
- Seek appropriate support groups and referrals to maintain psychosocial and physical well-being (8).
- Limit exercise to tolerance and allow rest periods between activities (9,10).
- Demonstrate breathing exercises that use accessory muscles (11).
- Describe behaviors that minimize infection (11).
- Notify appropriate health care provider of signs and symptoms of COPD (11).
- List ways to slow down the progression of the disease process (11).
- Stop smoking (11).
- Eliminate home environmental factors that aid in the progression of the disease (11).
- State importance of keeping follow-up appointments (11).

Other possible nursing diagnoses
Fluid volume excess; risk for infection; sexual dysfunction

Potential complications
Hypoxemia, atelectasis/pneumonia, tracheobronchial constriction, decreased cardiac output

Patient teaching

Slowing COPD progression
- Maintain natural resistance to illness (adequate nutrition, rest, exercise, clean living environment).
- Avoid persons with infections (especially URIs), crowds, and areas with poor ventilation.
- Avoid fatigue, extremes in temperature (keep warm and avoid chill), and alcohol intake.
- Avoid cigarette smoke, air pollution (dust, fumes, sprays, pollens, paint, aerosols), and allergens.
- Schedule follow-up appointment with doctor as directed and adhere to medical plan of care.
- Seek appropriate health resources to assist with maintenance of psychosocial and physical well-being (Meals on Wheels, physical therapy, occupational therapy).
- Seek local smoking cessation group to stop smoking.
- Ask doctor about need for immunization against influenza and pneumonia.
- Develop clear understanding of the disease process — know what to expect, how to treat, and how to live with COPD.
- Reinforce knowledge about COPD via reading materials, videos, and question and answer sessions with appropriate health care providers.
- Report evidence of respiratory infection promptly to doctor.
- Take prescribed antibiotic (keep supply available at home) at first sign of respiratory infection.
- Humidify indoor air in winter (30% to 50% humidity is best for lung function).
- Cough and expectorate sputum into tissue, then discard in plastic-lined trash container.

Signs and symptoms
- URIs
- Increase in breathing difficulty, amount and tenacity (thickness) of sputum
- Change in color of sputum from yellow to green to brown
- Lack of effective response to prescribed medications
- Elevated temperature (>101° F [38.5° C])
- Disorientation
- Sore throat, night sweats, chills
- Decrease in activity tolerance
- Change in pulse or feelings of heart palpitations
- Increase in use of O_2

Activity
- Explain importance of energy conservation.
- Limit exercise and activity to tolerance (avoid activities that produce shortness of breath, but do exercise to improve physical condition — seek the advice of doctor if unsure).
- Plan rest periods between activities.
- Avoid fatigue and adjust activities according to individual fatigue patterns.
- Limit visitation and avoid long conversations.
- Maintain pleasant and calm environment.
- Keep necessary items within easy reach of seating and sleeping areas.
- Avoid strenuous work (employment-related, heavy housework, straining or lifting).
- Seek vocational counseling for training in new job that is more sedentary in nature.

Medications
- Instruct on dosage, time of administration, purpose, and adverse effects.
- Explain need to avoid OTC drugs unless ordered by doctor; avoid alcohol use.
- Discuss dietary needs in relation to specific drug therapy.

Health care equipment
- Explain proper use and cleaning of vaporizer or humidifier in the home.

- Explain proper use of inhalers, nebulizers, and aerosols for medication administration, and instruct to perform oral hygiene after each treatment.
- Explain definition, purpose, and use of O_2 therapy in the home.
- Give directions related to prescribed flow rate and amount of O_2 to be delivered. Instruct patient and family not to alter flow rate or amount of O_2 unless ordered by doctor.
- Discuss and provide written communication about all safety issues related to O_2 therapy.
- Instruct patient and family to call O_2 equipment representative for specific instructions in relation to cleaning and changing O_2 equipment (tubing and humidifier).
- Instruct patient and family to list telephone number of electric company (in case of electrical outage) if using an O_2 concentrator that depends on electricity.
- Post "Oxygen in Use" sign in a window near the front door in the event of a fire so the fire department will know O_2 is in use.

Reducing bronchial secretions
- Use humidifier in room.
- Increase fluid intake to 2 to 3 L/day.
- Sleep with head of bed elevated 30° to 60°.
- Explain importance of postural drainage and controlled coughing after each postural position.
- Demonstrate postural drainage and controlled coughing techniques to patient and family.
- Teach the techniques of controlled breathing, diaphragmatic breathing, and pursed-lip breathing, and advise the patient to adhere to these techniques for a lifetime.
- Instruct patient to engage in exercise that maintains general body muscle tone, which enhances the ability to perform breathing exercises.

Nutrition
- Explain importance of maintaining a well-balanced diet.
- Perform oral hygiene before and after meals.
- Eat frequent, small meals (5 to 6 per day) to conserve energy.
- Avoid very hot and cold foods, and hard-to-chew foods, and do not eat when upset or angry.
- Drink at least 2 to 3 L/day unless contraindicated
- Weigh self daily and keep weight log.
- Eat foods high in protein and potassium, moderate in fats, low in carbohydrates and sodium.
- Take rest periods before and after meals if eating causes shortness of breath.

Critical thinking activities
1. Discuss how quality of life is affected by COPD.
2. List coping strategies that assist COPD patients in dealing with isolation and inactivity.
3. Explain which smoking cessation method, hypnosis or nicotine weaning, is most effective.
4. Identify and discuss psychosocial or motivational factors and smoking cessation activities utilized by COPD patients who exhibit long-term abstinence from smoking.
5. Identify and discuss effective nursing interventions to increase patient compliance with long-term therapeutic management of COPD.
6. Develop a teaching plan addressing nutritional needs for the patient with COPD.
7. Identify the effects of cigarette smoking directly associated with COPD.

Suggested research topics
- Coping strategies for COPD
- Effectiveness of smoking cessation methods and programs
- Compliance with therapy

Pneumonia

DRG: 90 Mean LOS: 4.3 days

Pneumonia is an inflammation of the distal lung, involving terminal airways, alveolar spaces, and interstitium. The inflammation can be caused by bacteria, viruses, mycoplasma organisms, fungi, protozoa (for example, *Pneumocystis carinii*), chemicals, dust, gases, and a variety of other organisms and materials. These agents can enter the lung via one of three ways: (1) aspiration from the nasopharynx or oropharynx, (2) inhalation of microbes present in the air, or (3) hematogenous spread from a primary infection in the body. Pneumonia is classified according to the causative organism and sometimes by the area and type of lung involvement.

Most cases of pneumonia occur when the body's defenses become incompetent or overwhelmed by the virulence or amount of infectious agent. Until the advent of penicillin and sulfa drugs, pneumonia was the leading cause of death in the United States. Despite progress in clinical medicine, the diagnosis of the disease remains difficult, and pneumonia is a major cause of death, especially in hospitalized patients.

Subjective assessment findings

Health history
Alcoholism, head injury, seizures, debilitating diseases, diabetes, smoking, chronic obstructive pulmonary disease (COPD), lung cancer, recent general anesthesia, exposure to air pollution and chemical toxins, drug overdose, burns

Medication history
Antibiotics, corticosteroids, chemotherapy, other immunosuppressants

Functional health patterns
Cognitive-perceptual: chest pain, painful respiration, headache, myalgia
Health perception–health management: fatigue, recent upper respiratory infection (URI)
Nutritional-metabolic: fever, chills, nausea, vomiting, anorexia
Activity-exercise: decreased mobility

Objective assessment findings

Physical findings
Cardiovascular: tachycardia
General: restlessness or lethargy, chest splinting over affected area
Neurologic: mental status changes, confusion to delirium
Integumentary: poor skin turgor, diaphoresis or dry skin, flushing, cyanosis or pallor
Respiratory: tachypnea; asymmetric chest movements or retraction; nasal flaring; decreased excursion; use of accessory neck and abdominal muscles; grunting; adventitious breath sounds; bronchial or absent breath sounds; pleural friction rub and dullness over consolidated areas on auscultation; tactile fremitus on percussion; scant to copious pink, rusty, purulent, green, yellow, or white sputum; tenacious cough; dyspnea

Diagnostic tests

Complete blood count, white blood cell count, arterial blood gases (ABGs), chemical profile with electrolytes, blood culture, sputum Gram stain with culture and sensitivity, chest X-ray (CXR), electrocardiogram, serologic studies, transtracheal aspiration, bronchoscopy with bronchoalveolar lavage

Related nursing diagnoses

1 Ineffective breathing pattern
2 Ineffective airway clearance
3 Impaired gas exchange
4 Pain
5 Anxiety
6 Sleep pattern disturbance
7 Ineffective management of therapeutic regimen: individual
8 Altered nutrition: less than body requirements
9 Activity intolerance
10 Self-care deficit
11 Risk for infection

Expected outcomes

The following expected outcomes pertain to the patient or family. Numbers in parentheses refer to related nursing diagnoses above.

- Exhibit respiratory rate of 12 to 18 breaths per minute, clear breath sounds, decreased or absent dyspnea, subsiding effective cough with expectoration of sputum, and normal ABGs and CXR (1,2,3).
- Demonstrate full chest excursion (1,2,3).
- Express decreased or absent chest pain and feeling of comfort (4).
- Have decreased anxiety (5).
- Verbalize feelings of being rested (6).
- State rationale to follow regimen (medication, activity schedule, fluid therapy) after discharge (7).
- Notify appropriate health care provider of the following after discharge: elevated temperature, diaphoresis/night sweats, chills, breathing difficulties, persistent cough, URIs (7).
- Perform breathing exercises four times daily for 6 to 8 weeks (7).
- State the importance of keeping follow-up appointments with health care provider after discharge from home care (7).
- Eliminate home environment factors contributing to disease recurrence (7).
- Maintain normal body weight (8).
- Maintain adequate nutritional and fluid intake (8).
- Cooperate with required activity (9).
- Limit exercise to tolerance and allow 2 to 3 rest periods per day (9).
- Be able to perform activities of daily living with assistance as necessary (10).
- Practice infection prevention measures (11).
- List ways to prevent recurrence and transmission of disease (11).

Potential complications

Hypoxemia, atelectasis/pneumonia, sepsis, respiratory failure

(Text continues on page 33.)

PLAN OF CARE	PREADMIT PHASE	INPATIENT CARE *Day 1*
DIAGNOSTIC TESTS	• Complete blood count (CBC) • White blood cell (WBC) count, chemical profile, and serum electrolytes (lytes) • Electrocardiogram • Chest X-ray (CXR)	• CBC • WBC count (leukocytes and neutrophils), chemical profile and lytes • Arterial blood gases • Blood culture, serology (titers and cold agglutinins, immune deficiency) • Pulse oximetry q 4 hr • Sputum Gram stain with culture and sensitivity (C & S) • Chest X-ray (CXR) • Physical assessment (PA & lateral [LAT]) • Transtracheal aspiration • Bronchoscopy
MEDICATIONS	• Assess current medications: prescription and over-the-counter.	• Antipyretics • Analgesics • Antibiotics • Antimicrobials • Expectorants/ mucolytics
PROCEDURES	• Take baseline vital signs (VS). • Evaluate I.V. access and oxygen (O$_2$) needs.	• Check VS q 4 hr. • Give respiratory therapy (RT): Nasal/mask O$_2$ to maintain O$_2$ saturation (O$_2$ sat) > 95%, humidification. • Provide artificial airway or mechanical ventilation support. • Provide nasopharyngeal or nasotracheal suctioning as needed. • Maintain I.V. of 5% dextrose in 0.225% sodium chloride (D$_5$ ¼ NS) and 20 to 30 mEq KCl as ordered. • Monitor I.V. site. • Elevate head of bed (HOB) 30° to 60°.
DIET	• Assess current diet, especially fluid intake. • Weigh patient.	• Push fluids as tolerated. • Weigh patient.
ACTIVITY	• Institute energy conservation measures. • Assess presence of chronic heart and lung disease and diabetes.	• Have patient get out of bed to chair as tolerated with bathroom privileges. • Keep HOB elevated 30° to 60°. • Have patient turn, cough, and deep breathe (TCDB) every 2 to 4 hours. • Initiate fall prevention measures.
ELIMINATION	• Assess presence of fever, diaphoresis, and tachypnea.	• Take temperature. • Measure intake and output.
HYGIENE	• Initiate medical asepsis. • Adhere to infection control guidelines.	• Give bed bath, and complete care.
PATIENT TEACHING	• Discuss need for inpatient care.	• Instruct about incentive spirometry. • Teach about disposal of contaminated tissue, and so forth. • Discuss hand washing. • Discuss deep-breathing (DB) exercises.
DISCHARGE PLANNING	*Social services consult:* • Determine needs for home care nursing and home health aide.	*Social services:* • Assess needs.

CLINICAL PATHWAY ■ Pneumonia

Day 2	Day 3	Day 4
• Pulse oximetry q 4 hr • Review C & S results. • Order additional testing as needed. • CXR	• Additional testing as needed • CXR if follow-up not already done	• Additional testing as needed
• Continue medications as ordered. • Assess effects of medications.	• Same as previous visit	• Same as previous visit
• Check VS q 4 hr. • Discontinue O_2 if O_2 sat 98% on room air • Give nasopharyngeal or nasotracheal suctioning as needed. • Give I.V. antibiotics (pending C & S). • Monitor I.V. site • DB exercises q.i.d. • Elevate HOB 30° to 60°.	• Check VS q 4 hr. • Give humidification. • Discontinue I.V. antibiotics and I.V. • DB exercises q.i.d.	• Check VS q 4 hr. • DB exercises q.i.d.
Dietitian consult: • Determine need for frequent small meals and diet supplements. • Push fluids • Weigh patient.	• Explain importance of diet maintenance. • Push fluids. • Weigh patient.	• Push fluids as tolerated. • Weigh patient.
• Have patient walk as tolerated. • Elevate HOB 30° to 60°.	• Encourage activity as tolerated. • Encourage frequent bed rest.	• Encourage activity as tolerated with 2 to 3 rest periods a day.
• Same as Day 1	• Same as Day 1	• Same as Day 1
• Assist as needed. • Encourage oral hygiene before meals.	• Same as previous day	• Have patient perform self-care as tolerated.
• Reinforce incentive spirometry instruction. • Reinforce disposal of contaminated tissue, and so forth. • Discuss hand washing. • Discuss DB exercises.	• Discuss infection control principles.	• Reinforce previous teaching.
Social services: • Arrange for home health, home O_2, and other medical equipment (vaporizer or humidifier).	*Home health:* • Visit patient and family while inpatient. • Assess ability to continue self-care at home.	• Assess patient's and family's knowledge of home health contact.

(continued)

PLAN OF CARE	HOME CARE Visit 1	Visit 2	Visit 3
DIAGNOSTIC TESTS	• Complete blood count • White blood cell count • Serum electrolytes	• Refer for chest X-ray (CXR) if indicated. • Review results of lab work with patient and family.	• Refer for CXR if indicated.
MEDICATIONS	• Evaluate effectiveness of medications. • Assess adverse effects of medication. • Evaluate compliance with drug regimen.	• Evaluate compliance with drug regimen. • Assess for positive and adverse effects of drug therapy. • Explain need to avoid over-the-counter (OTC) drugs without doctor approval.	• Evaluate compliance with drug regimen. • Assess for positive and adverse effects of drug therapy. • Explain need to avoid OTC drugs without doctor approval.
PROCEDURES	• Observe patient performing deep-breathing (DB) exercises and postural drainage. • Assess vital signs (VS), breath sounds, and thorax. • Assess proper and safe use of vaporizer or humidifier and oxygen (O_2).	• Reassess VS, thorax, and breath sounds. • Reassess proper and safe use of equipment and O_2. • Reassess DB exercises.	• Reassess VS, thorax, and breath sounds. • Reassess proper and safe use of equipment and O_2. • Encourage to continue DB exercises q.i.d. for 6 to 8 weeks.
DIET	• Weigh patient. • Have patient force fluids to 3 L/day unless contraindicated. • Assess nutritional intake (avoid high-calorie diet if overweight).	• Weigh patient. • Explain importance of diet maintenance and fluid intake.	• Reinforce previous visit. • Take 24-hour recall of food intake.
ACTIVITY	• Assess exercise tolerance. • Explain importance of 2 to 3 rest periods per day. • Evaluate O_2 needs.	• Same as previous visit	• Reinforce previous visit.
ELIMINATION	• Assess presence of fever, diaphoresis, night sweats, and persistent cough.	• Same as previous visit	• Same as previous visit
HYGIENE	• Evaluate home environment for recurrence factors (adequate heat/cooling, absence of persons with infections, fresh air).	• Same as previous visit	• Same as previous visit
PATIENT TEACHING	• Explain importance of gradual convalescence. • Explain need to prevent recurrence (keep warm, avoid chills and persons with infections, receive vaccinations for influenza and pneumonia as recommended by doctor). • Discuss symptoms to report to doctor (elevated temperature, chills, night sweats, diaphoresis, breathing difficulties, persistent cough). • Discuss medications (name, dosage, purpose, time and route of administration, adverse effects). • Explain methods of avoiding transmission of disease. • Teach O_2 use and safety and inhaler use if required.	• Discuss lifestyle modification and risk factor reduction (for example, smoking decrease/cessation, need for regular follow-up care).	• Reinforce and evaluate teaching sessions from previous home visits.
DISCHARGE PLANNING	• Assess home support and resource needs (for example, economic status for ability to purchase medication and equipment). • Refer to appropriate agency or social services as indicated.	• Assess home support and resource needs.	• Same as previous visit

Pneumonia (continued) · CLINICAL PATHWAY

Patient teaching

Preventing recurrence
- Maintain natural resistance to illness (adequate nutrition, rest, exercise).
- Avoid persons with infections, especially URIs.
- Avoid fatigue, extremes in temperature (keep warm and avoid chill), excessive alcohol intake, and overuse of over-the-counter (OTC) drugs.
- Avoid cigarette smoke, air pollution (dust, fumes, sprays, pollens, paint), and allergens.
- Schedule follow-up appointment with doctor as directed.
- Seek appropriate health resources to assist with maintenance of any chronic illnesses (diabetes, lung cancer, COPD, acquired immunodeficiency syndrome/human immunodeficiency virus infection, alcoholism, debilitating diseases).
- Seek local smoking cessation group to assist with smoking habit if patient willing.
- Ask doctor about need for immunization against influenza and pneumonia (especially if patient is age 50 or older or has chronic systemic diseases, COPD, or immunosuppression).

Reducing transmission
- Turn head away when coughing and cover mouth with tissue.
- Cover mouth and nose with tissue when sneezing.
- Cough and expectorate sputum into tissue.
- Use tissue only once and discard in trash container (preferably wax-lined paper bag or plastic-lined container).
- Wash hands after using tissue.
- Instruct family to use same techniques at home, especially to wash hands after direct contact with patient and his immediate environment (bedding, clothes, oral devices, trash containers).
- Avoid socialization with individuals who have URIs, lung diseases, and chronic illnesses; avoid socialization with individuals who are recovering from surgery and those who are immunosuppressed.

Signs and symptoms
- URIs
- Extreme sweating
- Night sweats
- Persistent cough (may be dry or productive with green-yellow or pink- to rusty-colored sputum)
- Difficulty breathing
- Changes in breathing rate (>14 to 18 breaths/min)
- Elevated temperature (>101° F [38.5° C])
- Chills
- Loss of appetite
- Chest pain (especially with breathing)
- Confusion

Activity
- Explain importance of increasing activity gradually.
- Limit exercise and activity to tolerance.
- Plan two to three rest periods per day.
- Avoid fatigue.
- Limit visitation and avoid long conversations.
- Maintain pleasant and calm environment.
- Keep necessary items within easy reach (tissue, appropriate trash container).
- Avoid strenuous work (employment-related, heavy housework, straining or lifting until approved by doctor).

Medications
- Instruct patient on dosage, time of administration, purpose, and adverse effects.
- Avoid OTC drugs and alcohol use.
- Discuss dietary needs in relation to specific drug therapy.
- Teach I.V. site care to patient and family if home I.V. antibiotics are ordered.

Health care equipment
- Explain proper use and cleaning of vaporizer or humidifier in the home.
- Explain proper use of inhalers if such medication is ordered.
- Explain definition, purpose, and use of oxygen (O_2) therapy if ordered for home use.
- Give directions related to flow rate and amount of O_2 to be delivered. Instruct patient and family not to alter flow rate or amount of O_2 unless ordered by doctor.
- Discuss and provide written communication about all safety issues related to O_2 therapy if ordered for home use.
- Instruct patient and family to call O_2 equipment representative for specific instructions in relation to cleaning and changing O_2 equipment (tubing and humidifier).
- Instruct patient and family to list telephone number of electric company (in case of electrical outage) if using an O_2 concentrator that depends on electricity.
- Post "Oxygen in Use" sign in window near the front door in the event of a fire so the fire department will know O_2 is in use.

Techniques to clear airway
- Instruct patient to splint chest when coughing if pleuritic pain is present.
- Have patient inhale slowly through nose, exhale, and then cough into tissue.
- Use humidifier in room.
- Increase fluid intake to 3 L/day.
- Sleep with head of bed elevated 30° to 60°.
- Explain importance of postural drainage and deep breathing (DB) exercises.
- Demonstrate postural drainage and DB techniques to patient and family.
- Instruct patient to continue DB exercises four times daily for 6 to 8 weeks.

Nutrition
- Explain importance of maintaining diet as tolerated.
- Perform oral hygiene before meals to remove foul taste of sputum and medications.
- Eat frequent, small meals to conserve energy.
- Avoid high-calorie diet if overweight.
- Drink at least 3 L/day unless contraindicated.
- Weigh daily and keep weight log 6 to 8 weeks.

Critical thinking activities
1. Compare the clinical manifestations of pneumonia and chronic bronchitis.
2. List interventions that a patient's significant others can engage in to prevent the spread of pneumonia.
3. Develop a care plan that addresses high risk for infection with pneumonia.
4. Develop a teaching plan addressing nutritional needs of the patient with pneumonia.
5. Identify the pathophysiologic changes associated with bacterial, viral, and fungal pneumonia.

Suggested research topics
- Compliance with therapy
- Strategies for reducing pneumonia among the elderly
- Effectiveness of hand washing for reducing pneumonia transmission

Tuberculosis

DRG: 80 Mean LOS: 5.3 days

Tuberculosis (TB) is a chronic infectious disease caused by the tubercle bacillus, *Mycobacterium tuberculosis,* an organism that invades the lung and can spread throughout the body if the disease is not treated. A worldwide problem, TB requires long-term treatment with a combination of drugs (as many as four agents). Administration of the drugs is based on disease resistance factors and patient compliance. If acute care is required, the in-hospital stay is brief.

The number of TB patients in the United States decreased with the introduction of drug therapy in the 1950s. Since 1984, the number of new cases has increased in several areas: inner cities with many instances of acquired immunodeficiency syndrome (AIDS) or large populations of homeless people; institutions with crowded living areas, such as prisons; and institutions with large populations of elderly, such as nursing homes. The incidence of TB is also high among the socioeconomically disadvantaged and medically underserved of all races. In the United States, the disease is most prevalent among Native Americans in some areas of Arizona and New Mexico.

Subjective assessment findings

Health history
TB, alcoholism, diabetes, AIDS/human immunodeficiency virus infection, prolonged steroid therapy, cancer, immunosuppressive therapy (organ transplants), chronic renal failure with hemodialysis, intestinal bypass for obesity, postgastrectomy, silicosis

Medication history
Steroids, immunosuppressive therapy

Functional health patterns
Activity-exercise: weakness, fatigue, prolonged bed rest or immobility, dyspnea, cough (dry or productive)
Nutritional-metabolic: anorexia
Cognitive-perceptual: headache, chest pain, painful lymph nodes

Objective assessment findings

Physical findings
Cardiovascular: tachycardia
General: malaise, fever, chills
Integumentary: diaphoresis (night sweats), pallor
Reproductive: irregular menses
Respiratory: productive cough with blood-streaked sputum or mucoid/mucopurulent sputum, enlarged lymph nodes, adventitious breath sounds (crackles over apex of lung, rhonchi), bronchial or absent breath sounds, difficulty breathing, hemoptysis, dyspnea, splinting of chest over affected lung area

(Text continues on page 39.)

Pulmonary tuberculosis (TB)

PLAN OF CARE	PREADMIT PHASE	INPATIENT CARE Day 1	Day 2
DIAGNOSTIC TESTS	• Complete blood count with differential • Arterial blood gases (ABGs) • Purified protein derivative (PPD) test • Multiple puncture tests • Sputum smear & culture (acid-fast bacilli) • Cultures (gastric washings, cerebro-spinal fluid, drainage from abscess) • Chest X-ray (CXR) • Fiberoptic bronchoscopy • Pleural needle biopsy	• White blood cell (WBC) count • ABGs • PPD analysis	• ABGs • Sputum and culture analyses • PPD analysis • CXR
MEDICATIONS	*Primary drugs:* • Isoniazid (INH) • Rifampin • Ethambutol • Streptomycin *Secondary drugs:* • Ethionamide • Capreomycin • Kanamycin • Pyrazinamide • Para-aminosalicylic (PAS) • Cycloserine	*Primary drugs:* • INH • Rifampin • Ethambutol • Streptomycin *Secondary drugs:* • Ethionamide • Capreomycin • Kanamycin • Pyrazinamide • PAS • Cycloserine	• Same as Day 1
PROCEDURES	• Administer antitubercular drugs. • Move to respiratory isolation.	• Check vital signs q 4 hr. • Maintain respiratory isolation (use high-efficiency particulate air [HEPA] mask). • Assess breath sounds, and weigh patient daily. • Elevate head of bed 30° to 60°.	• Same as Day 1
DIET	• Assess current diet.	• Force fluids to 2 to 3 L/day. *Dietary consult:* • Provide high-protein, high-carbohy-drate diet.	• Same as Day 1
ACTIVITY	• Institute energy conservation mea-sures.	• Encourage complete bed rest.	• Encourage bed rest with bath-room privileges.
ELIMINATION		• Measure intake and output (I & O). • Provide bedside commode.	• Measure I & O.
HYGIENE	• Protective isolation	• Give bed bath • Use protective isolation.	• Enforce hand washing and cough-ing into tissue. • Assist with activities of daily living. • Use protective isolation.
PATIENT TEACHING	• Discuss need for inpatient care.	• Explain respiratory isolation. • Emphasize avoiding close contact with others until doctor advises. • Instruct to cough into tissue, to turn head when coughing, and to avoid direct contact with sputum.	• Reinforce previous teaching. • Explain importance of frequent rest periods and diet mainte-nance.
DISCHARGE PLANNING	*Medical record consult:* • Report to Board of Health for follow-up on family and contacts. *Social services consult:* • Determine home care nursing needs.	*Social services:* • Assess needs, evaluate economic status for ability to purchase med-ication. Refer to appropriate agency or support group if indicated.	*Social services:* • Arrange for home health care.

Day 3	Day 4	Day 5
• WBC count • CXR	• CXR	• CXR
• Same as Day 1	• Same as Day 1	• Same as Day 1
• Same as Day 1	• Discontinue respiratory isolation or continue isolation, based on culture and sensitivity results.	• Same as previous day
• Explain importance of diet maintenance.	• Reinforce diet maintenance.	• Same as previous day
• Encourage frequent rest periods. • Have patient walk in room (use HEPA mask).	• Encourage frequent rest periods. • Have patient walk in hall (use HEPA mask).	• Same as previous day
• Same as previous day	• Same as previous day	• Same as previous day
• Enforce hand washing and coughing into tissue. • Perform self-care.	• Same as previous day • Discontinue protective isolation or continue, based on culture and sensitivity results	• Same as previous day
• Reinforce previous teaching.	• Reinforce previous teaching.	• Explain medications for home drug therapy and importance of continuing all prescribed drugs until doctor discontinues them. • Explain to avoid over-the-counter drugs until doctor advises.
Home health: • Visit patient and family while inpatient.	• Assess patient's and family's knowledge of home health and social services contacts.	• Same as previous day

(continued)

Pulmonary tuberculosis (TB) (continued)

CLINICAL PATHWAY

PLAN OF CARE	HOME CARE Visit 1	Visit 2	Visit 3
DIAGNOSTIC TESTS	• Complete blood count • Purified protein derivative (PPD) testing of family and contacts	• Review lab work with patient and family. • Refer to doctor for arterial blood gases (ABGs) if indicated. • Refer to chest X-ray (CXR) if indicated.	• Refer to doctor for ABGs if indicated. • Refer to CXR if indicated.
MEDICATIONS	• Evaluate for adverse effects of drug therapy. • Evaluate compliance with drug regimen. • Explain need to avoid over-the-counter medication without doctor approval.	• Reassess same as previous visit.	• Reassess same as previous visit.
PROCEDURES	• Check vital signs. • Assess breath sounds and signs of difficulty in breathing. • Assess presence of diaphoresis and night sweats. • Observe patient performing deep breathing exercises and postural drainage. • Assess maintenance of respiratory isolation. • Assess proper and safe use of any respiratory therapy equipment.	• Reassess same as previous visit.	• Reassess same as previous visit.
DIET	• Have patient force fluids to 2 to 3 L/day if tolerated. • Assess weight and nutritional intake. • Encourage high-protein, high-carbohydrate diet. • Refer to dietary consult if indicated.	• Reinforce previous visit. • Explain importance of diet maintenance. • Refer to dietary consult if indicated.	• Reinforce previous visit.
ACTIVITY	• Assess response to activity. • Explain importance of frequent rest periods.	• Reinforce previous visit.	• Reinforce previous visit.
ELIMINATION	• Evaluate fluid intake. • Instruct to keep daily weight and fluid intake log.	• Evaluate daily weight and fluid intake log.	• Evaluate daily weight and fluid intake log.
HYGIENE	• Assess home for sanitary equipment necessary for good hygiene: disposable waste bags and covered trash containers. • Assess home for sleeping conditions, crowding, persons with upper respiratory infections (URIs), children, elderly, and others susceptible to infection.	• Reassess same as previous visit.	• Reassess same as previous visit.
PATIENT TEACHING	• Discuss signs and symptoms to report to doctor • Discuss medication (name, dosage, purpose, time and route of administration, adverse effects). • Instruct patient to avoid close contact with others until doctor advises. • Instruct patient to avoid crowds and persons with URIs. • Teach respiratory isolation techniques. • Explain importance of hygiene measures and hand washing (coughing into tissue, avoiding direct contact with sputum, proper disposal of soiled tissue).	• Discuss causes and treatment of TB. • Reinforce previous teaching. • Evaluate maintenance of respiratory isolation. • Explain importance of regular follow-up care.	• Reinforce and evaluate teaching sessions from previous home visits.
DISCHARGE PLANNING	• Assess home support and resource needs (for example, economic status for ability to purchase medications and supplies and to maintain isolation in home until certain medication levels are attained). • Refer to appropriate agency or social services as indicated.	• Assess home support and resource needs.	• Reassess same as previous visit.

Diagnostic tests

Skin testing; cultures, such as of gastric washings, cerebrospinal fluid, drainage from abscess; sputum cultures and smears; pleural effusion or cavitation; fiberoptic bronchoscopy; pleural needle biopsy; white blood cell count, especially leukocytes

Related nursing diagnoses

1 Impaired gas exchange
2 Ineffective breathing pattern
3 Altered nutrition: less than body requirements
4 Altered health maintenance
5 Ineffective management of therapeutic regimen: individual
6 Activity intolerance
7 Risk for infection

Expected outcomes

The following expected outcomes pertain to the patient or family. Numbers in parentheses refer to related nursing diagnoses above.

- Exhibit improved breath sounds, less difficulty with breathing, temperature within normal limits, heart rate of 65 to 80 beats per minute, and decreasing night sweats (1,2).
- Adhere to a high-protein, high-carbohydrate diet (3).
- Maintain adequate nutritional and fluid intake (3).
- Explain the nature of the disease and the purpose of treatment (4).
- State the need for ongoing outpatient care (4).
- Report the following to doctor: hemoptysis, increased difficulty breathing, hearing loss, vertigo, night sweats, temperature elevation, and weight loss (4).
- Seek appropriate support groups and referrals to keep psychosocial and physical well-being (4).
- Comply with regimen, and avoid over-the-counter (OTC) drugs without doctor approval (5).
- Seek social services to assist with health maintenance (5).
- Adhere to prescribed drug therapy (5).
- State importance for ongoing outpatient care and need for frequent rest periods (6).
- Take appropriate measures to prevent spread of the disease (7).
- Name all contacts and close family members for follow-up by board of health (7).
- Maintain respiratory isolation until doctor advises (7).
- Practice good hygiene and hand washing to reduce transmission of disease (7).
- Avoid crowds, persons with upper respiratory infections (URIs), and close contact with others until doctor advises (7).

Potential complications

Hypoxemia, atelectasis, pneumonia, pneumothorax

Patient teaching

Preventing recurrence

- Maintain natural resistance (adequate nutrition, rest, exercise).
- Avoid persons with infections, especially URIs.
- Avoid fatigue, extremes in temperature, excessive alcohol intake, and use of OTC drugs.
- Keep follow-up appointments with doctor as directed (expect periodic sputum smears).
- Seek appropriate health resources (social services for financial assistance, alcoholic counseling, occupational therapy) to assist with health care needs.
- Continue taking prescribed medication therapy — stop only when doctor approves.

- Avoid job-related exposure to silicon (foundry work, rock quarry, sand blasting).
- Educate about the disease process — obtain the booklet *Understanding Tuberculosis Today: A Handbook for Patients* from the local American Lung Association.

Reducing transmission
- Turn head away when coughing and cover mouth with tissue.
- Cover mouth and nose with tissue when sneezing.
- Cough and expectorate sputum into tissue.
- Use tissue only once and discard in trash container.
- Wash hands after using tissue, and avoid direct contact with sputum.
- Instruct family to use same techniques at home, especially to wash hands after direct contact with patient and his immediate environment (bedding, clothes, oral devices, trash containers).
- Avoid socialization with those who have URIs, lung diseases, and chronic illnesses; those who are recovering from surgery; and those who are immunosuppressed.
- Maintain respiratory isolation until medication levels are obtained (follow doctor's orders).
- Avoid close contact with others until doctor advises.
- Promote purified protein derivative testing of family and contacts.

Signs and symptoms
- Hemoptysis (cough up blood), chest pain, increased difficulty in breathing, persistent cough
- Night sweats, elevated temperature (especially in afternoons), weight loss
- Hearing loss and vertigo (dizziness)

Activity
- Explain importance of gradually increasing activity.
- Limit exercise and activity to tolerance.
- Plan two to three rest periods per day. Avoid fatigue.
- Keep necessary items within easy reach (tissue, appropriate trash container).
- Avoid strenuous work until approved by doctor.

Medications
- Instruct patient on dosage, time of administration, purpose, and adverse effects.
- Avoid OTC drugs and alcohol use.
- Explain importance of drug therapy in relation to disease.

Nutrition
- Explain importance of maintaining high-protein, high-carbohydrate diet.
- Perform oral hygiene before meals to remove foul taste of sputum.
- Drink at least 3 L/day unless contraindicated.
- Weigh daily and keep weight log throughout treatment period.

Critical thinking activities
1. Create and test a health promotion program to reduce new TB cases in nursing homes.
2. Identify the structural and pathophysiologic changes of TB.
3. Develop a teaching plan addressing nutritional and rest needs of the TB patient.
4. Relate the clinical manifestation of TB to the pathophysiologic processes that occur.
5. List the interventions that significant others can do to prevent the spread of TB.

Suggested research topics
- Coping strategies for TB
- Compliance with therapy
- Effectiveness of TB education programs

PART 3

Cardiovascular problems

Coronary artery bypass surgery

Heart failure

Hypertension

Myocardial infarction

Coronary artery bypass surgery

DRG: 107 Mean LOS: 7.8 days

Cardiovascular diseases rank as the leading cause of death in the United States today. And coronary artery disease (CAD), in which fatty deposits partially or totally occlude one or more of the coronary arteries, is a cause of these diseases. The three major clinical manifestations of CAD are angina pectoris, acute myocardial infarction (MI), and sudden cardiac death.

The usual surgical treatment for CAD is myocardial revascularization. This may be accomplished by percutaneous transluminal coronary angioplasty (PTCA), in which the vessel is cannulated and dilated, or through the coronary artery bypass graft (CABG) — one of the most frequently performed surgeries in the United States. Candidates for CABG are patients who have not responded to CAD medical management, who have advanced CAD, or who have undergone an unsuccessful PTCA.

The CABG procedure uses a grafted blood vessel (usually the saphenous vein or internal mammary artery) to provide blood flow from the ascending aorta to the myocardial tissue distal to the stenosed portion of the coronary artery. Though a palliative treatment, not a cure, CABG provides patients with improved cardiovascular status.

Subjective assessment findings

Health history
CAD, MI, angina, heart failure, previous CABG

Medication history
Digitalis glycosides, diuretics, antiarrhythmics, anticoagulants, nonsteroidal anti-inflammatory drugs

Functional health patterns
Activity-exercise: dyspnea on exertion, paroxysmal nocturnal dyspnea, orthopnea, fatigue, syncope, smoking history
Sleep-rest: number of pillows used
Nutritional-metabolic: weight gain, edema, nausea
Cognitive-perceptual: behavioral changes, depression, dependency

Objective assessment findings

Physical findings
Cardiovascular: tachycardia, arrhythmias, abnormal heart sounds (S_3), jugular vein distention, peripheral edema
Integumentary: sacral and pedal edema
Neurologic: confusion, anxiety, restlessness
Respiratory: tachypnea, crackles, rhonchi, wheezes

Diagnostic tests

Cardiac catheterization, coronary arteriography, echocardiograms, stress test, nuclear imaging, arterial blood gases, Doppler studies (to evaluate peripheral perfusion), pulmonary function tests, thyroid studies, liver function tests

Related nursing diagnoses

1 Decreased cardiac output
2 Impaired gas exchange
3 Risk for injury

Expected outcomes

The following expected outcomes pertain to the patient or family. Numbers in parentheses refer to related nursing diagnoses above.

- Demonstrate improved cardiac output with vital signs within normal parameters, stable hemodynamic status (such as stable cardiac output, artery wedge pressure, and left ventricular end diastolic pressure), and absence of S_3 gallop (1).
- Demonstrate adequate ventilatory status with increased tolerance for activity, breath sounds clear bilaterally, and ability to expand chest fully on inspiration (2).
- Show no signs of infection, including no increase in temperature above baseline and no signs of wound infection at chest tube site, graft sites, or sternal incision site (3).

Other possible nursing diagnoses

Activity intolerance, anxiety, body image disturbance, pain

Potential complications

Decreased cardiac output, fluid and electrolyte imbalance, arrhythmias, pneumothorax or hemothorax, MI

Patient teaching

Complications

- Acute MI
- Arrhythmias
- Hemorrhage
- Pulmonary emboli
- Wound infection and fever
- Cerebral infarcts
- Acute respiratory distress syndrome
- Renal failure
- Depression

Stages of care

- Operating room
- Postanesthesia care unit
- Intensive care unit (ICU) or critical care unit (CCU)
- Step-down unit or post-ICU–CCU unit
- General care unit
- Cardiac rehabilitation

(Text continues on page 49.)

CLINICAL PATHWAY

PLAN OF CARE	PREADMIT PHASE	INPATIENT CARE Day 1	Day 2
DIAGNOSTIC TESTS	• Complete blood count (CBC) • Coagulation profile • Serum electrolytes (lytes) • Blood urea nitrogen (BUN) • Creatinine (Cr) • Cardiac enzymes • Serum chemistries • Magnesium (Mg) • Type and crossmatch • Urinalysis • Electrocardiogram (ECG) • Chest X-ray (CXR)	• CBC, lytes, BUN, Cr • Continuous ECG and hemodynamic monitoring • Pulse oximetry q 2 hr • CXR • Arterial blood gases (ABGs)	• Hemoglobin (Hgb) and hematocrit (Hct), lytes • Continuous ECG and hemodynamic monitoring • Pulse oximetry q 4 hr
MEDICATIONS	• Assess current medications: prescriptions and over-the-counter medications; discontinue (D/C) digoxin, diuretics, warfarin (Coumadin), acetylsalicylic acid (aspirin [ASA]), dipyridamole (Persantine), long-lasting insulin as ordered	• Diuretics with potassium (K) and Mg replacement as needed • I.V. antibiotics • ASA • Stool softener • Analgesics as needed	• Diuretics with K and Mg replacement as needed • ASA • Stool softener • Other analgesics as needed
PROCEDURES	• Stop smoking at least 1 week before surgery.	• Take vital signs (VS) every 30 minutes. • Endotracheal tube (ETT) to mechanical ventilation; extubate within first 8 hours per protocol based on ABG results. • After extubation, give oxygen (O_2) per nasal cannula 2 to 4 L/min to maintain O_2 saturation (O_2 sat) > 95%. • Suction as needed. • Perform incentive spirometry (IS), chest physiotherapy (CPT), cough, and deep breathing (DB) q 2 hr while awake. • Give pacing wire care (if present). • Give chest tube care. • Monitor I.V. infusions (peripheral and central lines). • Keep all incisions covered. • Apply antiembolic (TED) stockings.	• Take VS q 2 hr. • D/C nasal O_2 or use as needed if O_2 sat > 95% on room air. • Perform IS, CPT q 2 hr while awake. • Turn, cough, and perform DB q 2 hr while awake. • Give pacing wire care. • Give chest tube care. • D/C saline lock peripheral I.V. • Monitor I.V. infusions via triple-lumen central catheter (TL cath). • Remove dressings from leg incisions. • Keep all other wound sites covered. • Keep TED stockings on.
DIET	• Take baseline height and weight. • Evaluate current diet and nutritional status. • Give nothing by mouth (NPO) after midnight (MN).	• Nasogastric tube (NGT) to gravity; D/C NGT after extubation. • Give NPO until extubated, then ice chips. • Weigh patient.	• Give ice chips to clear liquids. • Weigh patient.
ACTIVITY	• Evaluate current activity capabilities.	• Turn q 2 hr. • Encourage bed rest; elevate head of bed 20°. • Assist patient to dangle legs at bedside while sitting. • Have patient start range-of-motion exercises.	• Have patient get out of bed (OOB) to chair with assistance. • Begin cardiac rehabilitation.

Coronary artery bypass surgery

Day 3	Day 4	Day 5	Day 6	Day 7
Hgb and Hct, lytes Continuous ECG monitoring D/C hemodynamic monitoring Pulse oximetry q 8 hr CXR ABGs	• Hgb and Hct, lytes, Mg, potassium (K) • D/C continuous ECG monitoring (2 to 3 hours after pacing wires D/C and no arrhythmia present) • Pulse oximetry q 12 hr	• CBC, BUN, Cr, lytes • D/C pulse oximetry if O_2 sat > 95% on room air. • ABGs	• Hgb and Hct, lytes • CXR	
ASA Stool softener Other noncardiac medications Laxative as needed Analgesics as needed	• ASA • Stool softener • Analgesics as needed	• ASA • Stool softener • Noncardiac medications	• Same as previous day	• Same as previous day
Take VS q 4 hr. Perform IS, CPT q 2 hr while awake. Turn, cough, and perform DB q 2 hr while awake. Give pacing wire care. If drainage < 30 ml/hr, D/C chest tubes per protocol; perform site care and apply dressing. Monitor I.V. infusions via TL cath. Change dressing. Give incision care b.i.d. Keep TED stockings on.	• Take VS q 4 hr. • Perform coughing and DB exercises q 4 hr. • D/C pacing wires per protocol if cardiac rhythm stable. • Give chest tube dressing care. • D/C TL cath per protocol; apply dressing. • Give incision care b.i.d. • Keep TED stockings on.	• Take VS q 4 hr. • Perform coughing and DB exercises q 4 hr. • D/C pacing wires per protocol if cardiac rhythm stable. • Give chest tube dressing care. • Give incision care b.i.d.	• Take VS q 4 hr. • Perform coughing and DB exercises q 4 hr. • Give chest tube dressing care. • Remove sternal staples. • Give incision care b.i.d.	• Take VS q 4 hr. • Perform coughing and DB exercises q 4 hr. • Give chest tube dressing care. • Evaluate all wounds and incisions before discharge.
Progress diet as tolerated Weigh patient.	• Give cardiac diet: low fat, low sodium, low cholesterol. • Weigh patient.	• Same as previous day	• Same as previous day	• Same as previous day
Have patient get OOB to chair t.i.d. to q.i.d. Progress cardiac rehabilitation. Have patient walk with assistance in room three times daily	• Walks in hall with assistance t.i.d. • Feeds self. • Gets up in chair in room t.i.d.	• Progress cardiac rehabilitation. • Increase walking in hall with assistance. • Feeds self; gets up in chair in room q.i.d.	• Increase walking in hall with assistance. • Feeds self. • Walks in room q.i.d.	• Walks in hall independently.

(continued)

PLAN OF CARE	PREADMIT PHASE	INPATIENT CARE Day 1	Day 2
ELIMINATION	• Evaluate for nocturia and frequency of urination.	• Measure urinary catheter output every hour. • Check NGT output every hour. • Check chest tube output every hour.	• D/C urinary catheter. • D/C NGT. • Measure urine output every shift. • Measure chest tube output q 4 hr.
HYGIENE	• Shower with bacteriostatic soap as ordered.	• Give bed bath; complete care.	• Assist with bed bath.
PATIENT TEACHING	• Explain autotransfusion and autologous blood donation, postop routine, pain relief/modulation.	• Reorient patient and family to unit routine. • Instruct on medications, wound care, and incentive spirometry.	• Instruct on lifestyle modifications and energy conservation.
DISCHARGE PLANNING	*Home health consult:* • Determine need and eligibility for home health services. *Social services consult:* • Evaluated need for placement after discharge (such as home, nursing home, assisted living facility). *Case manager consult:* • Evaluate progression of patient while on path.	• Evaluate discharge needs.	• Same as previous day

Day 3	Day 4	Day 5	Day 6	Day 7
D/C chest tube. Measure intake and output (I & O) every shift. Uses bedside commode with assistance.	▪ Measure I & O every shift.	▪ Same as previous day	▪ Same as previous day	▪ Same as previous day
Assist with hygiene.	▪ Have patient perform self-care with assistance as needed.	▪ Performs self-care. ▪ Assist as needed.	▪ Performs self-care.	▪ Performs self-care.
Dietary consult: Discuss diet. Discuss sodium, calorie, cholesterol, and saturated fat restrictions in diet as needed or ordered.	▪ Discuss medication effects and home monitoring. ▪ Instruct on carotid pulse measurement and wound care.	*Physical therapy (PT) consult:* ▪ Teach energy conservation techniques and progressive activity goals.	▪ Teach signs and symptoms of wound infection that should be reported.	*PT consult:* ▪ Reinforce home activity goals (increase in incremental fashion only with doctor approval).
Same as previous day	▪ Same as previous day	*Social services consult:* ▪ Arrange for home O$_2$, home medical equipment, and transportation.	*Home health consult:* ▪ Review schedule of home health nurse/aide visits.	▪ Discharge to home health.

(continued)

Clinical pathway 47

PLAN OF CARE	HOME CARE Visit 1	Visit 2	Visit 3
DIAGNOSTIC TESTS	▪ Draw blood for complete blood count, serum electrolytes, blood urea nitrogen, and creatinine level.	▪ Review results of previous lab with patient and family.	▪ Serum potassium (K) if on diuretic.
MEDICATIONS	▪ Assess compliance with drug regimen. ▪ Evaluate schedule of self-medication. ▪ Assess over-the-counter medication use.	▪ Evaluate cardiovascular and respiratory systems for adverse effects of drug therapy, including shortness of breath, edema, and rapid weight gain.	▪ Recommend to doctor medication increases or decreases in dosages as indicated per patient's physical status.
PROCEDURES	▪ Evaluate sternal wound, graft site(s), and previous chest tube sites for infection and stage of healing. ▪ Assess vital signs (VS) and peripheral pulses.	▪ Check VS. ▪ Evaluate surgical wound sites. ▪ Palpate peripheral pulses.	▪ Check VS. ▪ Review weight and heart rate logs. ▪ Palpate peripheral pulses.
DIET	▪ Give diet instructions with recall of cardiac diet: low-fat, low-sodium, low-cholesterol. ▪ Consult dietitian, as needed. ▪ Weigh patient.	▪ Reinstruct on foods low in cholesterol, saturated fat and sodium, and high in K. ▪ Weigh patient.	▪ Provide additional instructions on dietary choices and modifications within prescribed nutrient range. ▪ Weigh patient.
ACTIVITY	▪ Physical therapy evaluation. ▪ Progress cardiac rehabilitation (Phase 2: Outpatient Exercise Training).	▪ Review heart rate log. ▪ Determine level of compliance with prescribed exercise. ▪ Evaluate effects of prescribed exercise.	▪ Focus on increasing exercise capacity in activities such as walking, jogging, and weight training.
ELIMINATION	▪ Evaluate for nocturia and frequency of urination.	▪ Evaluate for constipation or straining at stool.	▪ Reassess need for diuretic, stool softener, and/or laxative.
HYGIENE	▪ Evaluate need for home health aide services.	▪ Assess as needed.	▪ Assess as needed.
PATIENT TEACHING	▪ Discuss early identification of medical problems, especially during exercise.	▪ Discuss patient's and family's risk reduction behaviors, such as smoking decrease/cessation.	▪ Discuss psychosocial needs of the patient and family to minimize episodes of anxiety and depression. ▪ Discuss need to resume sexual activities with doctor approval.
DISCHARGE PLANNING	▪ Investigate participation in community cardiac-related support groups and educational programs.	▪ Refer to occupational therapy as needed to assist in return to occupational and leisure activities.	▪ Provide patient and family with community support necessary for continuing lifestyle changes.

Postsurgical limitations
- Restrict driving for 4 to 6 weeks after surgery until approved by doctor.
- Restrict sexual activity for 2 to 4 weeks after surgery until approved by doctor.
- Restrict excessive exercise.
- Restrict lifting heavy objects or performing isometric exercises.
- Restrict sitting in the same position with feet dependent for long periods of time.

Activity
- Cough.
- Turn.
- Deep breathe.
- Splint incision.
- Use incentive spirometer.
- Avoid activities that produce shortness of breath, and limit activities during extreme hot or cold temperatures.
- Plan rest periods between activities.
- Avoid strenuous activities and work until doctor resuming these activities.
- Participate in a structured daily program of increasing activity and exercise.
- Stop activity if palpitations, shortness of breath, or severe fatigue occur.

Signs and symptoms
- Angina (chest pain)
- Dizziness
- Difficulty breathing
- Fast or irregular pulse
- Prolonged recovery time from exercise

Lifestyle modifications
- Eliminate smoking.
- Reduce weight.
- Moderate alcohol intake.
- Moderate stress.
- Take prescribed cardiovascular medications.

Nutrition
- Maintain low-sodium diet.
- Possibly reduce weight; maintain weight log.
- Follow doctor-prescribed diet.
- Refer to American Heart Association dietary recommendations to decrease fat and cholesterol intake.

Medications
- Instruct patient on dosage, time of administration, purpose, and adverse effects.
- Maintain up-to-date medication log.
- Follow dosage schedule.
- Understand food interactions and adverse effects of medications.
- Use over-the-counter drugs and alcohol cautiously; consult doctor before use.

Critical thinking activities
1. Describe how the activity progression after CABG varies to accommodate the physiologic limitations of elderly postsurgical patients.
2. List the most common home care needs of the patient following CABG surgery.

3. Determine the percentage of wound infections or other complications (for example, heart failure) requiring rehospitalization in CABG patients in "short-stay" inpatient environments. Determine the percentage for patients with longer inpatient stays. Compare the two figures.
4. In relation to postoperative exercise regimen and recovery, discuss the effect of using the radial artery instead of the saphenous vein for CABG bypass.
5. Describe the *typical* patient for whom percutaneous transluminal coronary angioplasty (PTCA, or balloon angioplasty) would be most successful.
6. A patient admitted for cardiac surgery inquires about alternative nonsurgical procedures that are available besides PTCA. Describe examples of other techniques used in the treatment of blocked coronary arteries.
7. List the postoperative complications of CABG surgery that occur most commonly in elderly patients.
8. Discuss the goal of rehabilitation after CABG surgery as the patient progresses from the In Hospital phase (Phase 1) to the Community Rehabilitation phase (Phase 3).
9. Discuss the reasons why PTCA and CABG may not be permanent solutions to the treatment of blocked coronary arteries.

Suggested research topics

- Rehospitalization rates
- Physiologic limitations of the elderly
- Postsurgery exercise programs
- Compliance with therapy
- Effectiveness of smoking cessation programs
- Effectiveness of weight reduction programs
- Effectiveness of stress reduction programs
- Coping with CABG surgery

Heart failure

DRG: 127 Mean LOS: 4.8 days

Also referred to as pump or cardiac failure, heart failure is the inability of the heart to pump enough blood to body tissues to meet oxygen and nutrient requirements. Heart failure can be classified as left-sided or right-sided. Causes of the disease include cardiac muscle disorders, coronary atherosclerosis (which can lead to myocardial infarction [MI]), and systemic or pulmonary hypertension; noncardiac causes include anemia, hypoxia, and increased metabolic rate.

Clinical features of heart failure vary with the side of the heart that has failed. For example, right-sided failure can cause edema of the feet and ankles, hepatomegaly, anorexia, nocturia, and weakness. Left-sided cardiac failure leads to pulmonary congestion, which results in dyspnea, orthopnea, paroxysmal nocturnal dyspnea, and cough.

Treatment includes pharmacologic therapy and dietary support. The drugs most commonly used for heart failure include cardiac glycosides such as digoxin, diuretics such as furosemide, angiotensin-converting enzyme inhibitors such as captopril, and vasodilators such as nitroglycerin. Dietary management usually includes restricting sodium intake to prevent, control, or eliminate edema and reducing fat and cholesterol intake to prevent worsening of atherosclerosis.

Subjective assessment findings

Health history
Coronary artery disease, MI, hypertension, arrhythmias, cardiomyopathy, cigarette smoking

Medication history
Diuretics, cardiac drugs, nonsteroidal anti-inflammatory drugs, corticosteroids

Functional health patterns
Activity-exercise: dyspnea, orthopnea, cough, palpitations, dizziness, syncope
Cognitive-perceptual: chest pain or heaviness, behavioral changes
Elimination: nocturia, decreased daytime urinary output, edema
Nutritional-metabolic: nausea, vomiting, anorexia, sodium intake, weight gain
Sleep-rest: fatigue, paroxysmal nocturnal dyspnea, number of pillows used

Objective assessment findings

Physical findings
Cardiovascular: tachycardia, S_3 and S_4 heart sounds, jugular vein distention, peripheral edema
Gastrointestinal: ascites, abdominal distention, right upper quadrant pain, hepatosplenomegaly
Integumentary: edema; cool, diaphoretic skin; cyanosis or pallor
Neurologic: confusion, restlessness, decreased attention span, memory problems
Respiratory: tachypnea; crackles; rhonchi; wheezes; frothy, blood-tinged sputum

Diagnostic tests
Serum electrolyte, blood urea nitrogen, and creatinine levels; liver function studies; chest X-ray; electrocardiogram; echocardiogram;, arterial blood gas analysis

(Text continues on page 55.)

PLAN OF CARE	PREADMIT PHASE	INPATIENT CARE Day 1	Day 2
DIAGNOSTIC TESTS	• Digitalis level • Complete blood count; electrolytes (lytes), blood urea nitrogen (BUN), and creatinine (Cr) levels; liver function tests; creatine kinase with isoenzymes; serum chemistries; and urinalysis • Urine-specific gravity • 12-lead electrocardiogram (ECG) • Chest X-ray (CXR)	• Lytes, BUN, and Cr levels • Arterial blood gas (ABG) analysis • Pulse oximetry q 4 hr • CXR • Continuous hemodynamic and ECG monitoring • Echocardiogram • Nuclear imaging	• Lytes, BUN, and Cr levels • ABG analysis • Pulse oximetry q 8 hr • CXR • If no arrhythmias, discontinue (D/C) continuous ECG monitoring.
MEDICATIONS	• Prescription and over-the-counter medications	• Cardiac glycosides, other inotropic agents, diuretics, angiotensin-converting enzyme (ACE) inhibitors, vasodilators, morphine sulfate • Potassium and magnesium supplements, as needed • I.V. drips via infusion pumps as ordered.	• Cardiac glycosides, other inotropic agents, diuretics, ACE inhibitors, vasodilators, morphine sulfate • Decrease or D/C I.V. inotropic therapy drips as ordered.
PROCEDURES	• Obtain baseline vital signs (VS). • Evaluate for I.V. access. • Determine baseline weight. • Determine code status and advance directives.	• Check VS every 1 to 2 hours. Evaluate for abnormal heart and breath sounds q 2 hr. • Maintain oxygen (O_2) via nasal cannula (NC) at 2-4 L/min or 40% O_2 via face mask to maintain O_2 saturation (O_2 sat) > 95%. • Evaluate for edema (pedal, ankle, pretibial, sacral, facial, and so forth) q 4 hr. • Monitor and record pulmonary artery (PA) catheter pressures q 2 hr and as needed. • Prepare for possible cardioversion, endotracheal intubation, mechanical ventilation, and intra-aortic balloon pump.	• Check VS q 4 hr. • Maintain O_2 via NC at 2 to 4 L/min or 40% O_2 via face mask to maintain O_2 sat > 95%. • Evaluate for abnormal heart and breath sounds q 4 hr. • Evaluate progression or diminishment of edema q 4 hr. • If PA wedge pressure improves, D/C PA catheter.
DIET	• Assess current diet.	• Institute sodium (Na) restriction (500 mg to 2 g/day). • Institute fluid restrictions. *Dietary consult:* Instruct on low-sodium diet.	• Continue Na restriction. • Continue fluid restrictions (moderate to severe heart failure). • Weigh patient.
ACTIVITY	• Institute energy conservation measures.	• Encourage bed rest in high Fowler's position. • Turn q 2 hr. • Have patient perform passive range-of-motion (ROM) exercises q 4 hr.	• Have patient get in chair and use bedside commode with help. • Turn q 2 hr while in bed. • Assist with performance of active and passive ROM exercises.
ELIMINATION	• Assess for nocturia and frequency of urination.	• Begin strict intake as directed. • Measure urine output every hour via urinary catheter.	• Continue strict input and output (I & O). • D/C catheter.
HYGIENE		• Give bed bath; provide complete care.	• Assist with hygiene needs.
PATIENT TEACHING	• Focus teaching on the reasons for hospitalization.	• Provide rationales for decreased Na and fluid intake. • Explain importance of energy conservation.	• Go over diet history and teach about diet, Na restriction, and need for taking daily weight. • Explain actions and adverse effects of medications. • Teach how to take carotid pulse.
DISCHARGE PLANNING	*Social services consult:* • Assess needs for home-care nursing and home-health aide.	*Social services:* • Assess needs. • As needed, arrange for pastoral care.	*Social services:* • Arrange for home health care, home O_2, and home durable medical equipment, if needed.

Day 3	Day 4	Day 5
■ Lytes, BUN, and Cr levels ■ Repeat digitalis level. ■ Pulse oximetry q 12 hr	■ Lytes, BUN, and Cr levels ■ CXR ■ Pulse oximetry q 12 hr	■ Lytes ■ D/C pulse oximetry.
■ Cardiac glycosides ■ Diuretics ■ ACE inhibitors, vasodilators ■ Saline lock I.V.	■ Cardiac glycosides ■ Diuretics ■ ACE inhibitors, vasodilators	■ Cardiac glycosides ■ Diuretics ■ ACE inhibitors, vasodilators ■ D/C saline lock.
■ Check VS q 4 hr. ■ Maintain O_2 via NC at 2 to 4 L/min or 40% O_2 via face mask to maintain O_2 sat > 95%. ■ Evaluate for abnormal heart and breath sounds q 8 hr. ■ Evaluate progression or diminishment of edema q 4 hr.	■ Check VS q 4 hr. ■ Maintain O_2 via NC at 2 to 4 L/min or 40% O_2 via face mask to maintain O_2 sat > 95%. ■ Evaluate for abnormal heart and breath sounds q 8 hr. ■ Evaluate saline lock I.V. site ■ Measure I & O every 8 hr.	■ Check VS q 8 hr. ■ D/C O_2 if O_2 sat > 95% on room air. ■ Evaluate for abnormal heart and breath sounds q 8 hr. ■ Evaluate progression or diminishment of edema q 4 hr.
■ Same as previous day	■ Same as previous day	■ Continue Na restriction. ■ Weigh patient.
■ Have patient walk with assistance and on O_2. ■ Turn q 2 hr while in bed. ■ Encourage bathroom privileges (BRP) with assistance.	■ Have patient walk in hall with assistance and on O_2 q 4 hr. ■ Encourage BRP with assistance.	■ Same as previous day
■ Measure I & O q 4 hr.	■ Measure I & O q 8 hr.	■ Same as previous day
■ Same as previous day	■ Have patient meet his own hygiene needs. ■ Evaluate tolerance of increased activity.	■ Performs self-care to meet hygiene needs ■ Evaluate tolerance of increased activity.
■ Continue teaching about Na restrictions. ■ Teach about weight reduction. ■ Teach about physical and occupational therapy. ■ Teach energy conservation and energy-efficient behaviors.	■ Evaluate patient's ability to take and log carotid pulse and daily weight accurately. ■ Teach patient and family how to assess for edema of feet, ankles, and pretibial and sacral areas; explain significance of edema.	■ Discuss signs and symptoms that call for contacting health care provider or going to emergency department. ■ Review home activity program as established.
Home health: ■ Arrange for visit with patient and family while patient still hospitalized.	■ Reevaluate progress toward discharge goals. *Social services:* ■ Reevaluate home care requirements.	

(continued)

PLAN OF CARE	HOME CARE Visit 1	Visit 2	Visit 3
DIAGNOSTIC TESTS	• Obtain blood urea nitrogen, creatinine, digoxin, and potassium levels.	• Review results of lab work with patient and family.	
MEDICATIONS	• Assess compliance with drug regimen. • Assess for positive and adverse effects of drug therapy.	• Assess compliance with drug regimen. • Assess for positive and adverse effects of drug therapy. • Reinforce permanence of drug regimen if necessary.	• Same as previous visit
PROCEDURES	• Perform comprehensive assessment to establish baseline.	• Reassess vital signs (VS), lungs, and cardiovascular and peripheral vascular systems. • Reassess mental status. • Reevaluate for the presence of edema. • Evaluate weight log. • Evaluate carotid pulse log.	• Same as previous visit
DIET	• Assess compliance with therapeutic diet. • Restrict sodium (Na) and fluids as necessary. • If patient on diuretic therapy, go over sources of potassium.	• Assess compliance with therapeutic diet.	• Same as previous visit
ACTIVITY	• Assess exercise tolerance. • Restrict activities if necessary. • Refer to physical or occupational therapy for energy conservation appraisal if needed.	• Assess exercise tolerance and tolerance of activities of daily living, including sexual activity.	• Same as previous visit
ELIMINATION	• Assess intake and output (I & O) patterns. • Assess for nocturia, urinary frequency, and constipation.	• Assess I & O patterns.	• Same as previous visit
HYGIENE	• Provide assistance as needed. • Evaluate for home health aide services.	• Assist as needed.	• Same as previous visit
PATIENT TEACHING	• Provide patient and family with written educational materials from sources such as the American Heart Association. • Teach lifestyle modifications and risk factor reduction, such as decreasing or stopping smoking. • Reinforce permanence of therapeutic regimen.	• Teach importance of regular follow-up visits with health care providers, effects of increased Na and fluid intake, and exercise and activity restrictions as necessary. • Teach patient about hidden sources of Na (such as antacids). • Teach food and drug interactions.	• Reinforce and evaluate teaching sessions from previous home visits.
DISCHARGE PLANNING	• Assess home support and resource needs, such as transportation needs for follow-up visits to health care providers, long-term durable medical equipment needs, and home health aide needs. • Make sure patient has an accurate scale for taking daily weight.	• Assess home support and resource needs.	• Same as previous visit

Heart failure (continued)

CLINICAL PATHWAY

Related nursing diagnoses

1 Activity intolerance
2 Fluid volume excess
3 Risk for impaired skin integrity
4 Impaired gas exchange
5 Anxiety
6 Self-care deficit
7 Ineffective management of therapeutic regimen: individual
8 Noncompliance

Expected outcomes

The following expected outcomes pertain to the patient or family. Numbers in parentheses refer to related nursing diagnoses above.

- Be able to tolerate activity to patient's satisfaction (1).
- Have reduced or no edema (2).
- Have no skin breakdown over edematous areas (3).
- Have decreased or no shortness of breath (4).
- Have clear lungs (4).
- Have decreased anxiety (5).
- Perform activities of daily living with assistance as necessary (6).
- Notify health care providers of the signs and symptoms of heart failure (7).
- Describe appropriate diet to decrease sodium intake and increase potassium intake (if taking a non-potassium-sparing diuretic) (7).
- State the importance of keeping follow-up appointments with health care providers (8).

Other possible nursing diagnoses

Ineffective individual coping, sleep pattern disturbance

Potential complications

Decreased cardiac output, cardiogenic shock, arrhythmias, adverse effects from medication, fluid and electrolyte imbalance, renal failure, respiratory failure

Patient teaching

Signs and symptoms

- Shortness of breath
- Chest pain
- Difficulty breathing when sleeping (needing more pillows)
- Fatigue
- Increased coughing and sputum production
- Voiding more frequently, especially at night
- Swelling of ankles, feet, or abdomen
- Weight gain of 1 to 2 lb (.5 to 1 kg) over a 2-day period
- Changes in heart rate and rhythm
- Nausea and vomiting

Nutrition

- Maintain low-sodium diet.
- Possibly reduce weight; maintain weight log.
- Follow doctor-prescribed diet.
- Refer to American Heart Association dietary recommendations to decrease fat and cholesterol intake.

Activity
- Plan for alternating periods of activity and rest.
- Gradually return to usual daily activity level.
- Avoid activities that can trigger fatigue.
- Stop activity if palpitations, SOB, or severe fatigue occur.
- Avoid strenuous activities and work until doctor resumption.

Medications
- Maintain up-to-date medication log.
- Follow dosage schedule.
- Understand food interactions and adverse effects of medications.
- Use over-the-counter drugs and alcohol cautiously; consult doctor before use.

Coping
- Understand the chronic nature of the disease.
- Adopt changes appropriate to the severity of the disease.
- Adopt positive strategies to cope with long-term disease management.

Critical thinking activities
1. Discuss factors that affect compliance with the therapeutic regimen in heart failure patients.
2. Describe how unrelieved anxiety and stress affect outcomes and convalescence.
3. Describe the energy conservation techniques that work best for heart failure patients.
4. Discuss the relationship between MI and heart failure.
5. Describe how increased preload can lead to decreased cardiac output and eventual heart failure. List conditions that may result in increased preload.
6. Diagram the etiology of left-sided and right-sided heart failure. Describe typical clinical manifestations of each type of failure.
7. Describe the effect of cardiac glycoside preparations on improving ventricular performance. Determine the cardiac conditions for which cardiac glycosides are contraindicated.
8. Develop a home teaching plan for the self-administration of a cardiac glycoside product by a newly diagnosed elderly heart failure patient.

Suggested research topics
- Coping strategies for heart failure
- Compliance with therapy
- Role of anxiety in heart failure
- Role of stress in heart failure

Hypertension

DRG: 134 Mean LOS: 3 days

Hypertension, also known as high blood pressure, is blood pressure (BP) in which the systolic reading is persistently greater than 140 mm Hg and the diastolic reading is greater than 90 mm Hg. Because of its insidious nature — that is, no symptoms are exhibited — hypertension is also called the "silent killer" and is a major health problem in the United States, especially among African Americans. Stress, obesity, diabetes mellitus, and a family history of hypertension all increase the likelihood of the disorder. Untreated hypertension can lead to heart and kidney failure as well as stroke.

Hypertension can be classified as essential, or primary hypertension, which has no identifiable medical cause, or as secondary hypertension, which has a specific cause, such as pregnancy or narrowing of the renal arteries. Ninety percent of adult hypertension is classified as essential.

Strategies for controlling hypertension include nonpharmacologic approaches, such as restriction of alcohol, tobacco products, and sodium; weight reduction; exercise; and relaxation. Pharmacologic therapy employs a stepped-care approach that begins with specific medications, then progresses to higher dosages or other medications as necessary.

Subjective assessment findings

Health history
Prior diagnosis of cardiovascular, renal, or peripheral vascular disease, diabetes mellitus, pheochromocytoma, disorders of the pituitary gland, structural disorders of blood vessels such as the aorta or renal arteries; patterns of alcohol and tobacco use

Medication history
Over-the-counter medications, antihypertensives, including compliance with therapy (past and present)

Functional health patterns
Nutritional-metabolic: total daily caloric intake, sodium and fat intake patterns, weight gain history
Coping–stress tolerance: stressful occurrences in family, social, or work environments
Cognitive-perceptual: frequent headaches, especially on rising in the morning; dizziness; syncopal episodes; blurred vision

Objective assessment findings

Physical findings
Cardiovascular: BP >140/90 mm Hg documented on more than one occasion, angina, palpitations, epistaxis, S_4 gallop
Musculoskeletal: muscle cramping
Ophthalmic: retinopathy
Peripheral vascular: absent pulses
Respiratory: dyspnea on exertion

PLAN OF CARE	PREADMIT PHASE	INPATIENT CARE *Day 1*
DIAGNOSTIC TESTS	• Serum electrolytes (lytes) • Blood urea nitrogen (BUN) • Creatinine (Cr) • Complete blood count (CBC) • Lipid profile • Fasting blood sugar • Urinalysis • Chest X-ray (CXR) • Electrocardiogram (ECG)	• Lytes • BUN • Cr • CBC • 12-lead ECG • Pulse oximetry every 1 to 2 hours • CXR • Computed tomography scan of head • Continuous ECG monitoring
MEDICATIONS	• None in early stage • Stepped approach to antihypertensives as required in later stages	• Parenteral antihypertensive (nitroprusside, labetalol) administered 2 to 5 minutes until BP stabilized; monitor for sudden hypotension. • Begin oral antihypertensives to wean off parenteral medications. • I.V. 5% dextrose in water at keep-vein-open rate.
PROCEDURES	• Periodic monitoring of blood pressure (BP) by health professional	• Check BP and other vital signs (VS) every 1 to 2 hours and as needed until stabilized. • Give oxygen (O_2) per nasal cannula 2 to 4 L/min to maintain O_2 saturation (O_2 sat) > 95%. • Analyses of ECG strip (rate, rhythm, and arrhythmia analysis). • Do neurologic checks (neuro checks) q 1 to 2 hr. • Evaluate pulmonary artery catheter pressures every hour and as needed (if present). • Monitor arterial line (if present).
DIET	• Weigh patient.	• Give nothing by mouth until BP stabilized *Dietary consult:* • Restrict sodium (Na) to < 2 to 3 g/day; decrease calories and fat. • Take diet history with 24-hour food recall.
ACTIVITY	• After physical exam, begin regular aerobic exercise 30 to 45 minutes, 3 to 5 times per week.	• Encourage complete bed rest until BP stabilized. • Place head of bed in high-Fowler's position (90°).
ELIMINATION	• Evaluate for presence of nocturia and hematuria.	• Measure intake and output (I & O) every hour until BP stabilized.
HYGIENE	• Assist as needed.	• Assist with all needs.
PATIENT TEACHING	• Discuss dietary management, smoking cessation, regular exercise, limiting alcohol, and medication effects and adverse effects. • Teach relaxation techniques. • Discuss stress reduction.	• Discuss the need for rapid decrease and stabilization of BP.
DISCHARGE PLANNING	• Schedule frequent monitoring of BP until stabilized; then monitor every 4 to 6 months.	*Case manager consult:* *Social services consult:* *Home health consult:* • Prepare patient for discharge from emergency department to intensive care unit or general care unit.

Day 2	Day 3
- Lytes - BUN - Cr - Pulse oximetry q 4 hr	- Lytes
- Monitor effects of oral medications: diuretics, adrenergic inhibitors, angiotensin-converting enzyme (ACE) inhibitors, calcium antagonists. - Perform saline lock I.V.	- Evaluate for adverse effects of medications: diuretics, adrenergic blockers, ACE inhibitors; calcium antagonists. - D/C saline lock.
- Check VS q 4 hr and as needed. - Discontinue (D/C) O_2 if O_2 sat > 95% on room air. - Do neuro checks every shift.	- Check VS. - D/C neuro checks.
- Give low-Na, low-fat, reduced-calorie diet as tolerated. - Restrict fluid if applicable.	- Give low-Na, low-fat, reduced-calorie diet as tolerated, as per nutritional therapy consult. - Weigh patient.
- Have patient walk in room with assistance.	- Have patient perform activities as tolerated.
- Measure I & O q 8 hr.	- Measure I & O every shift.
- Assist as needed.	- Assist as needed.
- Reinforce teaching on lifestyle and diet modifications. - Teach expected effects of new medications.	- Continue with instruction on lifestyle modifications. - Teach about possible adverse effects of new medication.
	- Refer to community BP screening programs as indicated.

(continued)

CLINICAL PATHWAY ■ **Hypertension**

PLAN OF CARE	HOME CARE Visit 1	Visit 2	Visit 3
DIAGNOSTIC TESTS	▪ Serum electrolytes (lytes) ▪ Blood urea nitrogen ▪ Creatinine	▪ Lytes	▪ Lytes
MEDICATIONS	▪ Validate antihypertensive medication type, dosage, and sequencing—diuretics, adrenergic inhibitors, angiotensin-converting enzyme inhibitors, calcium antagonists. ▪ Assess medication interactions with other drugs and with foods.	▪ Evaluate for expected effects of BP medications. ▪ Make recommendations to doctor for alterations in type and dose of medications if needed. ▪ Evaluate medications for adverse effects.	▪ Evaluate for adverse effects of BP medications (for example, depression, weakness, dry mouth, impotence, sedation, or orthostatic hypertension). ▪ Address interactions between BP medications and other medications or foods.
PROCEDURES	▪ Measure blood pressure (BP) carefully: take initially in both arms and subsequently in arm with the higher reading; measure BP in sitting, supine, and standing positions. ▪ Weigh patient.	▪ Measure BP carefully. ▪ Assess for edema of lower extremities. ▪ Weigh patient. ▪ Determine if BP medications have been taken as prescribed.	▪ Measure BP and note variance and trends from previous visits. ▪ Assess for edema. ▪ Weigh patient.
DIET	▪ Review prescribed diet. ▪ Establish dietary goals with patient and family for weight loss as necessary. ▪ Make sure family has use of a scale if needed.	▪ Take 24-hour recall of food intake. ▪ Review food choices which are appropriate or inappropriate as necessary.	▪ Review food in the home with patient and family for "hidden" sources of sodium and fat (for example, canned foods, processed foods, antacids, and so forth). ▪ Review "dining out" habits; stress need to avoid or eliminate "fast foods."
ACTIVITY	▪ Establish goals and parameters for incrementally increasing activity levels. ▪ Focus on goal of achieving long-term adherence.	▪ Review patient's participation in exercise since last visit. ▪ Revise activity goals if indicated.	▪ Encourage participation in aerobic exercises such as walking, biking, swimming, and so forth after evaluation by doctor.
ELIMINATION	▪ Evaluate for nocturia, hematuria, frequent urination, urine retention, and constipation.	▪ Evaluate urinary and bowel patterns.	▪ Evaluate urinary and bowel patterns.
HYGIENE	▪ Evaluate need for home health aide services.	▪ Assist as needed.	▪ Assist as needed.
PATIENT TEACHING	▪ Communicate BP reading to patient, and explain significance as necessary. ▪ Reinforce need for lifelong antihypertensive therapy. ▪ Review understanding of medication dosage and sequencing. ▪ Reinforce relaxation/stress management techniques.	▪ Instruct patient not to miss doses of medications, not to "double up" on doses, not to "borrow" BP medications from others, and not to abruptly discontinue medications. ▪ Discuss how to manage orthostatic hypertension: change positions slowly, do leg exercises, lie or sit down when dizzy.	▪ Teach patient that most adverse reactions to BP medication will diminish over time. ▪ Begin teaching patient or family member how to take BP measurements if willing, capable, and reliable.
DISCHARGE PLANNING	▪ Evaluate patient's financial resources necessary for compliance with antihypertensive therapy. ▪ Consult social services if financial resources appear inadequate to ensure long-term compliance with therapy.	▪ Begin to evaluate patient's and family's potential for long-term compliance with all aspects of therapy. ▪ Refer to smoking cessation courses as needed.	▪ Continue to evaluate patient for long-term lifestyle modification and medication compliance. ▪ Ensure that patient and family have written instructions related to medication therapy, diet therapy, and exercise instruction, and that they are following instructions.

Diagnostic tests

Serum electrolyte, blood urea nitrogen, and creatinine levels; fasting blood sugar; complete blood count; electrocardiogram; chest X-ray; urinalysis; cholesterol and triglyceride levels

Related nursing diagnoses

1 Ineffective management of therapeutic regimen: individual
2 Noncompliance
3 Altered nutrition: more than body requirements

Expected outcomes

The following expected outcomes pertain to the patient or family. Numbers in parentheses refer to related nursing diagnoses above.

- Have BP remain ≤ 140/90 mm Hg on return visits to health care professional (1).
- Be able to verbalize symptoms that require the attention of a health care provider: blurred vision, dizziness, epistaxis, angina, shortness of breath (1).
- Be aware of BP reading and understand the significance of the reading (1).
- Be able to correctly monitor BP and weight and record for review at the next home visit or doctor's office visit, if possible (1).
- Be aware of the correct type, dosage, and sequencing of BP medication as evidenced by verbal recall and by the correct number of BP medications left in the drug container (1).
- State the need for long-term compliance with lifestyle modification, such as weight loss; decrease in tobacco, alcohol, and sodium use; and antihypertensive therapy (2) to achieve or maintain normotensive status.

Other possible nursing diagnoses

Anxiety, ineffective denial, altered sexuality patterns

Potential complications

Cardiovascular; adverse effects of beta blocker, calcium channel blocker, or angiotensin-converting enzyme inhibitor therapy

Patient teaching

Definition of hypertension
- Hypertension, BP (include normal readings)
- Diastolic pressure, systolic pressure

Complications
- Cardiac, renal, peripheral vascular, cerebral vascular, retinal

Risk factors for essential hypertension
- Age, sex, race
- Family history
- Obesity, cigarette smoking, alcohol intake, dietary sodium
- Elevated serum lipids, diabetes
- Sedentary lifestyle, stress, socioeconomic status

Lifestyle modifications
- Restrict sodium intake to 2.3 g (<6 g of salt) per day.

- Restrict calorie and fat intake (total fat intake 30% or less of calories; saturated fatty acid < 10% of calories; cholesterol < 300 mg; restrictions may be tailored to patient, depending on obesity and cholesterol levels)
- Restrict alcohol intake to 1 ounce (oz) per day (equivalent of 24 oz beer, 8 oz wine, or 2 oz of 100 proof whiskey per day).
- Incorporate regular aerobic exercise, such as jogging, walking, and swimming, for 30 to 45 minutes, three to five times per week.
- Stop cigarette smoking.
- Incorporate stress management techniques into daily life.

Pharmacologic therapy
- Initial step, or first-line drugs, include monotherapy with either a diuretic or beta blocker.
- Subsequent steps include increases in dosage, adding another drug from a different class, or substituting a drug from a different class if BP is not controlled.

Coping
- Antihypertensive therapy is a long-term, often lifelong, therapy.
- Medications should never to be stopped abruptly because doing so can lead to hypertensive crisis.

Signs and symptoms
- Orthostatic hypotension (light-headedness on standing)
- "Racing" heartbeat, palpitations ("fluttering" in the chest)
- Blurred vision, dizziness
- Epistaxis, angina, shortness of breath

Critical thinking activities
1. List strategies that can be used to increase compliance with antihypertensive therapies among the elderly population.
2. Discuss how compliance strategies do and do not differ between the elderly and nonelderly hypertensive populations.
3. Observe a randomly selected sample of home health nurses. Record the number who are following the recommended guidelines for BP assessment: taking initial measurement in both arms, using a correct size cuff, using equipment that functions properly, and assessing the patient's BP in a sitting, lying, and standing position.
4. Discuss whether elderly patients being treated with the adrenergic inhibitors (blockers) are more likely to develop depression during treatment than nonelderly patients.
5. Discuss whether wellness and other education programs directed toward at-risk, young populations can decrease the incidence of hypertension.
6. Devise a chart that outlines the sequence of events leading to target organ damage as a result of hypertension.
7. Describe the physiologic factors that regulate BP in the short term (seconds to hours).
8. Discuss the role that stress plays in the development of hypertension.
9. Describe physiologically how hypertension leads to the development of transient ischemic attacks and brain attacks (stroke or cerebrovascular accident).

Suggested research topics
- Coping strategies for hypertension
- Compliance with therapy
- Effectiveness of smoking cessation, weight reduction, or exercise programs
- Depression and antihypertensive drugs

Myocardial infarction

DRG: 122 Mean LOS: 4.4 days

Myocardial infarction (MI)—also known as acute myocardial infarction, heart attack, and coronary occlusion—is the sudden occlusion of a coronary artery and the subsequent deprivation of blood and oxygen flow to the cardiac tissue distal to the blockage. MI leads to irreversible hypoxia and cellular death and is a leading cause of death in the United States, especially among individuals over age 65.

Risk factors for developing MI include factors that can be modified and those that cannot. Modifiable factors include physical inactivity; cigarette smoking; diet high in cholesterol, calories, and sodium; hypertension; and elevated serum cholesterol levels. Unmodifiable risks include age, sex, race, and heredity.

MI is an emergency, and patients experiencing symptoms should be transported immediately to a hospital. Emergency care includes prompt treatment of pain, initiation of oxygen therapy, continuous electrocardiograph (ECG) monitoring, and I.V. administration of medications, such as antiarrhythmics, anticoagulants, and thrombolytic agents, to help reestablish blood flow and limit the size of the infarct.

Subjective assessment findings

Health history
Hypertension, angina, previous MI, coronary artery disease, smoking history

Medication history
Antihypertensives, antianginal preparations, calcium channel blockers, diuretics

Functional health patterns
Cognitive-perceptual: severe, crushing chest pain unrelieved by rest or antianginal medications; pain radiating to jaw, back, neck, arms
Activity-exercise: weakness, fatigue, dyspnea, syncopal episodes, dizziness
Metabolic-nutritional: complaints of unrelieved severe indigestion, heartburn, nausea, vomiting, increased temperature
Coping–stress tolerance: feelings of anxiety, high level of stress, impending death

Objective assessment findings

Physical findings
Cardiovascular: arrhythmias, disturbances in rate (tachycardia or bradycardia), alterations in blood pressure (elevated initially, then decreased), jugular vein distention, S_3 gallop, murmurs, possible pericardial friction rub
Genitourinary: reduced urine output
Integumentary: cold, clammy, pale skin; diaphoresis
Respiratory: shortness of breath, tachypnea, presence of crackles

(Text continues on page 67.)

PLAN OF CARE	PREADMIT PHASE	INPATIENT CARE *Day 1*
DIAGNOSTIC TESTS	- MB isoenzyme of creatine kinase (CK-MB) fraction - Aspartate aminotransferase (AST) - Myoglobin - Lactate dehydrogenase (LD) and LD isoenzymes - Complete blood count (CBC) - Serum electrolytes (lytes) - Blood chemistry profile - Labs as per thrombolytic protocol - Urinalysis (UA) - Guaiac stool - Pulse oximetry - Chest X-ray and 12-lead electrocardiogram (ECG)	- CK with isoenzymes, lytes, activated partial thromboplastin time (APTT) if on heparin drip - UA - Guaiac stool - Pulse oximetry - 12-lead ECG - Continuous hemodynamic and ECG monitoring - 2D echocardiogram
MEDICATIONS	- Magnesium sulfate I.V. 2 to 4 mg/hr for pain - Lidocaine drip if thrombolytic therapy needed - Heparin therapy - I.V. nitroglycerin - I.V. 5% dextrose in water (D_5W) at keep-vein-open (KVO) rate - Acetylsalicylic acid (aspirin [ASA]) - Antiemetic if needed	- Heparin therapy if indicated - Nitroglycerin (NTG), beta blocker, calcium antagonist, angiotensin-converting enzyme inhibitor - ASA - Stool softener - Analgesic, sedative if needed - I.V. D_5W at KVO rate
PROCEDURES	- Check vital signs (VS) every 5 to 15 minutes and as needed. - Give oxygen (O_2) per nasal cannula (NC) 2 to 4 L/minute to maintain O_2 saturation (O_2 sat) > 95%. - Analyze ECG strip every hour and as needed (rhythm, ST-segment analysis, arrhythmia analysis). - Monitor complaints of chest pain: site, intensity (0 to 10 scale), quality, duration, radiation. Evaluate for abnormal heart and breath sounds every hour and as needed. - Evaluate pulmonary artery (PA) catheter pressures every hour and as needed. Monitor intra-arterial line if present. - Apply antiembolic (TED) stockings. - If patient has received thrombolytics, evaluate for signs of bleeding (I.V. sites, gums, hematuria). - Determine code status and advance directives.	- Check VS q 2 hr for first 8 hours, then q 4 hr. - Maintain O_2 per NC 2 to 4 L/min. - Analyze ECG strip q 4 hr and as needed. - Evaluate chest pain (0 to 10 scale). - Evaluate for abnormal heart and breath sounds q 4 hr. - Monitor and record PA catheter pressures q 4 hr and as needed. - Check TED stockings. - If patient has received thrombolytics, evaluate for signs of bleeding. - Enforce no I.M. injections.
DIET	- Give nothing by mouth. - Take baseline weight.	*Dietary consult:* - Give clear liquids; advance as tolerated. - Weigh patient.
ACTIVITY	- Encourage absolute bed rest (BR). - Place in high Fowler's position.	- Encourage BR with bedside commode. - Place in high Fowler's position.
ELIMINATION	- Monitor intake and output (I & O) every hour.	- Monitor I & O q 8 hr.
HYGIENE	- Assist with all needs.	- Assist with hygiene needs.
PATIENT TEACHING	- Discuss pain scale, need for frequent VS and other monitoring.	- Teach relaxation techniques; determine level of understanding and readiness to learn.
DISCHARGE PLANNING	- Report patient status to critical care unit staff. *Social services consult:* - Determine immediate psychosocial needs of patient and family. *Pastoral care consult:* - Assist patient and family to identify coping strategies.	*Social services:* - Assess discharge needs. *Cardiac rehabilitation consult:* - Determine need for services. *Home health consult:* - Check need and eligibility for home care.

Day 2	Day 3	Day 4	Day 5
CK with isoenzymes APTT (if on heparin), lytes Guaiac stool 12-lead ECG Continuous hemodynamic and ECG monitoring Radionuclide imaging Holter monitor, if needed	• CK with isoenzymes • APTT (if on heparin), lytes • Guaiac stool • Continuous ECG monitoring	• CK with isoenzymes (if still elevated • APTT (if on heparin) • Guaiac stool • Stress test	• APTT • CBC • Blood urea nitrogen • Creatinine
Heparin therapy NTG Beta blocker ASA Stool softener Analgesic, sedative if needed I.V. D_5W at KVO rate	• Same as previous day	• Same as previous day	• ASA • Stool softener • Beta blocker • Digoxin preparation if needed
Check VS q 4 hr. Maintain O_2 per NC 2 to 4 L/min. Analyze ECG strip q 8 hr. Evaluate chest pain every shift. Assess heart and lung sounds every shift.	• Same as previous day	• Check VS q 8 hr.	• Take routine VS. • Discontinue I.V. access.
Give diet low in sodium, cholesterol, and fat or American Diabetes Association (ADA) diet. Weigh patient.	• Continue with ordered diet. • Weigh patient.	• Same as previous day	• Continue with diet as ordered.
Gets out of bed to chair with assistance. Participates in activities of daily living.	• Assist with walking.	• Same as previous day	• Have patient walk independently. • Progress with level of physical activity.
Measure I & O every shift.	• Same as previous day	• Same as previous day	• Same as previous day
Same as previous day	• Same as previous day.	• Same as previous day.	• Have patient perform self-care.
Introduce need for dietary modifications. Begin cardiac teaching.	• Discuss stress testing. • Continue with cardiac teaching.	• Continue with cardiac teaching. • Begin home care instructions.	• Continue with cardiac teaching. • Discuss discharge medications.
Begin discharge teaching to move from coronary care unit to floor.	*Social services:* • Visit to arrange transport home, and to arrange for necessary home medical equipment. • Provide community resources list.		• Schedule for outpatient stress testing, cardiac catheterization, or angiography as indicated.

(continued)

Myocardial infarction *(continued)*

CLINICAL PATHWAY

PLAN OF CARE	HOME CARE Visit 1	Visit 2	Visit 3
DIAGNOSTIC TESTS	• Serum electrolytes • Blood urea nitrogen • Creatinine • Activated partial thromboplastin time • Digoxin level	• Review results of previous lab work with patient and family.	• Assist with scheduling of outpatient stress testing, cardiac catheterization, and so forth.
MEDICATIONS	• Assess medication compliance: aspirin, stool softener, beta blocker, digoxin, diuretic, analgesic as indicated.	• Assess for compliance with medication regimen. • Assist with modification in medications and dosage as needed. • Assess adverse effects of medications.	• Assess medication compliance. • Assess adverse effects of medications. • Reinforce permanence of medication regimen.
PROCEDURES	• Perform comprehensive admit assessment to establish home care baseline data set.	• Reassess vital signs (VS) and cardiovascular, respiratory, and peripheral vascular systems. • Evaluate for denial, anger, depression, fear, and despondency.	• Reassess VS and VS log if available. • Reassess cardiac and respiratory systems.
DIET	• Assess compliance with diet low in calories, sodium, and fat. • Weigh patient. • Consult dietitian as needed.	• Assess dietary compliance. • Weight patient. • Evaluate food choices and meal composition.	• Weigh patient and monitor for downward trend as indicated. • Reteach components as needed.
ACTIVITY	*Physical therapy and occupational therapy consult:* • Continue planned cardiac physical rehabilitation at home.	• Discuss activity limitations and planned rest periods. • Demonstrate home exercises.	• Reinforce consultation with doctor before resuming sexual activity, driving, work, and traveling.
ELIMINATION	• Assess intake and output patterns. • Assess for nocturia and constipation.	• Evaluate for edema in lower extremities.	• Evaluate for edema. • Evaluate consistency of stool.
HYGIENE	• Evaluate for home health aide services.	• Progress self-care activities as tolerated.	• Same as previous visit.
PATIENT TEACHING	• Assess level of understanding and compliance of previous cardiac teaching. • Assess ability to verbalize personal risk factors.	• Evaluate use of alcohol and tobacco products in home setting. • Stress need for permanent lifestyle changes.	• Reinforce teaching of symptoms that require immediate medical attention.
DISCHARGE PLANNING	• Assess home environment for stressors. • Determine need for home medical equipment, such as bedside commode, shower bench, and so forth.	• Determine need for assistance with transportation to attend outpatient cardiac rehabilitation and for follow-up visits to health care providers.	• Provide patient with information about local cardiac support groups, organizations, and services.

Diagnostic tests

Serum studies including cardiac enzymes and isoenzymes (creatine kinase [CK-MB], lactate dehydrogenase, aspartate aminotransferase), white blood cell (WBC) count, erythrocyte sedimentation rate, ECG, echocardiogram, chest X-ray, radionuclide blood pool scans, angiography

Related nursing diagnoses

1 Activity intolerance
2 Decreased cardiac output
3 Risk for injury
4 Pain
5 Ineffective management of therapeutic regimen: individual
6 Altered cardiopulmonary tissue perfusion

Expected outcomes

The following expected outcomes pertain to the patient or family. Numbers in parentheses refer to related nursing diagnoses above.

- Have vital signs within normal limits; can maintain blood pressure, pulse, and respirations within predetermined ranges during activity (1).
- Be actively involved in a structured daily program of increasing activity and exercise for long-term rehabilitation (1).
- Have cardiac output remain stable (2).
- Have decreased or absent cardiac arrhythmias (3).
- Verbalize absence of pain and appear relaxed (4).
- Notify appropriate health care provider of the following after discharge: resumption of chest pain or pressure, palpitation or irregular or rapid heart rate, dyspnea on exertion, any episode(s) of dizziness or fainting, edema of feet and ankles (5).
- Be able to recognize symptoms that require immediate medical attention: chest pain or pressure that is not relieved by nitroglycerin within 15 minutes (6).

Other possible nursing diagnoses

Anxiety, pain, ineffective individual coping, fear, altered sexuality patterns

Potential complications

Cardiovascular: decreased cardiac output, arrhythmias, adverse effects of antiarrhythmic therapy, pericarditis

Patient teaching

Phases of rehabilitation

- Phase 1, which begins in coronary care unit or intensive care unit
- Phase 2, which includes lifestyle modifications
- Phase 3, which includes gradual resumption of work, activities, and exercise
- Phase 4, which includes cardiac stability, goals, long-term conditioning, and unsupervised activities

Reducing risks

- Stop smoking.
- Reduce weight.
- Decrease stress.
- Increase exercise.
- Follow American Heart Association diet.

Signs and symptoms
- Resumption of chest pain or pressure
- Palpitation or irregular or rapid heart rate
- Dyspnea on exertion
- Dizziness or fainting
- Edema of feet and ankles
- Nausea and vomiting

Activity
- Avoid activities that produce shortness of breath, and limit activities during extreme hot or cold temperatures.
- Plan rest periods between activities.
- Avoid strenuous activities and work until doctor recommends resumption.
- Participate in a structured daily program of increasing activity and exercise.
- Stop activity if palpitations, shortness of breath, or severe fatigue occur.

Medications
- Instruct patient on dosage, time of administration, purpose, and adverse effects.
- Maintain up-to-date medication log.
- Follow dosage schedule.
- Understand food interactions and adverse effects of medications.
- Use over-the-counter drugs and alcohol cautiously; consult doctor before use.

Nutrition
- Maintain low-sodium diet.
- Possibly reduce weight; maintain weight log.
- Follow doctor-prescribed diet. Refer to American Heart Association dietary recommendations to decrease fat and cholesterol intake.

Critical thinking activities
1. Discuss the most common return-to-work issues confronting survivors of MI.
2. List and discuss the factors that lead to improved compliance with outpatient cardiac rehabilitation programs following MI.
3. Describe how the home environment should be altered to meet the needs of the patient following MI.
4. Discuss how the location and area of a myocardial infarct correlate with location of coronary artery lesions.
5. Compare and contrast the chest pain associated with angina and the chest pain associated with MI. Include chest pain characteristics, location, duration, severity, precipitating factors, related symptoms, and factors that may help to relieve the pain.
6. Obtain and review the laboratory reports and ECG readings of a patient recently diagnosed with acute MI. Describe how WBC and cardiac enzyme (and isoenzyme) levels correlate with ECG changes associated with MI.
7. Describe the type of home environment that would be the most conducive to facilitating early discharge from the hospital for a patient who has experienced an MI.

Suggested research topics
- Coping strategies for MI
- Effectiveness of smoking cessation, weight reduction, or exercise programs
- Compliance with therapy

PART 4

Metabolic function problems

Diabetes mellitus

Pain

Sepsis

Diabetes mellitus (type 2), newly diagnosed, uncontrolled

DRG: 294 Mean LOS: 4.3 days

Characterized by hyperglycemia, or elevated blood glucose level, diabetes mellitus (DM) results when either the pancreas partially or completely stops producing insulin or the patient develops an insulin resistance. It can be classified as one of four types: type 1, type 2, other specific type, or gestational.

Type 1 DM (immune-mediated or idiopathic) results from a functional defect or destruction of pancreatic beta cells, leading to absolute insulin deficiency and ineffective glucose transport across the cell membranes. The most common form of the disease, type 2 DM results when beta cells release insulin but cell membrane receptors are insulin-resistant. Diabetes classified by other specific types (genetic defect or drug- or chemical-induced) are distinguished from type 1 and type 2 DM by their different disease etiologies. Any degree of abnormal glucose levels during pregnancy is classified as gestational diabetes.

Long-term effects of diabetes include renal disease, eye disorders, and neuropathic complications. DM also plays a role in the occurrence of peripheral vascular disease, stroke, and myocardial infarction. Acute metabolic complications resulting from DM include diabetic ketoacidosis (DKA) and hyperosmolar hyperglycemic nonketotic syndrome (HHNS).

Initial treatment for a patient with type 2 DM may include lifestyle modifications in exercise and diet. If high blood glucose levels persist, the patient may receive oral hypoglycemic agents (OHAs). If OHAs do not control blood glucose adequately, the patient may need insulin therapy.

Subjective assessment findings

Health history
Recent infection, stress, surgery, or traumatic injury; pregnancy resulting in birth of infant weighing more than 9 lb (4 kg); chronic pancreatitis; history of alcoholism or gestational DM

Medication history
Use of glucocorticoids, diuretics, phenytoin; previous use of and compliance with OHAs or insulin preparations

Functional health patterns
Activity-exercise: muscle weakness, cramping
Cognitive-perceptual: changes in vision, numbness or tingling in hands and feet, decreased sensation in extremities, halo or fog seen around lights, headaches
Elimination: frequent urination, nocturia, incontinence
Nutritional-metabolic: obesity; excessive thirst or hunger; impaired healing, particularly in lower extremities; nausea
Sexuality-reproductive: decreased libido, impotence, recurrent vaginal infections and discharge

Objective assessment findings

Physical findings
Cardiovascular: peripheral vascular disorders (cool extremities and weak pedal pulses)

Integumentary: shiny, dry skin; evidence of recurrent skin infections; ulcers on legs or feet or both; decreased skin turgor
Musculoskeletal: muscle atrophy
Neurologic: altered sensation and reflexes
Other: fruity breath odor; dry, sticky mucous membranes (dehydration)

Diagnostic tests

Blood glucose tests; oral glucose tolerance and glycosylated hemoglobin tests; lipid profile; blood urea nitrogen, creatinine, and electrolyte levels; fasting triglyceride level; urinalysis; urine culture and sensitivity; urine analysis for microalbuminuria; urine glucose and acetone; neurologic and fundoscopic examinations

Related nursing diagnoses

1 Altered nutrition: more than body requirements or less than body requirements
2 Altered urinary elimination
3 Impaired skin integrity
4 Ineffective management of therapeutic regimen: individual
5 Noncompliance
6 Risk for infection
7 Risk for injury
8 Sensory/perceptual alterations (visual, tactile)

Expected outcomes

The following expected outcomes pertain to the patient or family. Numbers in parentheses refer to related nursing diagnoses above.
- Be able to select foods and menus that comply with prescribed dietary recommendations and healthy eating patterns (1).
- Maintain adequate fluid balance without evidence of polyuria or dehydration (2).
- Maintain skin integrity, especially in lower extremities (3).
- Be able to correctly monitor blood glucose levels (4).
- Be able to describe the interactions among diet, exercise, weight control, and insulin and blood glucose requirements (4)
- Be able to demonstrate accurate and safe self-administration of OHA, insulin, or both, as prescribed (4).
- Be able to describe adjustments to diet, exercise, and medication regimens required when patient is sick, under stress, or traveling (4).
- Be able to increase independent self-care incrementally (4).
- Comply with all components of the prescribed treatment plan (5).
- Practice routine foot and skin care (6).
- Maintain blood glucose and electrolyte levels within normal ranges before discharge (7).
- Be able to list signs and symptoms that may signal an impending hyperglycemic or hypoglycemic event and describe how to manage such an event (7).
- Be able to avoid extremes in blood glucose levels (hypoglycemia or hyperglycemia) after discharge (7).
- Recognize and avoid environmental hazards (8).

Other possible nursing diagnoses

Altered sexuality patterns, anxiety, ineffective denial, fatigue, fear, ineffective individual coping

(Text continues on page 75.)

PLAN OF CARE	PREADMIT PHASE	INPATIENT CARE Day 1	Day 2
DIAGNOSTIC TESTS	• Physical, fundoscopic, and neurologic examinations • Lipid profile, fasting blood sugar (FBS), glycosylated hemoglobin, blood urea nitrogen (BUN), and creatinine levels • Urinalysis (UA), urine analysis for microalbuminuria	• FBS; electrolyte (lytes), BUN, and creatinine levels • UA, urine osmolarity • Capillary blood glucose (CBG) checks q 6 hr	• FBS, lytes • CBG checks q 6 hr
MEDICATIONS	• Prescription and over-the-counter medications	• Insulin or oral hypoglycemic agents (OHA), or both as prescribed; evaluate effects of medications	• Insulin or OHA, or both as prescribed • Evaluate effects of medications: agents that prolong or enhance effects of OHA (anticoagulants, salicylates, alcohol).
PROCEDURES	• Obtain baseline vital signs (VS).	• Check VS. • Monitor I.V. site and rate if applicable.	• Check VS. • Monitor I.V. site and rate if applicable.
DIET	• Evaluate current diet. • Obtain baseline weight.	• Institute reduced-calorie, reduced-fat, increased-fiber diet based on American Diabetes Association (ADA) plan. • Weigh client.	• Continue ADA diet. • Weigh patient.
ACTIVITY	• Evaluate current activities; note self-imposed activity restrictions.	• Have patient walk ad lib.	• Have patient walk ad lib. • Discuss with patient need for regular exercise program.
ELIMINATION	• Assess for polyuria, nocturia, and constipation.	• Assess for polyuria, nocturia, and constipation.	• Same as Day 1
HYGIENE	• Evaluate care of feet and toes.	• Assist with foot care as needed.	• Demonstrate care of feet, toes, nails, and skin.
PATIENT TEACHING	• Teach patient about his specific form of diabetes mellitus. • Discuss goals of therapy. • Explain importance of inpatient care.	• Discuss goals of therapy (following prescribed diet, controlling weight, exercising, monitoring blood glucose, complying with medication regimen). • Demonstrate use of blood glucose monitoring device.	• Teach how to comply with prescribed meal plans and how to practice accurate portion control; stress importance of not delaying or skipping meals. • If possible, obtain blood glucose monitor patient will use at home. • Discuss injection site rotation.
DISCHARGE PLANNING	*Dietary consult:* • Evaluate need for dietary series. *Diabetic educator consult:* • Determine knowledge of disease, motivation, and readiness to learn about disease. • Coordinate learning needs of patient and family so all are met before discharge. *Case manager consult:* • Evaluate daily progress of patient while on path.	*Social services consult:* • Determine financial ability to pay for insulin and blood glucose monitoring supplies after discharge.	• Provide legible, educationally appropriate written sample meal plans and dietary instructions.

Day 3	Day 4
• Same as previous day	• Same as previous day
• Insulin or OHA, or both as prescribed • Evaluate effects of medications.	• Insulin or OHA, or both as prescribed • Evaluate effects of medication. • Note agents that decrease effects of OHA (thyroid medications, corticosteroids, thiazide diuretics).
• Monitor VS. • Saline lock I.V.	• Monitor VS.
• Same as previous day	• Same as previous day
• Have patient walk freely. • Arrange for physical therapy consult. • With doctor and patient, plan program of progressive exercise.	• Have patient walk freely. • Review details of exercise program (type, frequency, intensity).
• Same as Day 1	• Same as Day 1
• Same as previous day	• Request return demonstration of foot care.
• Request return demonstration of blood glucose monitoring device. • Teach effects of diet, exercise, and stress on insulin and blood glucose requirements.	• Provide written information on insulin and OHA, including care and storage of medications. • Teach insulin injection technique.
• Provide legible, detailed, written instructions on how to detect and prevent hypoglycemic and hyperglycemic events. *Home health nurse:* • Arrange to visit patient and family before discharge.	

(continued)

PLAN OF CARE	HOME CARE Visit 1	Visit 2	Visit 3
DIAGNOSTIC TESTS	• Review home glucose monitor use with patient as necessary.	• Same as previous visit	• Same as previous visit.
MEDICATIONS	• Observe patient's self-administration of insulin or oral hypoglycemic agent (OHA), or both.	• Same as previous visit	• Ask patient about episodes of hypoglycemia or hyperglycemia. • Ask patient about relationship of food intake to blood glucose fluctuations.
PROCEDURES	• Assess vital signs (VS). • Inspect skin and mucous membranes. • Palpate pedal pulses. • Perform neurologic assessment.	• Assess VS. • Inspect skin and mucous membranes. • Palpate pedal pulses.	• Same as previous visit
DIET	• Evaluate compliance with reduced-calorie, reduced-fat, increased-fiber diet as recommended by the American Diabetes Association. • Evaluate for alcohol intake. • Weigh patient.	• Review food and meal selections for previous week with patient and family. • Provide written instructions as necessary to reinforce previous dietary teaching or to add new concepts. • Weigh patient.	• Same as previous visit
ACTIVITY	• Evaluate compliance with prescribed activity plan. • Determine appropriateness of shoes patient uses for exercise. • Assess home safety.	• Review activity log if available. • Inspect lower extremities; if patient is bed-bound, inspect back.	• Same as previous visit
ELIMINATION	• Assess for constipation, frequent urination, and nocturia.	• Same as previous visit	• Same as previous visit
HYGIENE	• Assess need for home health aide.	• Assist as needed.	• Same as previous visit
PATIENT TEACHING	• Request demonstration of self-monitoring of blood glucose. • Reteach components as needed. • Establish daily schedule for testing. • Teach appropriate needle disposal and storage of insulin.	• Arrange for dietitian to teach patient advanced dietary management, such as reading and interpreting food labels, adjusting nutrients as needed, and eating away from home.	• Discuss with patient methods to prevent complications from diabetes. • Review blood glucose control up to this point.
DISCHARGE PLANNING	• Evaluate appropriateness, quantity, and correct storage of patient's diabetic supplies. • Evaluate patient's financial ability to purchase medical supplies and food. • Establish patient checklist and diabetes care record.	• Provide videotapes, audiotapes, and other education materials as necessary for home use. • Provide information about local diabetic support groups, screenings, and educational programs for the public. • Assess need for ongoing maintenance and custodial care; initiate referrals as needed.	• Help patient schedule routine medical check-ups and follow-up appointments for foot care, eye care, and dental care.

Potential complications

Hypoglycemia, hyperglycemia, negative nitrogen balance

Patient teaching

Pathophysiology and types of DM
- Type 1
- Type 2
- Gestational
- Other specific types

Signs and symptoms
- Polyuria
- Polydipsia
- Polyphagia
- Fatigue
- Skin wounds or ulcers
- Recurrent infections (such as vaginal infections)

Complications
- Neurologic
- Visual
- Cardiovascular
- Renal
- DKA
- HHNS

Lifestyle modifications
- Participate in a regular exercise program.
- Reduce stress.
- Develop coping strategies.
- Give up smoking.

Nutrition
- Control body weight.
- Reduce caloric intake.
- Reduce fat intake.
- Increase fiber intake.
- Follow American Diabetes Association guidelines for diet.

Medications
- OHAs
- Insulin

Managing DM
- Self-monitoring of blood glucose level
- Inspecting skin, particularly on feet and toes
- Detecting and managing hypoglycemic and hyperglycemic events
- Modifying therapeutic regimen to cope with travel and periods of increased psychological or physiologic stress
- Maintaining regular follow-up care, including dental, foot, and eye examinations
- Participating in support groups
- Monitoring for overall diabetes control (glycosylated hemoglobin test)

Critical thinking activities

1. Describe the best time to begin teaching a patient who has been newly diagnosed with type 2 DM about blood glucose level monitoring, insulin administration, and other self-care measures.
2. Discuss ways to increase a type 2 DM patient's compliance with lifestyle modifications, such as weight control and regular exercise.
3. Because hospital stays are shorter, home care has become increasingly important for the patient with DM. Discuss how the roles of multidisciplinary home care providers differ from the roles of inpatient care providers for the DM patient.
4. Compare and contrast etiology, risk factors, and distinguishing features of type 1 and type 2 DM.
5. Devise a chart that outlines the sequence of events leading to target organ damage as a result of DM.
6. What is the relationship between insulin resistance and insulin secretion in type 2 DM?
7. Discuss the value of the glycosylated hemoglobin blood test in evaluating long-term blood glucose control.
8. Describe the relationship between physical activity, dietary management, and use of medication in the management of DM.
9. What are the currently recommended nutritional guidelines for the individual with DM?
10. Discuss the chronic complications associated with DM.

Suggested research topics

- Compliance with therapy
- Coping strategies for DM
- Effectiveness of weight control programs
- Effectiveness of exercise programs

Pain

DRG: 464 Mean LOS: 2.8 days

A subjective experience, pain can be defined as whatever the person who is experiencing the pain says it is and exists whenever the person says it does. Pain is complex and multidimensional and is the most common reason people seek health care.

Pain can be categorized as acute or chronic. Characterized by recent onset and short duration (usually less than 3 months), acute pain may be accompanied by autonomic physiologic responses such as increased heart rate, blood pressure (BP), and respirations. Examples of acute pain include the pain associated with trauma or recent surgical procedures. Chronic pain usually has a longer duration (3 months or more), occurs continuously or intermittently, and usually does not trigger autonomic physiologic responses. Cancer pain, arthritis, and long-term back and neck pain are examples of chronic pain.

Whether acute or chronic, pain can be treated with drugs, nonpharmacologic techniques, or a combination of the two. The World Health Organization provides an "analgesic ladder" that can help health care providers determine what medications are appropriate for a particular patient. Such medications include nonopioid analgesics (aspirin and other salicylates, nonsteroidal anti-inflammatory drugs [NSAIDs], acetaminophen), corticosteroids, sedatives and antianxiety agents, tricyclic antidepressants, anticonvulsants, anxiolytics, and opioid drugs (morphine, fentanyl, and codeine). Counterirritants, such as ointments of oil of wintergreen or cloves, can help control local pain. Nonpharmacologic pain-control measures include positioning, cutaneous stimulation, acupuncture, biofeedback, behavior modification, distraction, imagery, relaxation, and hypnosis. Chronic, intractable, or uncontrollable pain can be decreased or eliminated by such neurosurgical procedures as neurectomy, sympathectomy, and rhizotomy.

Pain is often underdiagnosed and undertreated. The nurse must act as an advocate for pain management.

Subjective assessment findings

Health history
Biopathophysiologic causes, such as musculoskeletal disorders, visceral disorders, cancer, vascular disorders, inflammatory disorders; treatment-related causes, such as surgery, diagnostic tests, burns, accidents

Medication history
Pattern of opioid and nonopioid analgesic use; pattern of over-the-counter (OTC) medication, illicit drug, or alcohol use to moderate or alleviate pain

Functional health patterns
Activity-exercise: inability to participate in activities and exercise because of pain, muscle weakness and cramping, joint-disuse syndrome
Cognitive-perceptual: depression, apathy, anger, verbal and nonverbal expressions of pain
Elimination: constipation from narcotic use

(Text continues on page 81.)

PLAN OF CARE	PREADMIT PHASE	INPATIENT CARE *Day 1*
DIAGNOSTIC TESTS	• Perform comprehensive, multidisciplinary pain assessment and profile. • Perform complete physical examination.	• Evaluate feasibility of oral route for analgesic administration.
MEDICATIONS	• Begin analgesic administration using World Health Organization's analgesic ladder.	• Step I: For pain rated 1 to 3 on 0 to 10 scale, give nonopioid drugs, such as aspirin, nonsteroidal anti-inflammatory drugs, and acetaminophen, with or without adjuvants.
PROCEDURES	• Begin physical treatments such as massage, transcutaneous electrical nerve stimulation, and relaxation.	• Titrate analgesic dose to desired effect in consultation with patient and doctor.
DIET	*Dietary consult:* • Adjust patient's calorie intake as needed.	• Adjust patient's calorie and nutrient intake as prescribed.
ACTIVITY	*Physical therapy consult:* • Begin physical reconditioning slowly.	• Begin physical rehabilitation.
ELIMINATION	• Determine baseline patterns of urine and stool output.	• Monitor urinary and bowel output.
HYGIENE	• Evaluate patient's need for assistance.	• Assist as needed.
PATIENT TEACHING	• With patient, determine pain-management goals, such as pain control versus total elimination of pain.	• Select one pain-assessment tool and teach patient and family how to use it. • Teach preventive approach to pain management.
DISCHARGE PLANNING	*Multidisciplinary pain-management team consult:* • Address physiologic, affective, behavioral, and cognitive components of pain.	*Psychologist or psychiatrist consult:* • Evaluate need for psychologic counseling for patient and family.

Day 2

- Evaluate feasibility of alternative administration routes (epidural, intrathecal, transdermal, rectal, subcutaneous) if oral route not acceptable.

- Step II: For pain rated 4 to 5 on 0 to 10 scale, give Step I drugs in combination with opioids such as codeine or hydrocodone, with or without adjuvants.

- Same as Day 1

- Same as Day 1

- Advance physical rehabilitation as pain control allows.

- Assess patient taking opioids for constipation; begin stool softeners and laxatives.

- Assist as needed.

- Discuss concepts of addiction with patient and family; distinguish between physical dependence and addiction.

- Address needs of caregiver; refer caregiver to support groups and counseling.
- Evaluate patient's ability to use patient-controlled analgesia or other modalities at home.

Day 3

- Evaluate need for invasive relief strategies such as neural blocks or neurosurgical interventions.

- Step III: For pain that progresses to 6 to 10 on 0 to 10 scale, give such drugs as morphine or hydromorphone, with or without nonopioids or adjuvants.

- Same as Day 1

- Same as Day 1

- Continue to advance physical rehabilitation as pain control allows.

- Continue stool softeners and laxatives as needed.

- Assist as needed.

- Discuss the concept of equianalgesic dosing with patient and family.

Home health team consult:
- Assess need for continuing pain management in home setting.

(continued)

PLAN OF CARE	HOME CARE Visit 1	Visit 2	Visit 3
DIAGNOSTIC TESTS	• Determine blood levels of adjuvant medications, such as carbamazepine, as indicated.		
MEDICATIONS	• Assess effectiveness of prescribed pharmacologic pain regimen using 0 to 10 pain scale.	• Evaluate for evidence of over-dosing or underdosing of pain medications. • Assess pain using 0 to 10 pain scale	• Assess for adverse effects of pain regimen, such as overseda-tion, constipation, itching, respi-ratory depression, and nausea. • Assess pain using 0 to 10 pain scale.
PROCEDURES	• Check vital signs (VS). • Evaluate sleep and rest cycle.	• Check VS. • Evaluate sleep and rest cycle. • Assess for tolerance to pain medication.	• Check VS. • Evaluate sleep and rest cycle.
DIET	• Adjust patient's nutrient and caloric intake as prescribed. • Weigh patient.	• Ensure adequate fluid intake to prevent constipation. • Weigh patient.	• Weigh patient.
ACTIVITY	*Home physical therapy consult:* • Assess need for transcutaneous electri-cal nerve stimulation therapy, dermal stimulation, and heat and cold therapy.	• Progress with physical rehabili-tation as pain allows.	• Same as previous visit
ELIMINATION	• Evaluate pattern and consistency of bowel movements.	• Same as previous visit	• Same as previous visit
HYGIENE	• Assess need for home health aide.	• Assist as needed.	• Assist as needed.
PATIENT TEACHING	• Teach patient and family what type of pain patient should expect and how long pain is likely to last, emphasizing that pain is an individual experience.	• Teach how to use and store opi-oids safely, including effects of opioids on driving and operating equipment.	• If increasing doses of opioids are needed to tolerate pain, rein-force teaching related to the concept of tolerance.
DISCHARGE PLANNING	• Evaluate need for home medical equip-ment, such as canes, walker, and bed-side commode.	• Refer patient to local acute or chronic pain support groups.	• Ensure that patient and family understand importance of par-ticipating in outside activities to lessen preoccupation with pain and to provide distraction.

Nutritional-metabolic: inability to maintain total daily caloric intake, history of weight loss or gain, anorexia, nausea
Sleep-rest: restlessness, insomnia

Objective assessment findings

Physical findings
Autonomic responses (acute pain): increased BP, tachycardia, diaphoresis, dilation of pupils, changes in respiratory rate and depth
Behavioral responses: moaning, crying, pacing, self-focusing behaviors
Musculoskeletal: guarding behavior, alteration in muscle tone (flaccid to rigid)

Diagnostic tests
To confirm diagnoses, appropriate lab studies for the system causing the pain.

Related nursing diagnoses
1 Activity intolerance
2 Altered nutrition: more than body requirements or less than body requirements
3 Hopelessness
4 Ineffective individual coping
5 Ineffective management of therapeutic regimen: individual
6 Pain, chronic pain

Expected outcomes
The following expected outcomes pertain to the patient or family. Numbers in parentheses refer to related nursing diagnoses above.
- Identify measures that eliminate or control pain, such as positioning, immobilizing, or resting of the affected part; using hypnosis or distraction; and using appropriate pharmacologic agents (1).
- Be able to tolerate physical rehabilitation as prescribed (1).
- Maintain body weight as appropriate for height and body frame (2).
- Establish realistic goals related to pain relief or control (3).
- Express positive feelings about self (4).
- Begin pain-relief measures when pain first starts instead of waiting until pain becomes severe (5).
- Manage pain to patient's satisfaction (5).
- Accurately describe use of the pain assessment scale (5).
- Understand that addiction rarely results from use of opioids for pain (5).
- Understand that side effects of opioids lessen over time (5).
- Give information about the pain experience, including location, frequency, duration, and intensity of pain (on a 0 to 10 scale); measures that relieve pain; and measures that fail to relieve pain (6).

Other possible nursing diagnoses
Altered role performance, anxiety, confusion, constipation, fatigue, impaired physical mobility, powerlessness, risk for caregiver role strain, risk for disuse syndrome, self-care deficit, sensory/perceptual alterations, sexual dysfunction, sleep pattern disturbance, social isolation, spiritual distress

Potential complications
Adverse effects from medication therapy

Patient teaching

Five components of pain
- Affective, behavioral, cognitive, sensory, physiologic

Assessment tools
- Color tools (for children), visual analog scales, pain location charts, visual descriptor scales

Concepts
- Tolerance, dependence, addiction

Medications
- OTC nonopioid drugs such as aspirin, acetaminophen, and NSAIDs (used for mild pain)
- Opioid drugs such as codeine, oxycodone, and hydrocodone (used for moderate pain or persistent mild pain)
- Opioid analgesics such as morphine and fentanyl or hydromorphone (used for moderate to severe pain)
- Adjuvant drugs such as tricyclic antidepressants and anticonvulsants, steroids, and counterirritants

Adverse effects of opioids
- Constipation
- Sedation
- Nausea and vomiting
- Pruritus
- Respiratory depression

Nonpharmacologic measures
- Positioning
- Massage
- Acupressure
- Transcutaneous electrical nerve stimulation
- Heat or cold therapy
- Distraction
- Imagery
- Relaxation
- Biofeedback
- Behavior modification

Critical thinking activities
1. Describe in detail how pain should be assessed and managed in a nonverbal or confused elderly patient.
2. Discuss sociocultural factors that may influence an individual's response to pain.
3. Describe how alternative or complementary methods of pain control, such as acupuncture, massage, biofeedback, and therapeutic touch, work to relieve pain.
4. Compare and contrast the pharmacologic management of acute pain and chronic pain.
5. Discuss the concept of equianalgesic dosing.

Suggested research topics
- Effectiveness of nonpharmacologic pain control
- Coping strategies for chronic pain
- Effectiveness of pain assessment methods

Sepsis

DRG: 416 Mean LOS: 6.2 days

A metabolic emergency, sepsis occurs in response to a disseminated infection, usually of gram-negative bacteria. These bacteria release endotoxins and exotoxins into the bloodstream. Once released, the toxins activate the body's complement, kinin, and clotting systems. Fever; cardiovascular changes such as vasodilation; mental changes such as confusion, lethargy, and agitation; renal failure caused by acute tubular necrosis; and other pronounced metabolic, hematologic, and pulmonary complications can all result. Organisms that do not release endotoxins can also cause sepsis, but the complete sequence of events is not fully understood.

Risk factors for sepsis include burn injuries, human immunodeficiency virus infection, immunosuppression, major trauma, cancer, prolonged hospital stays (particularly in intensive care units), advanced age, and invasive I.V. lines or indwelling catheters. Aggressive avoidance or exposure to the risk factors for sepsis can help prevent the development of sepsis. If sepsis does develop, early detection and prompt treatment are essential.

Subjective assessment findings

Health history
Urinary, wound, or respiratory infection; burns; multiple trauma; cancer; acquired immunodeficiency syndrome; invasive lines or catheters; malnutrition; organ transplant; disseminated intravascular coagulation

Functional health patterns
Activity-exercise: dyspnea, palpitations, syncope, cough
Cognitive-perceptual: confusion, irritability, feeling of impending doom
Elimination: decreased urine output, concentrated urine, hematuria
Nutritional-metabolic: fever, anorexia, weight loss

Objective assessment findings

Physical findings
Cardiovascular: tachycardia, palpitations, arrhythmias, changes in blood pressure
Gastrointestinal: paralytic ileus, hypoactive bowel sounds, abdominal distention
Integumentary: warm extremities (in the initial stages), flushed appearance
Neurologic: confusion, anxiety, restlessness
Renal: oliguria, diminished response to diuretics
Respiratory: dyspnea, hypoxemia, hypercapnia, tachypnea

Diagnostic tests
Complete blood count with differential; blood culture and sensitivity; blood chemistries; electrolyte, blood urea nitrogen, and creatinine levels; coagulation profile; wound, urine, and stool cultures

(Text continues on page 87.)

PLAN OF CARE	PREADMIT PHASE	INPATIENT CARE Day 1	Day 2
DIAGNOSTIC TESTS	• Complete blood count with differential (CBC w/diff); blood urea nitrogen (BUN), creatinine (Cr), coagulation profile; blood chemistry profile; serum lactate level; liver function tests • Blood cultures (from peripheral and central lines before starting antibiotics) • Urinalysis (UA), urine culture, urine specific gravity, and wound and stool cultures. • Sputum for Gram stain and culture • Chest X-ray (CXR) • Arterial blood gas (ABG) analysis • Continuous electrocardiogram (ECG) and hemodynamic monitoring	• CBC w/diff • ABG analysis • Pulse oximetry q2hr • CXR • Continuous ECG monitoring and continuous hemodynamic monitoring • Serum chemistry • Coagluation profile	• Same as Day 1
MEDICATIONS	• Initiate broad-spectrum I.V. antibiotic therapy as soon as blood cultures are obtained. • Initiate I.V. isotonic fluid or volume expanders or both, as ordered.	• Administer broad-spectrum I.V. antibiotics (such as beta-lactams, aminoglycosides, cephalosporins). • Administer I.V. vasopressors, inotropics, and antiarrhythmics.	• Same as Day 1
PROCEDURES	• Take vital signs (VS) every 5 to 15 minutes and as needed. • Administer oxygen (O_2) to maintain O_2 saturation (O_2 sat) > 95%.	• Check VS every hour. • Give O_2 to maintain O_2 sat > 95%. • Have patient turn, cough, and deep-breathe (TCDB) and perform incentive spirometry (IS) q 2 hr. • Care for I.V. sites and central lines per hospital protocol. • Provide urinary catheter care. • Provide meticulous wound and skin care each shift and as needed.	• Check VS q 4 hr and report temperature spikes promptly. • Give O_2 to maintain O_2 sat > 95%. • Have patient TCDB and perform IS q 2 hr while in bed. • Care for I.V. sites and central lines per hospital protocol. • Provide meticulous wound and skin care each shift and as needed.
DIET	• Permit nothing by mouth. • Establish baseline weight.	• Initiate enteral feedings as tolerated. • Weigh patient.	• Continue enteral feedings. • Weigh patient.
ACTIVITY	• Bed rest (BR) in high Fowler's position. • If patient has low blood pressure, place head of bed down.	• BR in high Fowler's position. • Turn q 2 hr and perform passive range-of-motion exercises q 4 hr.	• Have patient get up in chair with assistance. • Turn q 2 hr while in bed.
ELIMINATION	• Measure intake and output (I & O) every hour. • Insert indwelling catheter.	• Measure I & O every hour. • Continue indwelling catheter.	• Measure I & O q 4 hr. • Discontinue (D/C) indwelling catheter.
HYGIENE		• Assist with all needs, including oral and perineal hygiene.	• Same as Day 1
PATIENT TEACHING	• Give emergency and inpatient care; no teaching.	• Discuss need for BR and energy conservation with limited visitors. • Teach hand-washing technique to patient and family.	• Explain results of cultures and need for aggressive pulmonary management.
DISCHARGE PLANNING		*Social services consult:* • Arrange for an evaluation. *Dietary consult:* • Plan initiation of enteral feedings. *Respiratory therapist consult:* • Initiate pulmonary management.	

Day 3	Day 4	Day 5	Day 6
• CBC w/diff, blood chemistry profile, coagulation profile • Serum levels of nephrotoxic drugs • ABG analysis • Pulse oximetry q 4 hr • CXR • MA • Continuous ECG monitoring and continuous hemodynamic monitoring	• Same as previous day	• CBC w/diff, blood chemistry profile • Serum levels of nephrotoxic drugs • Pulse oximetry every shift • D/C continuous ECG monitoring • Coagulation profile	• CBC w/diff, chemistry profile • D/C pulse oximetry • CXR
• Once culture results are obtained, administer I.V. antibiotics specific to the reported antimicrobial susceptibility as ordered.	• Maintain I.V. antibiotic administration as scheduled.	• Same as previous day	• Same as previous day
• Same as previous day.	• Check VS q 4 hr. • Administer O_2 to maintain O_2 sat > 95%. • Have patient TCDB and perform IS q 4 hr while patient is awake. • Establish I.V. saline lock. • Provide meticulous wound and skin care each shift and as needed. • Check routine VS.	• D/C O_2 therapy. • Continue IS q 4 hr while patient is awake. • Maintain saline lock. • Provide wound and skin care each shift and as needed.	• Check routine VS. • Continue IS q 4 hr while patient is awake. • D/C saline lock.
• Same as previous day	• Progress diet as tolerated (DAT); start clear or full-liquid diet. • Weigh patient.	• Progress DAT.	• Same as previous day
• Have patient walk with assistance. Turn q 2 hr while patient is in bed.	• Have patient walk with assistance. • Have patient get up in chair q.i.d. with assistance	• Have patient walk with assistance t.i.d. in hall.	• Have patient walk freely with assistance in hall and in room.
• Measure I & O q 4 hr.	• Measure I & O every shift.	• Same as previous day	• Same as previous day
• Same as Day 1	• Initiate self-care for oral and perineal hygiene.	• Continue self-care for oral and perineal hygiene.	• Same as previous day
• (If sepsis is related to immunosuppression, teach precautions to take [avoiding crowds, maintaining nutrition, practicing good handwashing technique]).	*Dietary consult:* • Teach the role of adequate nutrition in maintaining immune function.	• Stress importance of compliance with home antibiotic regimen, emphasizing importance of completing prescription and taking all medication as ordered.	• Provide detailed instruction on home antibiotic regimen. • Teach specific signs and symptoms to report to health care provider after discharge.
Social services: • Determine need for and financial eligibility for durable medical equipment at home.	*Social services:* • Initiate arrangements for transport home upon discharge.	*Home health service consult:* • Arrange for continuation of I.V. antibiotics at home. • Consider surgery consult for insertion of peripherally inserted central catheter.	• Discharge to home with home health services as provider.

(continued)

PLAN OF CARE	HOME CARE Visit 1	Visit 2	Visit 3
DIAGNOSTIC TESTS	▪ Complete blood count; electrolyte, blood urea nitrogen, and creatinine level.	▪ Review results of lab work with patient, family, and doctor.	
MEDICATIONS	▪ Administer I.V. anti-infectives as pre-scribed or assess compliance with oral anti-infectives.	▪ Same as previous visit	▪ Same as previous visit
PROCEDURES	▪ Perform comprehensive assessments to establish baseline.	▪ Assess vital signs, particularly temperature. ▪ Evaluate any wounds for signs of infection. ▪ Evaluate I.V. site if present. ▪ Assess for cough, sputum.	▪ Assess vital signs, particularly temperature. ▪ Evaluate any wounds for signs of infection. ▪ Evaluate I.V. site if present. ▪ Assess for cough, sputum. ▪ Reassess vital signs, lungs, and cardiovascular systems. ▪ Assess mental status.
DIET	▪ Assess compliance with diet high in protein, carbohydrate, and calories. ▪ Weigh client.	▪ Assess for anorexia, nausea, vomiting. ▪ Determine weight change. ▪ Assess compliance with diet.	▪ Same as previous visit.
ACTIVITY	▪ Evaluate tolerance for exercise and activities of daily living.	▪ Same as previous visit.	▪ Same as previous visit.
ELIMINATION	▪ Assess for urinary tract infection.	▪ Same as previous visit.	▪ Same as previous visit.
HYGIENE	▪ Evaluate need for home health aide ser-vices.	▪ Assist as needed.	▪ Same as previous visit.
PATIENT TEACHING	▪ Teach about anti-infective therapy (take as prescribed, follow dosage schedule, do not skip doses).	▪ Provide teaching specific to patient's risk for sepsis. ▪ Discuss importance of comply-ing with medication regimen, diet, and exercise.	▪ Reinforce and evaluate teaching sessions from previous home visits.
DISCHARGE PLANNING	▪ Assess home support and resource needs (financial ability to purchase anti-infectives; medical equipment needs).	▪ Assess home support and resource needs.	▪ Reinforce importance of keeping follow-up appointments.

Related nursing diagnoses

1 Decreased cardiac output
2 Hyperthermia
3 Ineffective management of therapeutic regimen: individual, families
4 Noncompliance
5 Risk for injury
6 Sensory/perceptual alterations: tactile

Expected outcomes

The following expected outcomes pertain to the patient or family. Numbers in parentheses refer to related nursing diagnoses above.

- Maintain cardiac and urine output and oxygen saturation within normal limits (1).
- Maintain vital signs within normal limits (2).
- List events that can trigger sepsis and describe how to detect and prevent sepsis in the future (3).
- Recognize and report signs of infection (3).
- Follow careful hand-washing technique to prevent spread of infection (4).
- Comply with anti-infective therapy (4).
- Have laboratory values, including white blood cell count, return to normal ranges (5).
- Resolve anxiety and feelings of impending doom (6).

Other possible nursing diagnoses

Acute confusion, altered nutrition: less than body requirements, altered thought processes, altered tissue perfusion (peripheral), fear, impaired gas exchange, impaired tissue integrity, ineffective breathing pattern, ineffective thermoregulation, social isolation, spiritual distress

Potential complications

Decreased cardiac output, arrhythmias, hypoxemia

Patient teaching

Preventing recurrence

- Follow good hand-washing technique.
- Take protective measures when susceptibility is high: Stay away from large crowds, such as in malls or shopping centers, and limit visitors at home, particularly young children with colds or other communicable diseases.
- Follow meticulous personal hygiene: Take steps to prevent skin irritation, breakdown, and disruption and use an electric razor to minimize the risk of cuts.
- Eat and drink enough healthy food and fluids.
- Take time to rest to minimize fatigue.
- Do not use tobacco or drink alcohol.
- Minimize use of enemas and suppositories, and do not take temperature rectally.
- Vaccinate against influenza and pneumonia.

Signs and symptoms

- Know how to read a thermometer accurately, preferably a digital thermometer.
- Recognize signs and symptoms of infection to report to health care provider.
- Understand that in periods of pronounced immunosuppression, the usual signs and symptoms of infection may not occur.

Activity
- Explain importance of increasing activity gradually.
- Limit exercise and activity to tolerance.
- Plan two to three rest periods per day.
- Avoid fatigue.
- Limit visitation and avoid long conversations.
- Maintain pleasant and calm environment.
- Keep necessary items within easy reach (tissue, appropriate trash container).
- Avoid strenuous work (employment-related, heavy housework, straining or lifting until approved by doctor).

Medications
- Instruct patient on dosage, time of administration, purpose, and adverse effects.
- Avoid over-the-counter drugs and alcohol use.
- Discuss dietary needs in relation to specific drug therapy.
- Teach I.V. site care to patient and family if home I.V. antibiotics are ordered.

Nutrition
- Explain importance of maintaining diet as tolerated.
- Eat frequent, small meals to conserve energy.
- Eat diet high in protein and carbohydrates; maintain weight.
- Drink at least 3 L/day unless contraindicated.
- Weigh daily and keep weight log for 6 to 8 weeks as directed.

Critical thinking activities
1. Discuss the effectiveness of discharge teaching in preventing infection in high-risk patients.
2. Discuss how well discharged high-risk hospital patients comply with anti-infective therapy when they do not receive follow-up home health care.
3. List and describe the factors that need to be controlled to decrease the occurrence of sepsis in hospitalized elderly patients.
4. Describe the types of continuing education programs related to aseptic technique that would be most beneficial to health care personnel.
5. List the most common organisms responsible for wound infections.
6. Discuss risk factors for the development of sepsis in hospitalized individuals.
7. Describe assessment findings related to septicemia.
8. Explain why the mortality rate from septic shock is so high.
9. Describe the etiology of the warm shock stage, which is associated with the early stages of septic shock.

Suggested research topics
- Compliance with therapy
- Rates of sepsis in hospitalized patients
- Effectiveness of discharge teaching

PART 5

Cancer

Acute myelogenous leukemia (adult)

DRG: 473 Mean LOS: 7.9 days

Classified as acute or chronic, leukemia refers to a group of hematologic malignancies that primarily affect bone marrow and lymph tissue. Half the cases are acute; half, chronic. Acute leukemia produces excessive numbers of immature cells and usually presents as an acute illness. Chronic leukemia is the proliferation of excessive mature white blood cells (WBCs) and has an insidious onset. The two most common types of leukemia in adults are acute myelogenous leukemia (AML) and chronic lymphocytic leukemia. The etiology of leukemia is unknown; however, genetic predisposition, drugs, viruses, and exposure to radiation and chemicals have been implicated.

Clinical manifestations of leukemia include bone marrow and systemic effects. Excessive malignant cells cause lymphadenopathy and hepatosplenomegaly. Too many immature leukocytes in the bone marrow lead to the crowding out of other marrow components, a condition that results in anemia, thrombocytopenia, and granulocytopenia. Most patients present with bleeding or infection as their chief complaint at diagnosis. Other common symptoms include fatigue, weakness, dizziness, and bone pain. Additional symptoms vary with the type of leukemia. Antileukemic treatment includes chemotherapy and sometimes bone marrow transplantation, which is performed after remission with chemotherapy has been achieved. Treatment rarely includes radiation therapy.

AML, specifically, presents as an acute illness with large numbers of immature WBCs (blasts) in both bone marrow and serum. As the serum count rises, so does the risk of leukostasis (the occlusion of microvasculature), especially in the brain and lungs. Leukostasis results in thromboses, intracranial events such as cerebrovascular accident, and hypoxemia. In treating AML, rapid lysis of WBCs may occur, resulting in a rapid spilling of internal tumor components into the circulation, causing tumor lysis syndrome. Tumor lysis causes hyperkalemia, hyperphosphatemia, hypocalcemia, hyperuricemia, and excess serum uric acid, which may result in renal tubular obstruction and renal failure.

Subjective assessment findings

Health history
Exposure to radiation or radioactive substances, chemicals (including chemotherapy), Epstein-Barr virus, human immunodeficiency virus

Medication history
Use of prescription and over-the-counter (OTC) drugs, especially chloramphenicol, phenylbutazone, and drugs that interfere with clotting (aspirin [ASA], nonsteroidal anti-inflammatory drugs, histamine-2 blockers)

Functional health patterns
Nutritional-metabolic: unexplained weight loss, anorexia, nausea, night sweats, fever, chills, prolonged bleeding episodes, easy bruising
Elimination: hematuria, melena, constipation, diarrhea
Cognitive-perceptual: abdominal pain, tenderness over lymph nodes, headache

Activity-exercise: fatigue, dyspnea on exertion (DOE) or at rest, weakness, lethargy
Health perception–health management: family history of leukemia or other cancer

Objective assessment findings

Physical findings
Cardiovascular: tachycardia, palpitations, arrhythmias
Integumentary: pallor, cyanosis, jaundice, petechiae, skin infections, ecchymoses, rashes
Neurologic: confusion, disorientation, papilledema, seizure, dizziness, pupillary reactions
Respiratory: shortness of breath, DOE, abnormal breath sounds
Other: lymphadenopathy, splenomegaly, hepatomegaly, pain, malaise, weight loss, fever

Diagnostic tests
Complete blood count, coagulation profile, cytogenetic analysis, bone marrow aspiration, arterial blood gases, lumbar puncture, computed tomography scans (chest, abdomen, head), chest X-ray, electrocardiogram, electrolytes, serum chemistries

Related nursing diagnoses
1 Risk for caregiver role strain
2 Pain and discomfort
3 Ineffective individual coping
4 Altered family processes
5 Risk for infection
6 Risk for injury

Expected outcomes
The following expected outcomes pertain to the patient or family. Numbers in parentheses refer to related nursing diagnoses above.
- Be aware of community support agencies and services available to patients diagnosed with leukemia (1,2,3).
- Have pain managed to patient's satisfaction (2).
- Reduce frequency and severity of nausea and vomiting to a tolerable level for the patient (2).
- Display no evidence of mucositis or stomatitis (2).
- Be aware of the long-term nature of this disease process and its treatment (3,4).
- Have psychosocial concerns and needs addressed to patient's satisfaction (1,3).
- Present no evidence of infection (5).
- Have minimal exposure to environmental pathogens (5).
- Have vascular access device (VAD) site free of infection (5).
- Be proficient in the home care of VAD before discharge (1,3,5).
- Be able to verbally list signs and symptoms of anemia, leukopenia, and thrombocytopenia that need to be reported to a health care provider (5,6).
- Be aware of importance of postdischarge follow-up appointments with health care providers (5,6).
- Be able to verbally list signs and symptoms that may indicate relapse of the leukemia (5,6).

Other possible nursing diagnoses
Ineffective management of therapeutic regimen

Potential complications
Sepsis, thrombocytopenia, negative nitrogen balance, electrolyte imbalances, adverse reactions to medication therapy

(Text continues on page 95.)

Acute myelogenous leukemia (adult)

PLAN OF CARE	PREADMIT PHASE	INPATIENT CARE Day 1	Day 2
DIAGNOSTIC TESTS	• Complete blood count (CBC) • Coagulation profile • Cytogenetic analysis • Bone marrow aspiration • Arterial blood gases (ABGs) • Lumbar puncture • Computed tomography scan (chest, abdomen, head) • Chest X-ray • Electrocardiogram • Electrolytes (lytes) • Serum chemistries	• CBC, lytes and magnesium (Mg) levels b.i.d. • Serum chemistries • Pulse oximetry	• CBC, lytes, and Mg levels t.i.d. • Coagulation studies every day (disseminated intravascular coagulation [DIC] screen) • Serum chemistries, including uric acid levels • Pulse oximetry
MEDICATIONS	• Over-the-counter and prescription medications • Sedation or pain medication before scans, punctures, aspirations	• I.V. chemotherapy induction therapy • Electrolytes replacement	• Same as Day 1
PROCEDURES	• Perform complete physical assessment.	• Perform baseline oral inspection. • Insert VAD. • Provide VAD site care. • Perform complete physical assessment. • Initiate chemotherapy precautions.	• Perform complete physical assessment. • Monitor for occurrence of tumor lysis syndrome (development of acute hyperuricemia, hyperkalemia, hyperphosphatemia, and hypocalcemia, with or without acute renal failure). • Provide VAD site care. • Perform assessment of venous patency before, during, and after vesicant chemotherapy administration. • Continue with chemotherapy precautions.
DIET	*Nutrition consult:* • Determine calorie count. • Determine weight loss.	• Give neutropenic diet or nothing by mouth (NPO) as ordered. • Assess for signs of fluid overload during chemotherapy; institute fluid restriction as indicated. • Weigh patient.	• Same as Day 1
ACTIVITY	*Physical therapy (PT) consult:* • Evaluate joint pain and swelling.	• Have patient walk in room with assistance.	• Same as Day 1
ELIMINATION	• Evaluate for baseline data: hematuria, melena, and constipation.	• Start strict intake and output, which includes emesis. • Evaluate for and report hematuria, melena, and constipation.	• Same as Day 1
HYGIENE	• Assist with care.	• Assist with meticulous oral and perineal hygiene.	• Same as Day 1
PATIENT TEACHING	• Discuss disease process, need for chemotherapy and/or radiation therapy, effects and adverse effects of therapy, and need for a vascular access device (VAD).	• Reinforce previous teaching. • Teach self-care of VAD. • Teach patient to monitor blood counts if willing and able. • Prepare patient for alopecia and other physical changes.	• Teach patient about chemotherapy effects and adverse effects, expected nadir, long-term nature of process, transfusions, and transfusion reactions.
DISCHARGE PLANNING	*Social services consult:* *Home health consult:* *Pastoral care consult:* • Evaluate home environment and caregiver abilities.	• Determine financial eligibility for future therapies, including the possibilities of bone marrow transplantation.	• Consult psychologist or psychiatrist for psychologic counseling of patient and family as needed.

Day 3	Days 4 to 5	Days 6 to 7
• Same as previous day	• CBC, lytes b.i.d. • Serum chemistries • Culture blood, sputum, urine, VAD as needed for temperature spike • ABGs as needed for respiratory distress • Coagulation studies every day	• CBC, lytes • Cultures if temperature spikes
• Same as Day 1	• Packed red blood cells (PRBCs) and platelets as ordered • I.V. antibiotics as ordered	• Same as previous day
• Same as previous day	• Same as previous day	• Perform complete physical assessment. • Provide VAD site care. • Perform assessment of venous patency before, during, and after vesicant chemotherapy administration. • Continue with chemotherapy precautions.
• Same as Day 1	• Give neutropenic diet unless mucositis is severe. • Weigh patient.	• Same as previous day
• Same as Day 1	*PT:* • Assist with active and passive range-of-motion exercises as tolerated.	*PT:* • Same as previous day
• Same as Day 1	• Same as Day 1	• Same as Day 1
• Same as Day 1	• Assist with meticulous oral and perineal hygiene. • Inspect mucous membranes carefully.	• Same as previous day
• Teach patient about neutropenic precautions and neutropenic diet; need to remain in room or wear a mask outside the room.	• Discuss before discharge information related to anemia, leukopenia, thrombocytopenia, and reportable signs of bleeding.	• Same as previous day
• Help patient and family identify community support services and agencies, such as American Cancer Society, Leukemia Society, and CanSumount.	*Home health nurse:* • Visit patient and family while inpatient. • Provide verbal and written discharge instructions on signs and symptoms of anemia, leukopenia, and thrombocytopenia.	• Evaluate recall of discharge teaching.

(continued)

PLAN OF CARE	HOME CARE Visit 1	Visit 2	Visit 3
DIAGNOSTIC TESTS	• Complete blood count • Electrolytes • Blood chemistries	• Same as first visit	• Same as first visit
MEDICATIONS	• Administer chemotherapeutic agents as ordered. • Evaluate effects and adverse effects of prescription and over-the-counter (OTC) medications.	• Same as first visit	• Same as first visit
PROCEDURES	• Perform in-depth physical assessment as baseline. • Evaluate vascular access device (VAD) site and patient compliance with home maintenance of VAD. • Check vital signs (VS).	• Evaluate for signs and symptoms of infection, neutropenia, anemia, and thrombocytopenia. • Assess VAD site and site care. • Check VS. • Weigh patient and compare to baseline.	• Same as previous visit
DIET	• Encourage diet as tolerated to maintain enough calories for metabolic needs.	• Determine amount and calories consumed in 24-hour diet recall. • Adjust plan of care based on findings.	• Encourage diet high in protein, vitamins, minerals, and fluids.
ACTIVITY	• Evaluate level of fatigue and impact on activity.	• Encourage progressive activity.	• Same as previous visit
ELIMINATION	• Evaluate for constipation or diarrhea as chemotherapy adverse effects.	• Same as first visit	• Same as first visit
HYGIENE	• Inspect oral and perineal areas to determine patient's ability to maintain hygiene.	• Inspect oral and perineal areas to determine patient's ability to maintain hygiene. • Consider contacting home health aide services.	• Same as previous visit
PATIENT TEACHING	• Discuss medication and VAD care as needed. • Reinforce schedule of follow-up visits and therapy. • Teach home chemotherapy precautions and home safety needs.	• Discuss with patient and family psychosocial concerns (for example, fear of recurrence, changes in family roles, survivorship issues, reproductive concerns, sexuality issues).	• Same as previous visit
DISCHARGE PLANNING	*Social worker:* • Perform a comprehensive needs assessment related to financial, occupational, social, psychological, and spiritual needs.	*Social services:* • Refer to vocational counseling. • Refer to occupational therapy. • Refer to psychological counseling. • Refer to community support agencies and groups.	*Social services:* • Same as previous visit

Patient teaching

Complications
- Immunosuppression
- Deficiency of WBCs (neutropenia)
- Deficiency of red blood cells (anemia)
- Deficiency of platelets (thrombocytopenia)
- Deficiency of all three cellular blood elements (pancytopenia)

Reducing risks of infection
- Emphasize good hand washing with soap, water, and friction for all health care personnel and family who come in contact with the patient.
- Be certain caregivers understand the importance of meticulous oral care, perineal care, and skin care to prevent infection.
- Discuss the need for a neutropenic diet—cooked foods only, no raw fruits or vegetables.
- Discuss the importance of removing all standing and potentially stagnant sources of water, including denture cups, water pitchers, humidifiers, cut flowers, and live plants from the patient's environment. Make sure patient understands that water must be changed daily, particularly in respiratory equipment.
- Review the need to limit admittance of ill family or health care personnel to the room.
- Teach why the patient's temperature must be checked frequently and why a spike in temperature should be reported promptly.
- Discuss the need to avoid rectal temperatures, enemas, suppositories, and I.M. injections.
- Explain why soft toothbrushes or sponges are preferred for oral care.
- Tell patient to avoid ASA-containing products.
- Explain the need to observe stool, urine, and other body fluids for blood.

Signs and symptoms
- Infection (redness, swelling, fever, drainage, sore throat, cough, and fever >101° F [38° C])
- Blood in urine, stools, and so forth
- Usual signs of infection may not be present in severe immunocompromised states

Activity
- Limit exercise and activity to tolerance.
- Plan rest periods before and after activity; allow recuperation for future activities.
- Avoid fatigue.

Nutrition
- Explain importance of maintaining ideal weight.
- Discuss the need for a neutropenic diet—cooked foods only, no raw fruits or vegetables.

Medications
- Instruct patient on dosage, time of administration, purpose, and adverse effects.
- Avoid OTC drugs.
- Explain importance of drug therapy.

Critical thinking activities
1. Discuss the most prevalent quality of life issues for adult leukemia patients who have experienced bone marrow transplantation.
2. Interview adult leukemia patients and their families to determine how much they know about neutropenic and other precautions that should be adopted in the home setting.
3. Define surveillance cultures and discuss whether they are helpful in the management of infections in acute adult leukemia.

Suggested research topics
- Coping with leukemia
- Compliance with therapy
- Preventing infections
- Coping with leukemia treatments

Breast cancer

DRG: 260 Mean LOS: 1.6 days

Breast cancer ranks as the most common malignancy in American women. A new case is diagnosed every 3 minutes, the disease affects one in eight postmenopausal women, and the incidence has increased steadily over past decades. Mortality from breast cancer is second only to that of lung cancer among women. In recent years, mortality appears to be declining among white women, but it continues to increase among black women, and they are more than twice as likely to die from breast cancer as white women.

Risk factors for developing breast cancer include being female, being age 55 or older, never having had children (nulliparity) or experiencing a first full-term pregnancy after age 30, and experiencing the onset of menarche before age 12 or onset of menopause at age 55 or older. Other significant risk factors include having a family history of breast cancer in a maternal first-degree relative (particularly premenopausal) and a personal history of breast, colon, endometrial, or ovarian cancer. A history of obesity also appears to increase the risk for developing breast cancer.

Early detection of the disease plays a major role in the potential for cure. Current recommended screening methods include: (1) monthly breast self-examination (BSE) beginning by age 20, (2) clinical breast examinations by a trained health professional at least every 3 years between ages 20 and 40 and every year after age 40, (3) screening mammography for asymptomatic women every 1 to 2 years between the ages of 40 and 49 and every year after age 50.

Currently, a wide variety of treatments for breast cancer exists. Therapy should consider the stage of the disease, the woman's age and menopausal status, and the possible disfiguring effects of the surgery. The most common surgical interventions include breast conservation surgery followed by radiation therapy and modified radical mastectomy with axillary node dissection.

Subjective assessment findings

Health history
Previous cancer history, including personal history of breast, ovarian, colon, or endometrial cancer; history of fibrocystic breast disease; menstrual cycle history (age at menarche and age at menopause); history of nulliparity; age when first child born; history of obesity; history of exposure to radioactive substances

Medication history
Use of oral contraceptives and estrogen replacement therapy

Functional health patterns
Nutritional-metabolic: obesity, intake of alcohol, fat intake, unexplained loss of greater than 10% of body weight
Sexuality-reproductive: palpable lump in breast, breast asymmetry, nipple discharge or retraction, change in size or contour of breast
Health perception–health management: genetic predisposition to breast cancer, particularly in first-degree female relative (mother, sister); method of breast lump discovery; BSE-mammogram practices

(Text continues on page 101.)

PLAN OF CARE	PREADMIT PHASE	INPATIENT CARE *Day 1*
DIAGNOSTIC TESTS	• Complete blood count (CBC) • Calcium levels • Electrolytes (lytes) • Alkaline phosphatase levels • Liver function tests (LFTs) • Prothrombin time and international normalization ratio • Activated partial thromboplastin time • Chest X-ray (CXR) • Liver scan • Bone scan • Electrocardiogram	• CBC • Lytes • CXR
MEDICATIONS	• Outpatient medications evaluation • Acetylsalicylic acid (aspirin) or other anticoagulants to be discontinued (D/C) as directed by doctor • Estrogen evaluation	• I.V. medications for pain • Nausea medication • Antibiotics as prescribed • Resumption of preadmission medications postoperatively
PROCEDURES	• Take baseline weight. • Take baseline vital signs (VS). • Establish I.V. access.	• Check VS q 4 hr. • Monitor I.V. fluids and site. • Evaluate pain using pain scale. • Evaluate surgical site and drains. • Assess breath sounds.
DIET	• Give diet as tolerated (DAT).	• Give nothing by mouth. • Give DAT after surgery.
ACTIVITY	• Walk without restriction.	• Assist with walking. • Restrict movement of affected arm.
ELIMINATION		• Measure intake and output, including output from drains.
HYGIENE	• Ad lib	• Assist
PATIENT TEACHING	• Discuss turning, coughing, and deep breathing exercises. • Teach about postoperative arm exercises. • Explain recovery period.	• Begin teaching about home care of drains. • Teach about breast self-examination and need for mammogram and follow-up care.
DISCHARGE PLANNING	• Evaluate family support structure. • Consider need for home health referral. • Address psychosocial concerns.	• Refer to support groups and programs such as Reach for Recovery and Y-ME.

CLINICAL PATHWAY ■ Modified radical mastectomy

Day 2

- CBC
- Lytes

- Pain medications by mouth.
- Nausea medication
- Antibiotics and preadmission medications

- Check VS every shift.
- D/C I.V.
- Evaluate pain using pain scale.
- Evaluate surgical site and drains.

- Advance as tolerated.

- Same as previous day

- Same as previous day

- Same as previous day

- Teach about precautions for mastectomy site and care of affected side.
- Instruct about dressing change.

- Discharge to home with home health follow-up.

(continued)

PLAN OF CARE	HOME CARE Visit 1	Visit 2	Visit 3
DIAGNOSTIC TESTS	• Complete blood count • Electrolytes		
MEDICATIONS	• Evaluate preoperative medications. • Evaluate need for and frequency of pain medications. • Determine adverse reactions to medications.	• Determine adverse reactions to medications.	• Same as previous visit
PROCEDURES	• Inspect surgical wound and surgical dressing. • Inspect suture line. • Inspect drain site(s).	• Inspect surgical wound for wound infection, flap necrosis, and seroma formation.	• Same as previous visit
DIET	• Encourage high-protein diet as tolerated (DAT). • Evaluate for nausea or anorexia.	• Encourage DAT.	• Same as previous visit
ACTIVITY	*Physical therapy (PT) consult* • Evaluate need for postmastectomy exercise and for ways to decrease lymphedema if present.	• Progress postmastectomy exercises as prescribed by PT. • Monitor lymphedema levels.	• Same as previous visit
ELIMINATION	• Assess drainage from surgical drain.	• Assess for constipation.	• Same as previous visit
HYGIENE	• Assist with hygiene needs as required. • Assess caregiver abilities.	• Same as first visit	• Same as first visit
PATIENT TEACHING	• Discuss concerns related to sexuality, resumption of sexual intercourse, and other psychosocial needs. • Discuss prosthesis and reconstruction. • Discuss safe home environment.	• Provide information related to planned adjuvant therapies, such as chemotherapy and radiation therapy or tamoxifen therapy.	• Teach about new symptoms that should be reported: new back pain, weakness, shortness of breath, confusion, constipation (may indicate metastasis).
DISCHARGE PLANNING	• Reinforce schedule of follow-up visits with surgeon. • Discuss schedules for radiation therapy and chemotherapy as needed.	• Encourage participation in community support programs such as I Can Cope, Look Good Feel Better, and Reach to Recovery. • Discuss potential referrals for lymphedema management if needed in future.	• After 6 weeks and with doctor's approval may begin aerobics, water exercise, and overall fitness program.

Objective assessment findings

Physical findings
Breast examination: palpable breast lump most commonly found in upper outer quadrant
Examination of lymph node status: axillary and supraclavicular lymphadenopathy

Diagnostic tests
Positive results on mammography, fine-needle aspiration or surgical biopsy, evidence of metastatic disease on chest X-ray, liver scans, bone scans, calcium and phosphate levels, complete blood count

Related nursing diagnoses
1 Pain and discomfort
2 Risk for ineffective individual coping
3 Risk for infection
4 Risk for injury
5 Risk for ineffective management of therapeutic regimen
6 Impaired physical mobility
7 Situational low self-esteem

Expected outcomes
The following expected outcomes pertain to the patient or family. Numbers in parentheses refer to related nursing diagnoses above.
- Verbalize absence or control of nausea to patient's satisfaction (1).
- Verbalize absence or control of pain to patient's satisfaction (1).
- Be able to identify ways of reexerting control of the situation to positively influence outcome (2).
- Show no evidence of mastectomy incision infection (3,5).
- Show no evidence of mastectomy incision hematoma (4).
- Have drainage from surgical drains decrease daily (3,4).
- Verbalize correct care of wound at the time of discharge (3,5).
- Verbalize postdischarge exercise responsibilities (5,6).
- Be able to identify positive aspects of self (7).

Other possible nursing diagnoses
Anxiety, body image disturbance, risk for altered family processes, fatigue, fear, anticipatory grieving, altered nutrition (less than body requirements or more than body requirements), altered role performance, self-care deficit (bathing/hygiene, feeding, dressing/grooming, toileting), sensory-perceptual alterations, altered sexuality pattern, spiritual distress, impaired tissue integrity

Patient teaching

Complications
- Lymphedema
- Symptoms: swelling of the arm on the affected side, heaviness of the arm, pain, numbness in the arm and fingers, impaired mobility of the arm

Care after axillary lymph node dissection
- Do not have blood pressure measurements, blood sampling, injections, or vaccinations on the affected arm.
- Avoid dependent arm positions (positions in which the arm is lower than the level of the heart); elevate the hand and the arm on a pillow to facilitate drainage of lymph.

- Wear protective clothing and heavy gloves when gardening or whenever there is a risk of arm or hand injury.
- Protect the arm and hand on the affected side from burns, such as when removing food from hot ovens or when ironing.
- Avoid any clothing or jewelry that is too tight on the affected arm and hand.
- Try to avoid cuts and scratches to the affected side. Monitor all breaks in the skin for signs of infection. Contact a doctor immediately if signs of infection occur.
- Be consistent with exercises that prevent arm swelling or lymphedema.

Signs and symptoms
- Temperature >101° F (38° C)
- Warmth, redness, excessive bruising, unusual pain, tenderness, or swelling at incision site
- Swelling of the arm

Activity
- Perform range-of-motion exercises as directed.
- Discuss overall fitness programs.

Medications
- Chemotherapy
- Radiation therapy
- Lymphedema prevention

Nutrition
- Maintain appropriate body weight.
- Continue high-protein diet as tolerated while the incision heals.

Critical thinking activities
1. Describe the similarities and differences between breast cancer screening practices of women at high risk for the development of breast cancer because of family history or ethnicity and those of women not at high risk because of family history or ethnicity.
2. Discuss whether the physical and psychosocial concerns of women treated for breast cancer in "short stay" inpatient programs are addressed to the women's satisfaction.
3. Discuss whether the fears of recurrence of breast cancer for women treated with breast conservation surgery followed by radiation therapy differ from those of women treated by modified radical mastectomy.
4. Describe the cancers, other than breast cancer, that have been linked to genetic, hereditary, or familial predisposition.
5. In collaboration with an older relative, compile a cancer pedigree (family tree) for your family.
6. Determine whether screening of women at high risk for development of breast cancer (BRAC 1 and BRAC 2) is available in your community. If so, determine who can refer patients for screening, the average cost of screening, and whether counseling is available.

Suggested research topics
- Coping strategies for breast cancer
- Compliance with therapy
- Effectiveness of screening programs

Lung cancer

DRG: 82 Mean LOS: 5.7 days

Even though most cases can be prevented, lung cancer is the leading cause of death from cancer worldwide. In the United States, more women die annually from lung cancer than from breast cancer, and it is the number one cause of death from malignant disease among American males. As much as 80% of cases of the disease can be attributed to a single cause—cigarette smoking. Other risk factors for lung cancer include occupational exposure to potential and known carcinogens, exposure to air pollution, and exposure to passive, or second-hand, tobacco smoke. Genetics may also play a role.

Primary lung cancers are classified into two major histologic types: small-cell lung cancer (SCLC) or non-small-cell lung cancer (NSCLC). The long-term survival rate for either type is dismal—only 10% of patients live 5 years—partly because the early stages are usually asymptomatic so the disease is generally advanced by the time symptoms (cough, hemoptysis, hoarseness, or weight loss) appear. At this time, no large-scale screening or early-detection method for lung cancer is available.

Treatment of SCLC and NSCLC depend on the stage of disease at the time of diagnosis. Because of the aggressive metastatic nature of SCLC, surgery is not usually an option for this form of lung cancer, which is responsive to chemotherapy and radiation therapy. Surgery, radiation therapy, and chemotherapy may be used to treat NSCLC. The preferred treatment option for resectable tumors is almost always surgical excision.

Subjective assessment findings

Health history
Smoking history, including number of years smoked, number of cigarettes smoked per day, level of tar and nicotine in brands of cigarettes smoked, attempts to stop smoking; exposure to second-hand smoke; occupational exposure to potential and known carcinogens; exposure to pollutants; previous diagnosis of acute or chronic lung conditions

Medication history
Prescription and over-the-counter (OTC) inhalers, cough medications

Functional health patterns
Activity-exercise: weakness, bone pain, fatigue, dyspnea on exertion, dizziness, shortness of breath (SOB) at rest, persistent cough, hemoptysis
Nutritional-metabolic: unexplained weight loss, anorexia, taste changes, fever, chills, night sweats
Cognitive-perceptual: pain, forgetfulness, memory loss or lapses, headaches, inability to learn, seizure activity (late sign)
Health perception–health management: patterns of respiratory infections and illnesses; family history of cancer, particularly lung cancer; attitudes toward tobacco use

(Text continues on page 107.)

PLAN OF CARE	PREADMIT PHASE	INPATIENT CARE Day 1	Day 2
DIAGNOSTIC TESTS	• Sputum cytology • Cultures • Bronchoscopy • Computed tomography scan • Percutaneous needle biopsy • Chest X-ray • Blood chemistries • Coagulation studies • Pulmonary function tests • Arterial blood gases (ABGs) • Electrocardiogram	• Pulse oximetry q 4 hr • ABGs • Complete blood count (CBC) • Electrolytes (Lytes) • Serum chemistries	• Pulse oximetry q shift • ABGs • CBC • Lytes • Serum chemistries
MEDICATIONS	• Evaluation use of prescription and over the-counter (OTC) medications. • Discontinue (D/C) aspirin 5 to 7 days and anticoagulants (with doctor's order) 36 hr before surgery. • Possible initiation of bronchodilator.	• Analgesics (magnesium sulfate or fentanyl) • I.V. antibiotics • Resumption of preadmission medications as ordered; I.V. fluids with lytes and peripheral nutrition • Bronchodilator as needed	• Same as Day 1
PROCEDURES	*Respiratory therapy (RT) consult:* • Initiate postural drainage, deep breathing and coughing techniques.	• Check vital signs (VS) q 4 hr. • Monitor chest tube. • Provide oxygen (O_2) to maintain O_2 saturation (O_2 sat) > 94%. • Provide pulmonary hygiene. • Suction carefully as needed. • Assess breath sounds q 4 hr.	• Check VS q 4 hr. • Monitor chest tube. • Provide O_2 to maintain O_2 sat >94%. • Have patient TCDB at least q 2 hr. • Suction carefully as needed. • Assess breath sounds every shift.
DIET	• Give diet as tolerated (DAT).	• Nothing by mouth until extubated; then give ice chips, progressive diet. • Weigh patient.	*Nutrition consult:* • Give DAT; determine calorie count • Weigh patient.
ACTIVITY	*Pulmonary rehabilitation consult:* • Evaluate effects of disease on pulmonary capacity and potential for rehabilitation post operation.	• Keep patient on complete bed rest. • Elevate head of bed (HOB). • Have patient avoid lying on operative side for prolonged periods.	• Dangle feet and legs on side of bed. • Have patient get out of bed to chair one time, elevate HOB. • Have patient avoid lying on operative side for prolonged periods.
ELIMINATION	• Evaluate need for assistance post operation.	• Measure intake and output (I & O), including chest tube drainage, q 4 hr.	• Same as Day 1
HYGIENE	• Evaluate need for postoperative help.	• Assist with all needs.	• Same as Day 1
PATIENT TEACHING	• Discuss need to curtail smoking prior to surgery. • Discuss turning, coughing, and deep breathing (TCDB) exercises, and postoperative pain control. • Discuss expectations after surgery.	• Discuss pain assessment scale and need for frequent VS and other monitoring. • Discuss splinting the incision line during coughing (C) and deep breathing (DB).	• Discuss pain assessment scale, need for frequent VS and other monitoring. • Discuss splinting incision line during C and DB. • Discuss activity increase.
DISCHARGE PLANNING	*Social services consult:* *Home health consult:* *Pastoral care consult:* *Smoking cessation program consult:* • Evaluate effects of disease on pulmonary capacity and potential for postoperative rehabilitation.	*Social services:* • Assess discharge planning needs (home O_2, ambulation assistive devices). • Evaluate need for vocational counseling.	• Refer to community support services and programs for patient and family (for example, American Cancer Society, American Lung Association programs).

Day 3	Day 4	Day 5
• Same as previous day.	• Pulse oximetry	• ABGs • CBC • Lytes • Pulse oximetry
• Convert analgesics to by mouth (P.O.). • I.V. antibiotics	• Same as previous day	• Convert all medications to P.O.
• Check VS q 4 hr. • Monitor chest tube. • Provide O_2 to maintain sat >94%. • Encourage TCDB at least q 2 hr. • Suction as needed. • Assess breath sounds every shift. • Monitor for right-sided heart failure from pulmonary hypertension.	• Check VS q 8 hr. • D/C chest tube (by doctor) when drainage decreased. • Continue to encourage TCDB. • Assess breath sounds every shift.	• Check VS q 8 hr. • Continue to encourage TCDB. • Assess breath sounds every shift.
• Give DAT. • Weigh patient.	• Same as previous day	• Same as previous day
• Have patient get up in chair with assistance in the morning and afternoon. • Elevate HOB.	• Assist with walking and up in chair.	• Same as previous day
• Measure I & O, including chest tube drainage, q 8 hr. • Evaluate for constipation.	• Measure I & O.	• Same as previous day
• Same as Day 1	• Same as Day 1	• Same as Day 1
• Begin teaching about need for follow-up care and need for chemotherapy and radiation therapy if needed. • Teach about chest tube site care and signs and symptoms of respiratory infection.	• Reinforce need for adjuvant therapies. • Emphasize importance of smoking cessation.	• Discuss need to avoid contact with persons with respiratory infections. • Discuss need for flu vaccine.
Social services: • Evaluate need for home O_2 and durable medical equipment such as hospital bed, shower bench, bedside commode. • Address and emphasize importance of smoking cessation plan with patient and family.	*Home health nurse:* • Visit patient and family prior to discharge to evaluate home needs. • Discuss plans for follow-up.	• Discharge to home.

(continued)

PLAN OF CARE	HOME CARE *Visit 1*	*Visit 2*	*Visit 3*
DIAGNOSTIC TESTS	• Pulse oximetry • Complete blood count • Electrolytes • Blood chemistries	• Pulse oximetry	• Same as previous visit
MEDICATIONS	• Inspect medications: prescription and over-the-counter medications (bronchodilators, aspirin). • Evaluate effects of pain medications. • Assess for adverse reactions to medications.	• Same as first visit	• Same as first visit
PROCEDURES	• Evaluate breath sounds carefully and compare to baseline data. • Evaluate for hoarseness. • Weigh patient. • Examine oxygen (O_2) delivery system and services. • Assess for right-sided heart failure: note signs and symptoms such as peripheral edema, weight gain, edema of dependent body parts, jugular vein distention.	• Evaluate breath sounds, hoarseness, and O_2 delivery system. • Weigh patient.	• Same as previous visit
DIET	• Evaluate for dysphagia as baseline. • Evaluate whether calorie consumption is appropriate for metabolic needs.	• Same as first visit	• Same as first visit
ACTIVITY	*Physical therapy (PT) and occupational therapy (OT):* • Evaluate need for assistive devices such as canes, walkers, wheelchairs, and mobile O_2 devices.	• *PT and OT:* Teach patient and family use of prescribed assistive devices.	• *PT and OT:* Same as previous visit
ELIMINATION	• Assess for constipation.	• Same as first visit	• Same as first visit
HYGIENE	• Evaluate need for home health aide services.	• Encourage use of bedside commode or shower bench as needed.	• Same as previous visit
PATIENT TEACHING	• Reinforce previous teaching about smoking cessation, adequate food and fluid intake, and need for follow-up appointments. • Teach about operating and troubleshooting home devices.	• Discuss specifics related to chemotherapy and radiation therapy prescribed for the patient as adjuvant therapy.	• Teach patient and family signs and symptoms to report that could indicate progression of the disease. • Reinforce teaching related to chemotherapy and radiation therapy.
DISCHARGE PLANNING	• Refer to OT, PT, and pulmonary rehabilitation as needed. • Evaluate knowledge and use of community support services. • Investigate possibility of living will.	• Refer to community programs, such as I Can Cope, CanSurmount, and others. • Refer to vocational counseling as appropriate.	• Refer to community hospice program if indicated.

Objective assessment findings

Physical findings

Cardiovascular: tachycardia, swelling of face, neck, and upper extremities (superior vena cava syndrome)
Integumentary: cool, clammy skin; pallor; diaphoresis
Neurologic: arm weakness, facial asymmetry (Bell's palsy)
Respiratory: SOB, increased sputum production, hemoptysis, cough, dyspnea, stridor, wheezing, hoarseness (damage to recurrent laryngeal nerve), decreased breath sounds, chest or shoulder pain, use of accessory muscles to breathe, unequal chest excursion

Diagnostic tests

Sputum cytology, cultures, bronchoscopy, computed tomography scan, percutaneous needle biopsy, chest X-ray, blood chemistries, pulmonary function tests, arterial blood gases, electrocardiogram

Related nursing diagnoses

1 Activity intolerance
2 Impaired gas exchange
3 Risk for infection
4 Noncompliance with treatment regimen
5 Pain

Expected outcomes

The following expected outcomes pertain to the patient or family. Numbers in parentheses refer to related nursing diagnoses above.

- Know that fatigue may persist after discharge and that progressive activity is recommended (1).
- Be free of pulmonary congestion before discharge (2).
- Be able to list symptoms, such as fever, cough, and purulent secretions, that indicate a respiratory infection (2,3).
- Be aware of signs and symptoms indicating disease progression that should be reported immediately to a health care provider: increasing pain, seizure activity, hoarseness, edema of face and upper extremities, increasing SOB or difficulty breathing (2).
- Have an incision line that is free of infection (3).
- Know importance of smoking cessation; have been referred for appropriate assistance (4).
- Know importance of postdischarge follow-up appointments with health care providers (4).
- Have pain managed to patient's satisfaction (5).

Other possible nursing diagnoses

Anxiety, body image disturbance, ineffective breathing pattern, ineffective individual coping, fatigue, fear, anticipatory grieving, risk for caregiver role strain, impaired home maintenance management, ineffective management of therapeutic regimen (community, family, individual), altered nutrition: less than body requirements, impaired physical mobility, self-care deficit (bathing/hygiene, feeding, dressing/grooming, toileting), spiritual distress

Potential complications

Hypoxemia, atelectasis, pneumonia

Patient teaching

Nicotine polacrilex gum (Nicorette, Nicorette DS)
- Therapeutic outcome: to lessen withdrawal effects when decreasing cigarette smoking; to decrease cigarette use
- Adverse effects: nausea, vomiting, anorexia, indigestion
- Contraindicated in pregnant women, patients who experience severe angina pectoris, and patients in the acute period after myocardial infarction (MI)
- Onset is rapid; peak action in ½ hour
- Drug to drug interaction: increases the effects of acetaminophen and caffeine, furosemide, propranolol, and other drugs.
- Cautions: Do not exceed chewing thirty 2-mg pieces of gum/day; discontinue after 6 months.

Nicotine transdermal system (Habitrol, Nicoderm, Nicotrol, Prostep)
- Therapeutic outcome: to decrease cigarette smoking; to lessen withdrawal effects when decreasing cigarette smoking
- Adverse effects: burning, itching, redness at the site of patch application, headache, insomnia
- Contraindicated in pregnant women, nonsmokers, patients with severe arrhythmias, patients with severe angina, and patients in the acute post-MI period
- Onset is rapid; peak action in ½ hour
- Drug to drug interactions: increases the effects of acetaminophen and caffeine, furosemide, propranolol, and other drugs
- Cautions: Some patches are to be worn only during waking hours; some patches can be worn 24 hours; patches should be protected from heat sources.

Signs and symptoms
- Temperature above 101° F (38° C)
- Warmth, redness, excessive swelling, purulent drainage from the incision

Activity
- Increase exercise under the direction of a physician.
- Recognize limitations in activity levels after lung resection.

Coping
- Discuss support services and agencies available in the community.
- Encourage progress with smoking reduction and cessation attempts.

Critical thinking activities
1. Discuss the impact, if any, of OTC smoking-cessation aids, such as nicotine gum, on decreasing the incidence of cigarette smoking.
2. As part of a clinical project, you have been asked to teach about the hazards of smoking to a group of 9- to 12-year-old school children. Outline the most important aspects to be covered with this particular age-group.
3. Describe systemic manifestations of paraneoplastic syndromes associated with SCLC.
4. Discuss why there are no effective mass screening tests for early detection of lung cancer.
5. Discuss the metastatic potential of the four major types of lung neoplasms (epidermoid, adenocarcinoma, large cell, and small cell). Describe implications for patient and family education.

Suggested research topics
- Coping strategies for lung cancer
- Effectiveness of smoking cessation programs or aids
- Compliance with treatment for lung cancer

Renal disorders

Acute renal failure

DRG: 316 Mean LOS: 5.4 days

Acute renal failure is a clinical syndrome characterized by sudden, severe impairment of renal function. When acute renal failure occurs, substances normally eliminated in the urine—nitrogenous waste products, such as blood urea nitrogen (BUN) and serum creatinine (Cr)—begin to accumulate in body fluids. This accumulation, known as azotemia, progresses to a symptomatic state of uremia that, in turn, leads to a disruption in homeostatic, endocrine, and metabolic functions. Acute renal failure is usually associated with a decrease in urine output (<400 ml/day [oliguria]); however, output may be normal or increased. Acute renal failure may develop over hours or days with progressive elevations of BUN, Cr, and potassium (K), regardless of urine output.

Causes include the following: (1) reduction in renal blood flow (prolonged hypotension, cardiogenic and septic shock, burns, hemorrhage, hypovolemia); (2) contact with a nephrotoxic agent (infection, drugs, chemicals, blood transfusion); (3) trauma; (4) obstructive lesions; and (5) postoperative complications or complications of extensive surgery in elderly patients. The most common cause is reduction in renal blood flow, which accounts for 50% to 70% of all cases.

Acute renal failure is generally reversible; however, recovery varies with the underlying illness, the general health and age of the individual, the length of the oliguric phase, and the management of the individual during the illness. If the kidneys do not recover, the individual progresses to chronic renal failure (CRF). The mortality rate is 5% to 25% higher in the elderly than in younger persons, and death is usually caused by infection, GI hemorrhage, or myocardial infarction.

Subjective assessment findings

Health history
Sepsis; dehydration; trauma; obstructive lesions; volume depletion secondary to hemorrhage, shock, burns, and hypotension; exposure to nephrotoxic agents (lead, mercury, X-ray media); cardiac and vascular conditions; cardiopulmonary bypass; multiple blood transfusions; surgery of aorta, renal vessels, and biliary tree; extensive surgery in elderly; diabetes; recurrent urinary tract infection (UTI); acute nephritis or nephrotic syndrome; lupus; hypertension; hyperparathyroidism

Medication history
Anesthetics such as pipecuronium bromide, antibiotics such as aminoglycosides and cephalosporins, cyclosporines, analgesic abuse

Functional health patterns
Activity-exercise: weakness, immobility, muscle cramps
Nutritional-metabolic: anorexia, fever, nausea, thirst, weight loss or gain
Cognitive-perceptual: inability to concentrate, metallic taste in mouth, headache, irritability, confusion
Sleep-rest: interrupted sleep, insomnia
Coping–stress tolerance: fear, anxiety, emotional distress
Role-relationships: decreased self-esteem, intimacy dysfunction, personality changes

Objective assessment findings

Physical findings

Cardiovascular: hypertension, hypotension, anemia, dry mucous membranes, decreased venous filling, edema, arrhythmias, heart failure, altered clotting mechanisms
Gastrointestinal: vomiting, weight loss or gain, anorexia, nausea, ulcers, hiccoughs, hemorrhage, diarrhea, constipation, bleeding
General: malaise or fatigue, lethargy
Genitourinary: anuria, oliguria, bladder distention, diuresis
Integumentary: pruritus, bruising, pallor, decreased skin turgor, thin, brittle hair and nails
Neuromuscular: peripheral neuropathy, seizures, coma, fatigue, sleep disorders, muscle twitching, mental status abnormalities
Respiratory: Kussmaul breathing, pleural effusions, pulmonary edema

Diagnostic tests

Urine studies (pH, osmolality, specific gravity, sodium, Cr, urine sediment), complete blood count, BUN, serum phosphate, magnesium, K, calcium, sodium (Na), renal ultrasound, retrograde pyelography, excretory urography, renal scan, renal biopsy, electrocardiogram, magnetic resonance imaging

Related nursing diagnoses

1 Fluid volume deficit or excess
2 Altered renal tissue perfusion
3 Altered nutrition: less than body requirements
4 Risk for injury
5 Risk for infection
6 Self-care deficit (bathing/hygiene, feeding, dressing/grooming, or toileting)
7 Risk for impaired skin integrity
8 Anxiety
9 Ineffective management of therapeutic regimen (community, family, individual)

Expected outcomes

The following expected outcomes pertain to the patient or family. Numbers in parentheses refer to related nursing diagnoses above.
- Excrete metabolic wastes (1,2).
- Maintain acid-base equilibrium (1,2).
- Be able to minimize nausea and maintain stable weight (1,2,3).
- Comply with diet plan (3,6).
- Sustain no injuries (4,7).
- Be free of infection (5).
- Avoid persons with respiratory infection (5).
- Practice good hand-washing techniques (5).
- Have good skin turgor (5,6,7).
- Perform activities of daily living independently (6).
- Monitor blood pressure, daily weight, and intake and output (6,9).
- Seek appropriate support groups and referrals to maintain well-being (6,8,9).
- Recognize signs and symptoms (S/S) to report to doctor (9).
- Comply with the medical health management plan and drug therapy (9).

(Text continues on page 117.)

PLAN OF CARE	PREADMIT PHASE	INPATIENT CARE Day 1	Day 2
DIAGNOSTIC TESTS	▪ Serum electrolytes (lytes) ▪ Complete blood count (CBC) ▪ Prothrombin time and International Normalized Ratio ▪ Activated partial thromboplastin time ▪ Blood urea nitrogen (BUN) ▪ Serum creatinine (Cr) ▪ Magnesium (Mg) ▪ Calcium (Ca) ▪ Phosphate ▪ Protein ▪ Albumin ▪ Lipids ▪ Urinalysis, culture and sensitivity, and osmolality ▪ 24-hour urine for creatinine clearance ▪ Arterial blood gases ▪ Chest X-ray ▪ Computed tomography scan of abdomen and renal structures ▪ Electrocardiogram (ECG)	▪ Lytes ▪ BUN ▪ Cr ▪ Hematocrit (Hct) ▪ Hemoglobin (Hgb) ▪ Guaiac stools ▪ Possible retrograde pyelography ▪ ECG	▪ Lytes ▪ BUN ▪ Cr ▪ Hct ▪ Hgb ▪ Guaiac stools ▪ ECG
MEDICATIONS	▪ Diuretics if indicated ▪ Alkalinizing agents if indicated ▪ Potassium-lowering agents (sodium polystyrene sulfonate [Kayexalate], I.V. insulin, sodium bicarbonate, or calcium gluconate) if needed ▪ Antihypertensives (calcium channel blockers, angiotensin-converting enzyme [ACE] inhibitors) ▪ Anti-infectives ▪ Phosphate-binding agents (Tums, PhosLo) ▪ Histamine-2 (H$_2$) blockers if indicated ▪ Multivitamins ▪ Ferrous sulfate ▪ Antiemetics	▪ Diuretics if indicated ▪ Alkalinizing agents if indicated ▪ Potassium-lowering agents if needed ▪ Antihypertensives ▪ Anti-infectives ▪ Phosphate-binding agents ▪ H$_2$ blockers if indicated ▪ Multivitamins ▪ Ferrous sulfate ▪ Antiemetics ▪ Stool softener	▪ Diuretics if indicated ▪ Antihypertensives ▪ Anti-infectives ▪ Phosphate-binding agents ▪ Multivitamins ▪ Ferrous sulfate ▪ Antiemetics ▪ Stool softener
PROCEDURES	▪ Check baseline vital signs (VS). ▪ Obtain I.V. access ▪ Prepare for dialysis if needed.	▪ Use aseptic technique for all procedures. ▪ Use safety precautions with restraints if necessary. ▪ Check VS q 4 hr. ▪ Encourage patient to use incentive spirometry q 2 hr while awake. ▪ Assess heart and breath sounds b.i.d. ▪ Monitor I.V. rate. ▪ Initiate dialysis if necessary.	▪ Same as Day 1
DIET	*Dietary consult:* ▪ Give high-fat, high-carbohydrate, low-protein diet. ▪ Restrict sodium (Na) and potassium (K). ▪ Restrict fluid based on lytes and losses during oliguric phase (usually 400 to 500 ml/24 hours). ▪ Give total parenteral nutrition (TPN) if necessary	▪ Give high-fat, high-carbohydrate, low-protein diet. ▪ Restrict Na and K ▪ Restrict fluid based on lytes and losses during oliguric phase. ▪ Give tube enteral feeding, or TPN if necessary. ▪ Weigh patient daily.	▪ Same as Day 1

Acute renal failure ■ CLINICAL PATHWAY

Day 3	Day 4	Day 5
• Lytes • BUN • Cr • CBC • Mg • Phosphate • Ca • Albumin • Protein • Guaiac stools	• BUN • Lytes • Cr • Urine studies (osmolality, Cr, pH)	• BUN • Lytes • Cr • Urine studies (osmolality, Cr, pH)
• Same as previous day	• Same as previous day	• Same as previous day
• Same as Day 1	• Same as Day 1	• Check VS q 4 hr. • Assess heart and breath sounds.
• Same as Day 1	• Same as Day 1	• Same as Day 1

(continued)

PLAN OF CARE	PREADMIT PHASE	INPATIENT CARE Day 1	Day 2
ACTIVITY	• Institute energy conservation measures.	• Encourage bed rest. • Have patient perform range of motion (ROM) exercises q 4 hr while awake. • Have patient turn, cough, and deep-breathe (TCDB) q 2 hr.	• Have patient get out of bed (OOB) with assistance as tolerated. • Encourage ROM exercises.
ELIMINATION	• Assess fluid excess or deficit.	• Assess effects of diuretics. • Maintain strict intake and output (I & O).	• Same as Day 1
HYGIENE	• Assess for presence of infection.	• Encourage oral hygiene before and after meals. • Massage and lubricate skin. • Provide emollient baths for pruritus.	• Same as Day 1
PATIENT TEACHING	Discuss need for inpatient care.	• Explain cause of acute renal failure episode if known. • Explain reason for dietary and fluid restrictions. • Teach about ordered medications and adverse effects. • Explain importance of turning, changing position, and ambulating. • Teach how to measure blood pressure (BP). • Instruct patient to avoid contact with persons who have respiratory infections. • Explain dialysis if needed. • Teach importance of rest. • Advise to avoid over-the-counter drugs	• Reinforce previous teaching. • Provide renal failure management or prevention information if cause of acute renal failure is identified.
DISCHARGE PLANNING	*Social services consult:* • Determine homecare and support group needs.	*Psychological consult:* • Assess coping. *Social services:* • Assess needs.	• Assess abilities to perform activities of daily living (ADLs).

Day 3	Day 4	Day 5
• Have patient get OOB as tolerated. • Have patient walk in room as tolerated.	• Same as previous day	• Have patient walk as tolerated
• Same as Day 1	• Same as Day 1	• Same as Day 1
• Same as Day 1	• Same as Day 1	• Same as Day 1
• Reinforce previous teaching. • Instruct patient to weigh self daily using same scale at same time of day. • Teach how to collect and measure urine output daily. • Teach signs and symptoms (S/S) of acute renal failure. • Teach S/S of urinary tract infection. • Evaluate patient's performance of daily weighing, BP, and I & O procedures.	• Reinforce previous teaching. • Evaluate patient performance of daily weighing, BP, and I & O procedures.	• Continue to provide prevention and management information on acute renal failure.
• Assess abilities to perform ADLs. • Arrange for home health.	*Home health:* • Visit patient and family while inpatient.	• Assess patient's and family's knowledge of home health and support group contacts.

(continued)

PLAN OF CARE	HOME CARE Visit 1	Visit 2	Visit 3
DIAGNOSTIC TESTS	• Blood urea nitrogen • Complete blood count • Serum electrolytes • Urine and serum creatinine • Osmolality	• Repeat as indicated.	• Repeat as indicated.
MEDICATIONS	• Monitor effectiveness of medications. • Evaluate compliance with drug regimen.	• Monitor effectiveness of medications. • Evaluate compliance with drug regimen. • Observe for positive and adverse effects of drug therapy.	• Reassess same as previous visit.
PROCEDURES	• Check vital signs. • Assess breath and heart sounds. • Evaluate mental status. • Evaluate coping and family processes.	• Same as first visit	• Same as first visit
DIET	• Assess nutritional intake. • Assess compliance with dietary restrictions (increased calories, decreased protein, potassium, and sodium) • Weigh patient.	• Reinforce previous visit. • Refer to nutrition consult if indicated.	• Same as previous visit
ACTIVITY	• Assess sleep activity. • Assess ability to perform activities of daily living.	• Reinforce first visit.	• Reinforce first visit.
ELIMINATION	• Assess presence of edema. • Evaluate intake and output (I & O).	• Reinforce first visit.	• Reinforce first visit.
HYGIENE	• Assess dialysis site if present. • Assess skin integrity. • Encourage oral hygiene before and after meals.	• Reinforce first visit.	• Reinforce first visit.
PATIENT TEACHING	• Discuss signs and symptoms to report to doctor • Teach importance of avoiding persons who have respiratory infections. • Discuss importance of good hand-washing techniques for patient and others in close contact with patient. • Teach how to measure blood pressure (BP), and instruct to check BP daily at same time. • Advise patient to avoid over-the-counter drugs without doctor approval. • Encourage daily rest periods. • Teach I & O procedure. • Instruct to weigh daily in same clothing, at same time, and using same scale. • Discuss medications (name, dosage, purpose, time and route of administration, and adverse effects.). • Teach healing process and inspection and aseptic cleaning of dialysis site if present.	• Teach definition and factors that cause acute renal failure episodes. • Teach prevention of acute renal failure: control of BP, limiting exposure to industrial chemicals and nephrotoxic drugs, and adequate hydration. • Teach about need for regular follow-up care.	• Reinforce and evaluate teaching sessions from previous home visits.
DISCHARGE PLANNING	• Assess home environment for hygienic measures. • Refer to appropriate agency or social services as indicated.	• Assess home and support resource needs. • Refer to psychological counselor if indicated.	• Assess home and support resource needs.

Other possible nursing diagnoses

Altered family processes, sensory-perceptual alteration (visual, auditory, kinesthetic, gustatory, tactile, or olfactory) altered thought processes, constipation

Potential complications

Arrhythmias, hyperkalemia, metabolic acidosis, renal insufficiency, pericarditis, coagulation defects, GI bleeding

Patient teaching

Preventing recurrence

- Maintain natural resistance (adequate nutrition, fluid intake, rest, exercise).
- Avoid persons with infections, especially upper respiratory and streptococcal infections.
- Seek medical care at earliest S/S of UTIs or other infections.
- Avoid exposure to various nephrotoxins (majority of drugs are excreted by the kidneys).
- Avoid over-the-counter (OTC) drugs because many are nephrotoxic (for example, nonsteroidal anti-inflammatory drugs).
- Avoid chronic analgesic (for example, narcotics) abuse; interstitial nephritis may result.
- Seek prompt medical attention for care of wounds and burns; these may lead to sepsis.
- Monitor urine output and report decreased urine production to doctor as early as possible.
- Seek treatment for any conditions (for example, blood loss or use of antihypertensive agents) that may produce long periods of hypotension.
- Learn about medications that are nephrotoxic.
- Make sure that the correct blood transfusion is administered.
- Be aware of industrial and agricultural chemicals and products (insecticides, cleaning agents, organic solvents) that may be nephrotoxic.
- Schedule diagnostic studies requiring dehydration (nothing by mouth) so that there are "rest days" between treatments. This is especially important for an older adult who may not have adequate renal reserve.
- Keep follow-up appointments with doctor as directed.
- Seek appropriate health resources to assist with health care needs: social services for financial assistance, National Kidney Foundation for health information, pharmacist for pharmacologic consultation, dietitian for nutrition consultation, doctor for medical consultation if diabetic or receiving cancer therapy especially chemotherapeutic drugs, psychologist for psychological consultation.
- Wash hands after bathroom use, before and after eating, after direct contact with persons with infections, and before and after cleaning self as well as before and after cleaning any wounds.
- Instruct family to use good hand-washing techniques at home.
- Clean and lubricate skin to prevent breakdown.

Signs and symptoms

- Oliguria (decrease in urine output)
- Edema
- Hypotension, hypertension, tachycardia
- Nausea and vomiting
- Fatigue, lethargy
- Pruritus
- Diuresis
- Kussmaul breathing (deep, gasping respirations)
- Muscle weakness
- Weight gain of > 2 lb (0.9 kg) per day

- Infection (local with chills, redness, swelling, fever, drainage; UTI with dysuria, urgency, frequency, foul-smelling urine, and fever >101° F [38° C])
- Decreased attention and memory span.
- Behavior and mood changes, such as withdrawal, depression

Activity
- Explain importance of gradual convalescence (3 to 12 months may be necessary).
- Limit exercise and activity to tolerance without fatigue.
- Plan rest periods throughout the day.

Medications
- Instruct patient on dosage, time of administration, purpose, and adverse effects.
- Tell patient to avoid OTC drugs.
- Explain importance of drug therapy in relation to disease.

Nutrition
- Explain importance of maintaining high-calorie, low-protein diet (may change in accordance with renal function).
- Restrict K and Na as directed.
- Perform oral hygiene before meals to remove metallic taste and decrease the incidence of ulceration or thrush.
- Drink at least 3 qt (3 L) per day unless contraindicated.
- Weigh daily and keep weight log throughout treatment period; report extreme weight loss or gain (more than 2 lb per week)

Critical thinking activities
1. Identify coping strategies that assist acute renal failure patients to deal with depression.
2. Describe the most effective measures to ensure compliance with follow-up care and therapy in patients with acute renal failure.
3. Determine and discuss whether patients with acute renal failure who use resource and support groups for ongoing health promotion experience more or less CRF than patients who do not use the services.
4. Describe the most effective measures for preventing infection in the elderly patient with acute renal failure living in a nursing home or community-based elder home.
5. Explain the causes and descriptions of laboratory and urinary changes during the oliguric and diuretic phases of acute renal failure.
6. Explain the rationale for restricted protein, Na, and K during acute renal failure.
7. Explain the pathophysiologic processes of acute renal failure related to prerenal, intrarenal, or postrenal causes.
8. Identify age-related factors that increase the mortality rate when acute renal failure occurs and that increase the older patient's risk of acute renal failure.
9. Identify whether and how the acute renal failure that developed in a specific patient could have been prevented.
10. Explain how carbohydrates and fats are modified to prevent protein catabolism in patients with acute renal failure.

Suggested research topics
- Coping strategies for acute renal failure
- Compliance with therapy
- Effectiveness of instruction on infection prevention

Chronic renal failure

DRG: 316 Mean LOS: 5.4 days

Chronic renal failure (CRF) is a progressive deterioration of kidney function that ends in uremia (an excess of urea and other nitrogenous wastes in the blood). Kidney nephrons are destroyed and replaced by scar tissue, leading to physiologic changes in all major organ systems. Uremia is fatal unless dialysis or a kidney transplant is performed. Causes of CRF include: diabetes, hypertension, nephrotoxins (antibiotics), mechanical obstruction (prostate cancer, benign prostatic hyperplasia, calculi, trauma, hemorrhage). In the United States, the primary causes are diabetic nephropathy (34%), hypertensive disease (29%), and glomerulonephritis (12%).

The stages of CRF are characterized by decreased renal reserve, renal insufficiency, renal failure, and uremia, or end-stage renal disease (ESRD). Symptoms resulting from increasing blood urea nitrogen (BUN) and creatinine (Cr) levels (fatigue, weakness, headache, nausea, pruritus, nocturia, and polyuria), start to appear during the renal insufficiency stage. Few symptoms develop until after more than 75% of glomerular filtration is lost. (Progressive destruction of nephrons limits the glomerulus's ability to filter wastes.) Because of the progressive nature of symptoms during ESRD, individuals are generally not able to function without assistance.

Maintenance dialysis and renal transplantation have helped to prevent many CRF deaths since 1973. In the United States, the incidence of individuals being treated for ESRD is rising by an average of 8% per year, with older individuals the fastest growing group. This increased incidence is believed to be attributed to the increased mean age of the population, coupled with the associated increased incidences of diabetes and hypertension.

Subjective assessment findings

Health history
Acute renal failure, polycystic kidney disease, chronic pyelonephritis, chronic urinary obstruction, hypertensive nephropathy, diabetic nephropathy, gouty nephropathy, chronic glomerulonephritis, lupus, neoplasms (metastatic or primary), sarcoidosis, amyloidosis, Goodpasture's syndrome, arteriosclerosis, atherosclerosis

Medication history
Anesthetics, cyclosporines, antibiotics such as aminoglycosides and cephalosporins, analgesic abuse

Functional health patterns
Activity-exercise: weakness, immobility, history of pathologic fractures
Nutritional-metabolic: anorexia, fever, nausea, thirst, weight loss or gain, stomatitis
Cognitive-perceptual: inability to concentrate, metallic taste in mouth
Sleep-rest: interrupted sleep, insomnia
Coping–stress tolerance: fear, anxiety, emotional distress, depression, withdrawal
Role-relationships: decreased self-esteem, intimacy dysfunction, personality changes

(Text continues on page 125.)

PLAN OF CARE	PREADMIT PHASE	INPATIENT CARE Day 1	Day 2
DIAGNOSTIC TESTS	• Serum electrolytes (lytes) • Complete blood count (CBC) • Blood urea nitrogen (BUN) • Serum creatinine (Cr) • Magnesium • Calcium • Phosphate • Arterial blood gases • Protein, albumin, lipids • Urine Cr • Urine culture • Urinalysis and osmolality • Cr clearance levels • Guaiac stools • Computed tomography scan • Renal scan • Ultrasound • Electrocardiogram (ECG)	• Lytes • BUN • Cr (urine & serum) • CBC • Lipids • Platelet count • Guaiac stools • ECG	• Same as Day 1
MEDICATIONS	• Diuretics • Alkalinizing agents • Potassium-lowering agents (sodium polystyrene sulfonate [Kayexalate], I.V. insulin, glucose, and calcium gluconate) • Antihypertensives (calcium channel blockers, angiotensin-converting enzyme inhibitors) • Anti-infectives • Phosphate-binding agents (Tums, PhosLo) • Histamine-2 (H_2) receptor agents • Multivitamins • Antianemics • Antipruritics • Antiemetics	• Diuretics • Alkalinizing agents • Potassium-lowering agents (sodium polystyrene sulfonate [Kayexalate], I.V. insulin, glucose, and calcium gluconate) • Antihypertensives (calcium channel blockers, angiotensin-converting enzyme inhibitors) • Anti-infectives • Phosphate-binding agents (Tums, PhosLo) • Histamine-2 (H_2) receptor agents • Multivitamins • Antianemics • Antipruritics • Antiemetics	• Same as Day 1
PROCEDURES	• Take baseline vital signs (VS). • Initiate I.V. access • Perform dialysis.	• Check VS q 4 hr. • Encourage use of incentive spirometry q 2 hr while awake. • Assess heart and breath sounds q 4 hr. • Monitor I.V. rate. • Monitor patency of dialysis access device. • Initiate measures that decrease trauma or bleeding at access device site. • Initiate safety precautions with restraints if necessary. • Use aseptic technique for all procedures.	• Same as Day 1
DIET	*Nutrition consult:* • Give high-calorie diet. • Restrict protein. • Restrict sodium and potassium. • Restrict fluid (depends on losses and daily urine output). • Weigh patient daily.	*Nutrition consult:* • Give high-calorie diet. • Restrict protein. • Restrict sodium and potassium. • Restrict fluid (depends on losses and daily urine output). • Weigh patient daily.	• Same as Day 1

Day 3	Day 4	Day 5
• Same as Day 1	• Same as Day 1	• Same as Day 1
• Same as Day 1	• Same as Day 1	• Same as Day 1
• Same as Day 1	• Same as Day 1	• Same as Day 1
• Same as Day 1	• Same as Day 1	• Same as Day 1

(continued)

PLAN OF CARE	PREADMIT PHASE	INPATIENT CARE Day 1	Day 2
ACTIVITY	▪ Institute energy conservation measures	▪ Encourage bed rest. ▪ Have patient perform range-of-motion exercises q 4 hr while awake. ▪ Have patient turn, cough, and deep breathe (TCDB) q 2 hr.	▪ Assist to chair for 30 min to 1 hr t.i.d. ▪ Have patient TCDB q 2 hr.
ELIMINATION	▪ Assess for fluid excess. ▪ Assess for edema.	▪ Monitor for diarrhea and constipation ▪ Institute strict intake and output (I & O) measurements.	▪ Same as Day 1
HYGIENE	▪ Assess for presence of infection.	▪ Encourage oral hygiene before and after meals (ac & pc). ▪ Massage and lubricate skin. ▪ Control pruritus. ▪ Avoid soap in bath. ▪ Use emollients.	▪ Oral hygiene ac & pc. ▪ Massage and lubricate skin. ▪ Control pruritus.
PATIENT TEACHING	▪ Discuss need for inpatient care.	▪ Explain cause of chronic renal failure if known. ▪ Explain reason for dietary and fluid restrictions. ▪ Teach about ordered medications. ▪ Teach measures that relieve itching. ▪ Explain importance of turning, changing position, and ambulating. ▪ Teach how to measure blood pressure (BP). ▪ Instruct patient to avoid contact with persons who have respiratory infections. ▪ Explain dialysis. ▪ Teach importance of rest. ▪ Advise patient to avoid over-the-counter drugs. ▪ Discuss maintenance of safe environment to prevent injury or fractures.	▪ Reinforce previous teaching.
DISCHARGE PLANNING	*Social services consult:* ▪ Discuss home care and support groups.	*Psychological consult:* ▪ Assess coping. *Social services:* ▪ Assess support and resource needs (for example, economic status to purchase medication, equipment, and proper foods). ▪ Refer to appropriate agency or social services as needed. ▪ Assess abilities to perform activities of daily living.	▪ Assess home support and resource needs.

Day 3	Day 4	Day 5
• Have patient get out of bed as tolerated. • Have patient walk in room as tolerated.	• Same as previous day	• Same as previous day
• Same as Day 1	• Same as Day 1	• Same as Day 1
• Same as previous day	• Same as previous day	• Same as previous day
• Reinforce previous teaching. • Instruct patient to weigh self daily wearing same clothes, using same scale at same time of day. • Teach signs and symptoms (S/S) of infection, hyperkalemia, peripheral neuropathy, and excess fluid volume. • Teach S/S of urinary tract infection. • Evaluate patient performance of daily weighing, BP, and I & O procedures.	• Reinforce previous teaching.	• Reinforce previous teaching.
Home health: • Visit patient and family while inpatient.	• Assess patient's and family's knowledge of home health and support groups.	• Same as previous day

(continued)

PLAN OF CARE	HOME CARE Visit 1	Visit 2	Visit 3
DIAGNOSTIC TESTS	• Blood urea nitrogen • Complete blood count • Serum electrolytes • Urine and serum creatinine • Osmolarity • Urinalysis • Electrocardiogram	• Repeat as indicated.	• Repeat as indicated.
MEDICATIONS	• Assess effectiveness of medications. • Assess compliance with drug regimen.	• Assess effectiveness of medications. • Assess compliance with drug regimen. • Assess for positive and adverse effects of drug therapy.	• Same as previous visit
PROCEDURES	• Check vital signs. • Assess breath and heart sounds. • Evaluate mental status. • Observe coping and family processes.	• Same as previous visit	• Same as previous visit
DIET	• Assess nutritional intake. • Evaluate compliance with dietary restrictions (protein, potassium, sodium). • Assess presence of nausea, vomiting, and anorexia (conditions that cause loss of needed nutrients). • Refer to nutrition consult if indicated. • Weigh patient.	• Reinforce first visit. • Weigh patient.	• Same as previous visit
ACTIVITY	• Assess sleep activity. • Assess ability to perform activities of daily living. • Instruct patient to turn, cough, and deep breathe q 2 hr if immobile.	• Reinforce first visit.	• Reinforce first visit.
ELIMINATION	• Assess intake and output (I & O). • Assess for presence of edema. • Encourage exercise and sufficient dietary bulk.	• Reinforce first visit.	• Reinforce first visit.
HYGIENE	• Assess dialysis site. • Assess skin integrity. • Encourage oral hygiene before and after meals.	• Reinforce first visit.	• Reinforce first visit.
PATIENT TEACHING	• Discuss signs and symptoms (S/S) to report to doctor. • Teach importance of avoiding persons who have respiratory infections. • Teach importance of good handwashing techniques for patient and others in close contact with patient. • Teach how to measure blood pressure (BP), and instruct to check BP daily at same time; keep daily record and report changes to doctor. • Advise patient to avoid over-the-counter drugs without doctor's approval.	• Teach definition and factors that cause chronic renal failure. • Teach S/S of edema, hyperkalemia, hyperphosphatemia, hypermagnesemia, and hypocalcemia. • Teach purpose of dialysis. • Teach care of dialysis access device or catheter. • Discuss measures that decrease risk of injury and infection of dialysis access device or catheter. • Instruct to report S/S of redness, pain swelling or drainage from dialysis access device or catheter to doctor.	• Reinforce and evaluate teaching sessions from previous home visits. • Observe patient and family performing dialysis access device or catheter care, BP, and I & O procedures.

PLAN OF CARE	HOME CARE Visit 1	Visit 2	Visit 3
	• Encourage daily rest periods. • Discuss medications (name, dosage, purpose, time and route of administration, and adverse effects) • Teach I & O procedure, and instruct to report changes in output to doctor. • Instruct patient to weigh self daily wearing same clothing, at same time, and using same scale. • Instruct patient to avoid laxatives and antacids that contain magnesium. • Advise use of stool softeners to avoid straining during bowel movements.	• Teach S/S of urinary tract infection (dysuria, foul-smelling urine, fever), and instruct patient to report them to doctor. • Teach S/S of pericarditis (pericardial friction rub and chest pain). • Tell patient not to measure BP or allow venipuncture in the arm that has dialysis access device in place.	• Assess home environment for hygienic measures. • Refer to appropriate agency or social services as indicated.
DISCHARGE PLANNING	• Assess home and support resource needs. • Refer to psychological counselor if indicated.	• Assess home/support resource needs.	

Objective assessment findings

Physical findings
Cardiovascular: hypertension, anemia, arrhythmias, heart failure, hyperlipidemia, pericarditis, hyperkalemia, hypocalcemia, pericardial effusion, pitting edema, engorged neck veins, paradoxical pulse, palpitations

Gastrointestinal: vomiting, anorexia, nausea, ulcers, hiccoughs, diarrhea, constipation alternating with diarrhea, bleeding, stomatitis

General: malaise/fatigue, lethargy

Genitourinary: anuria, oliguria, polyuria, nocturia

Integumentary: pruritus, bruising, pallor, decreased skin turgor, yellow skin color, petechiae, ecchymoses, thin brittle nails and hair

Neuromuscular: peripheral neuropathy, headache, seizures, coma, fatigue, sleep disorders, muscle twitching, altered mental abilities, osteomalacia, osteitis fibrosa, metastatic calcification, nocturnal leg cramps, asterixis

Reproductive: infertility, decreased libido, sexual dysfunction, amenorrhea in females, atrophy of testicles in mates, gynecomastia

Respiratory: Kussmaul breathing, pleural effusions, pulmonary edema, dyspnea, pleurisy

Diagnostic tests
Urine studies (pH, osmolality, specific gravity, sodium, Cr, urine sediment), complete blood count, BUN, serum Cr, Cr clearance, serum phosphate, magnesium, potassium (K), calcium, and

sodium (Na); renal ultrasound; retrograde pyelography; excretory urography; renal scan; magnetic resonance imaging; renal biopsy; electrocardiogram, arterial blood gases

Related nursing diagnoses

1 Fluid volume excess
2 Altered renal tissue perfusion
3 Altered nutrition: less than body requirements
4 Risk for injury
5 Activity intolerance
6 Risk for infection
7 Self-care deficit (bathing/hygiene, feeding, dressing/grooming, or toileting)
8 Ineffective management of therapeutic regimen (community, family, or individual)
9 Sensory-perceptual alteration (visual, auditory, kinesthetic, gustatory, tactile, or olfactory)
10 Risk for impaired skin integrity
11 Anxiety
12 Anticipatory grieving
13 Self-esteem disturbance
14 Pain

Expected outcomes

The following expected outcomes pertain to the patient or family. Numbers in parentheses refer to related nursing diagnoses above.
- Maintain acid-base and electrolyte balance (1,2,3).
- Maintain normal bowel function (1,2,3).
- Have no signs and symptoms (S/S) of excess fluid after dialysis treatment (1,2).
- Have normal breath and heart sounds (1,2).
- Maintain stable weight (1,2).
- Comply with diet restrictions (3,7).
- Sustain no injuries (4).
- Perform activities of daily living (ADLs) independently (5,7,13).
- Be free of infection (6).
- Avoid persons with respiratory infection (6,7).
- Practice good hand-washing techniques (6,7).
- Monitor blood pressure (BP), daily weight, and intake and output (7,8).
- Maintain intact I.V. access device (8).
- Assess patency of dialysis access device by checking for thrills and skin care as instructed (7,8).
- Reduce frequency and severity of nausea to a tolerable level for the patient (14).
- Recognize S/S to report to doctor: infection, hyperkalemia, peripheral neuropathy, and excess fluid volume (4,6,8,9).
- Comply with the medical health management plan and drug therapy (8,9).
- Seek assistance from resource and support groups and referrals to maintain well-being (8,9,12,13).
- Have skin integrity remain intact (10).
- Verbalize feelings related to CRF, its treatment, and prognosis (11,12,13).

Other possible nursing diagnoses

Altered family processes, sexual dysfunction, altered thought processes, constipation

Potential complications

Arrhythmias, hyperkalemia, hypertension, peripheral neuropathy, GI bleeding, anemia, pericarditis, pulmonary edema, accelerated atherosclerosis

Patient teaching

Health promotion and maintenance

- Maintain natural resistance (adequate nutrition, fluid intake at least 2 qt (2 L)/day, rest, exercise to tolerance level).
- Avoid persons with infections, especially upper respiratory infections and streptococcal infections.
- Seek medical care at earliest S/S of urinary tract infection (UTI) or other infections.
- Avoid exposure to various nephrotoxins (a majority of drugs are excreted by the kidneys); if prescription nephrotoxic drugs are necessary for treatment of other conditions, renal function must be monitored by BUN and Cr determinations.
- Avoid over-the-counter (OTC) drugs because many are nephrotoxic.
- Weigh daily and observe for S/S of edema.
- Seek medical attention for care of wounds, burns, and so forth; these may lead to sepsis.
- Monitor urine output and report decreased urine production to doctor as early as possible.
- Seek treatment for any conditions that may produce long periods of hypotension or hypertension.
- Learn about medications that are nephrotoxic.
- Be aware of industrial and agricultural chemicals and products in immediate environment (insecticides, cleaning agents, organic solvents) that may be nephrotoxic.
- Learn about medications that are high in magnesium.
- Learn about renal dialysis, transplantation, and causes of CRF.
- Keep follow-up appointments with doctor as directed.
- Take BP daily; record and report hypertension or hypotension to doctor.
- Seek appropriate health resources: social services for financial assistance, National Kidney Foundation for health information, dietitian for nutrition information, psychologist for psychological assistance, and doctor and nurses for health care needs.
- Wash hands after bathroom use, before and after eating, after direct contact with persons with infections, and before and after cleaning self as well as before and after cleaning wounds.
- Instruct family to use good hand-washing techniques at home.
- Provide skin care with tepid water, bath oils, and creams to prevent breakdown, drying, and itching.
- Keep environment safe to reduce risk of injury, and avoid risk-taking activities.

Signs and symptoms

- Hyperkalemia (muscle weakness, arrhythmia, tachycardia, paresthesia, intestinal colic, diarrhea)
- Fluid volume excess (edema, weight gain >2 lb [.9 kg], dyspnea, elevated BP)
- Hypertension (headache, dizziness, shortness of breath, chest pain, edema, elevated BP)
- Peripheral neuropathy (restlessness of legs, loss of muscle strength, footdrop, muscle cramps, numbness and burning of feet, decreased sensation in feet)
- Anemia (fatigue, lethargy, low hematocrit and hemoglobin, bleeding, inability to perform ADLs)
- Pruritus, redness, and skin breakdown
- Infection (local with chills, redness, swelling, fever, drainage, sore throat, cough; UTI with dysuria, urgency, frequency, foul-smelling urine, fever >101° F [38° C])
- Diarrhea and constipation
- Depression, withdrawal, behavior and mood changes
- Mental confusion, decreased attention and memory span
- Hypocalcemia (muscle pain, limited mobility of joints, demineralization of bone, elevated serum phosphate levels, deposition of calcium-phosphate in joints and other places, fractures)
- Decreased urine output, inability to void

Activity
- Take iron and erythropoietin between meals as ordered.
- Limit exercise and activity to tolerance.
- Plan rest periods before and after activity; allow recuperation for future activities.
- Avoid fatigue.
- Avoid straining during bowel movements; take stool softeners or laxatives as needed.

Medications
- Instruct patient on dosage, time of administration, purpose, and adverse effects.
- Avoid OTC drugs, especially laxatives or antacids that contain magnesium.
- Explain importance of drug therapy in relation to CRF.

Nutrition
- Explain importance of maintaining ideal weight.
- Instruct patient about high-calorie, high-carbohydrate diet with protein, phosphate, K, and Na restriction as prescribed.
- Perform oral hygiene before meals to remove metallic taste.
- Suck on hard candy to increase carbohydrate intake.
- Eat small, frequent meals or snacks.
- Limit fluid intake as ordered; instruct patient to suck on lemon or ice cube to relieve thirst.
- Weigh daily and keep weight log; report extreme weight loss or gain >2 lb (.9 kg).

Dialysis care
- Reinforce use of good hand-washing techniques before access site care and sterile technique when performing dialysis exchanges.
- Encourage verbalization of fears, concerns and anxieties related to dialysis.
- Encourage discussions about kidney transplantation, if indicated; seek appropriate resource information.

Care of hemodialysis access device
- Instruct patient to hold medications until after dialysis treatment.
- Palpate for thrills and report absence of thrills at access site.
- Report pain or change in color of affected extremity.
- Avoid BP measurement in affected extremity.
- Keep sterile dressings on site.
- Do not carry heavy objects on arm with access device.
- Wear plastic sleeve over extremity when exposed to water.
- Carry clamp at all times to stop bleeding in case shunt separates.
- Report redness, pain, swelling, or drainage from access site.
- Reinforce use of good hand-washing techniques before access site care and sterile technique when cleaning access site.

Peritoneal dialysis access device
- Protect catheter from damage.
- Wash catheter insertion site gently with soap and water; rinse well and pat dry.
- Keep sterile cap and dressing in place.
- Report turbid, cloudy, malodorous, bloody, or feces-stained dialysate immediately.
- Report redness, pain, swelling, or drainage from catheter insertion site.

Critical thinking activities

1. Investigate whether there is a relationship between cultural factors and evidence that African-Americans have better outcomes on chronic dialysis than Caucasians.
2. Develop a detailed protocol to assist a patient and family with the ethical dilemma of whether to continue chronic dialysis.
3. Taking the part of a legal nurse expert, explain in writing for a court of law who should get an available donor kidney: the next individual on the transplant list or the individual with the best matched tissue type to the donor organ.
4. Discuss whether coping strategies can be identified to assist patients with CRF to deal with feelings of depression and isolation.
5. Describe how stresses for the elder patient on dialysis differ from those of younger patients.
6. Discuss the quality of life for a patient on chronic dialysis.
7. Explain the effects of uremia on the urinary system, metabolic processes, electrolyte and acid-base balance, and psychologic function.
8. Identify the daily nutrient requirements of patients receiving conservative, hemodialysis, and peritoneal dialysis treatments.
9. Compare and contrast hemodialysis and peritoneal dialysis in terms of advantages, disadvantages, indications, contraindications, complications, and effectiveness.
10. List the pros and cons of organ donation by family members of the patient with CRF.
11. Identify problems and interventions for the patient with CRF that are different from those common to the patient with acute renal failure.

Suggested research topics

- Coping strategies for CRF
- Compliance with therapy
- Coping with transplant and donor organ issues

Transurethral resection of the prostate

DRG: 337   Mean LOS: 2.3 days

Transurethral resection of the prostate (TURP) is a surgical procedure used to remove part or most of the prostate gland via a resectoscope inserted through the urethra. TURP is the most common type of surgery for treatment of benign prostatic hyperplasia (BPH), a condition in which the prostate gland enlarges and prevents the bladder from emptying. The procedure is recommended for individuals with moderate enlargement of the prostate and for elderly or debilitated individuals. Postoperative complications, such as penile erectile dysfunction or long-term incontinence, are less common with TURP than with other types of prostate surgery. Indications for TURP include obstructive uropathy, acute urine retention, bladder complications, and urinary tract infections (UTIs) related to BPH.

BPH is related to endocrine changes associated with aging that initiate hyperplasia of both glandular and cellular prostate tissue. To detect and treat problems early, the American Cancer Society and the American Urological Association recommend a yearly medical history and digital rectal examination for men older than age 40. After age 50, if symptoms of BPH become more evident, further diagnostic study and screening is recommended.

Subjective assessment findings

Health history
Prostate cancer, obstructive uropathy, acute urine retention, bladder complications or UTI related to BPH

Medication history
Estrogen or testosterone supplementation

Functional health patterns
Nutritional-metabolic: adequate fluid intake
Elimination: diminution in caliber and force of urinary stream, hesitancy in starting urination, dribbling after voiding, urine retention, incontinence
Sleep: nocturia
Self-perception: anxiety
Cognitive-perceptual: bladder discomfort, sensation of incomplete voiding

Objective assessment findings

Physical findings
General: older adult male
Genitourinary: smooth, firm, elastic enlarged prostate; palpable bladder

Diagnostic tests
Urinary analysis, urine culture and sensitivity, blood urea nitrogen, serum creatinine, serum electrolytes, complete blood count, cystoscopy, excretory urography, ultrasonography

Related nursing diagnoses

1 Altered urinary elimination
2 Ineffective management of therapeutic regimen (community, family, or individual)
3 Risk for fluid volume deficit
4 Risk for infection
5 Altered sexuality patterns
6 Anxiety
7 Pain

Expected outcomes

The following expected outcomes pertain to the patient or family. Numbers in parentheses refer to related nursing diagnoses above.

- Achieve bladder control (1).
- Have catheter remain patent while in place (2,4).
- Establish a regular voiding pattern after catheter is removed (1,2).
- Void clear yellow urine before discharge (1,4).
- Show no signs and symptoms (S/S) of UTI or hemorrhage (1,4).
- List S/S of UTI and gross hematuria (2,3).
- Engage in daily Kegel exercises (2).
- Have a balanced input and output (3).
- Be free of infection (4).
- Have vital signs that are within normal limits (3,4).
- Express fears, feelings, and concerns related to sexuality (5,6).
- Report diminished discomfort on urination (7).

Potential complications

Hemorrhage, infection, urinary incontinence

Patient teaching

Preventing recurrence of UTI

- Drink at least 2 to 3 qt (2 to 3 L), or 8 to 10 glasses, of fluids per day, and include drinks that promote systemic flushing such as water and cranberry juice.
- Avoid caffeinated drinks and alcohol.
- Seek medical care at earliest S/S of UTI (pain or burning, dysuria, foul smelling urine, fever >101° F [38° C])
- Avoid over-the-counter (OTC) drugs.
- Urinate at first desire to do so; empty bladder every 2 to 3 hours.
- Monitor urine output and report decreased urine production to doctor as early as possible.
- Keep follow-up appointments with doctor as directed.
- Wash hands before and after bathroom use.
- Keep urinary meatus area clean and dry.
- Shower instead of bathing.
- Void before and after sexual intercourse.

Signs and symptoms

- Bleeding
- Urinary incontinence
- Dysuria
- Fever >101° F (38° C)

(Text continues on page 135.)

PLAN OF CARE	PREADMIT PHASE	INPATIENT CARE Day 1
DIAGNOSTIC TESTS	• Serum electrolytes (lytes) • Complete blood count, type, and screen • Blood urea nitrogen • Serum creatinine • Prothrombin time and International Normalized Ratio • Activated partial thromboplastin time • Prostate-specific antigen • Urinalysis (UA) • Chest X-ray • Electrocardiogram	• As indicated
MEDICATIONS	• Antibiotics	• Antibiotics • Antispasmodics • I.M. analgesics
PROCEDURES	• Check vital signs (VS). • Start I.V. fluids. • Insert indwelling urinary catheter. • Apply antiembolism (TED) stockings. • Measure intake and output (I & O).	• Check VS q 4 hr. • Assess for signs and symptoms (S/S) of infection (urinary tract infection [UTI] and incision). • Monitor for complications: hemorrhage, hyponatremia, bladder perforation. • Assess catheter for drainage, hematuria, obstruction. • Apply TED stockings. • Keep catheter taped to abdomen and thigh and allow for straight catheter flow. • Implement pain management. • Irrigate catheter.
DIET	• Give nothing by mouth after midnight. • Encourage high fluid intake. • Give high acid ash-producing foods.	• Give clear fluids when awake.
ACTIVITY	• Have patient walk as tolerated.	• Have patient get out of bed (OOB) as tolerated postanesthesia. • After epidural anesthesia, have patient remain flat in bed for 8 hours; then raise head of bed. • Have patient perform leg exercises b.i.d.
ELIMINATION	• Use urethral catheter.	• Continue catheter. • Maintain strict intake and output (I & O).
HYGIENE	• Assess ability to perform activities of daily living (ADLs).	• Assist with care if needed.
PATIENT TEACHING	• Explain surgical procedure. • Orient to hospital and unit. • Teach about urinary catheter, leg exercise, pain relief, types of anesthesia, and turning, coughing, and deep breathing (TCDB). • Explain reason for ordered blood transfusion. • Review plan of care with patient and family.	• Teach about doing leg exercises. • Allow opportunities for patient and family to discuss concerns about sexuality • Review TCDB. • Discuss incentive spirometry. • Explain reason for checking postvoid residual.
DISCHARGE PLANNING	*Social services consult:* • Discuss home care and support groups	*Social services:* • Assess abilities to perform ADLs.

■ Transurethral resection of the prostate

CLINICAL PATHWAY

Day 2	Day 3

Day 2

- Hemoglobin
- Hematocrit
- Lytes
- UA
- Urine culture and sensitivity if indicated

Day 3

- As indicated

Day 2

- Antibiotics if needed
- Antispasmodics
- I.M. analgesics
- Analgesics by mouth (P.O.)
- Stool softeners if needed

Day 3

- Antibiotics if needed
- Antispasmodics
- P.O. analgesics
- Stool softeners if needed

Day 2

- Check VS q 4 hr.
- Assess for bladder spasms.
- Assess for spontaneous voiding after catheter removal.
- Continue TED stockings.
- Institute progressive urine collection.
- Continue to monitor for complications, including UTI.
- Remove catheter.

Day 3

- Check VS q 4 hr.
- Assess for bladder spasms.
- Continue TED stockings.
- Continue to monitor for complications, including UTI.

Day 2

- Give diet as tolerated.
- Reduce spicy food and caffeine intake.
- Encourage fluids to 2 qt (2 L)/day unless contraindicated.

Day 3

- Same as previous day

Day 2

- Have patient get OOB and walk as tolerated.
- Have patient alternate activity with rest periods.
- Have patient keep legs elevated when sitting.

Day 3

- Same as previous day

Day 2

- Continue progressive urine collection.
- Continue I & O.

Day 3

- Continue I & O.

Day 2

- Have patient perform self care.

Day 3

- Have patient perform self-care.

Day 2

- Teach about Kegel exercises.
- Teach S/S of UTI to patient and family.
- Instruct patient to avoid strenuous exercise for 2 to 3 weeks after surgery.
- Demonstrate good hand-washing techniques
- Teach about care of incision if present.
- Provide information about expectation of return of sexual functioning.

Day 3

- Reinforce previous teaching.
- Teach about medication: name, dosage, schedules, purpose, and adverse effects
- Instruct patient and family to call doctor if pain becomes severe, gross hematuria occurs, or is unable to void.
- Instruct patient and family to seek psychological counseling for sexuality concerns or problems.

Day 2

Social services:
- Assess support and resource needs (such as ability to purchase supplies).
Psychological consult:
- Contact if necessary.

Day 3

- Refer to home health as needed.
- Arrange for follow-up visit with doctor.

(continued)

PLAN OF CARE	HOME CARE Visit 1	Visit 2	Visit 3
DIAGNOSTIC TESTS	• Hemoglobin • Hematocrit • Urinalysis • Culture and sensitivity if indicated	• As indicated	• As indicated
MEDICATIONS	• Give stool softeners if indicated. • Give antibiotics if indicated.	• Same as first visit	• Same as first visit
PROCEDURES	• Assess vital signs. • Assess for bladder spasms. • Catheterize for postvoid residual if indicated.	• Same as first visit	• Same as first visit
DIET	• Encourage diet as tolerated. • Encourage fluid to 2 qt (2 L)/day if tolerated.	• Same as first visit	• Same as first visit
ACTIVITY	• Encourage activity as tolerated. • Teach Kegel exercises. • Instruct patient to avoid straining and heavy lifting. • Tell patient to keep legs up when sitting.	• Same as first visit	• Same as first visit
ELIMINATION	• Teach about intake and output. • Explain use of voiding diary if necessary. • Assess color and characteristics of urine.	• Same as first visit	• Same as first visit
HYGIENE	• Assess skin irritation around urinary meatus site and perineal area.	• Same as first visit	• Same as first visit
PATIENT TEACHING	• Teach about medications: name, dosage, schedule, and adverse effects. • Teach prevention of urinary tract infection (UTI). • Teach signs and symptoms (S/S) of UTI. • Instruct to report S/S of UTI to doctor. • Instruct to avoid over-the-counter drugs without doctor's approval.	• Evaluate previous teaching.	• Evaluate previous teaching.
DISCHARGE PLANNING	• Emphasize importance of ongoing outpatient care. • Consult psychological counselor for sexual functioning concerns and problems.	• Reinforce first visit.	• Reinforce first visit.

- Continued burning on urination
- Continued cloudy urine
- Foul-smelling urine
- Decrease in size of urinary stream

Activity
- Avoid straining and strenuous activities and exercises.
- Take stool softeners and laxatives to prevent straining during bowel movements.
- Resume sexual activity in 6 to 8 weeks.
- Perform Kegel exercises 10 to 20 times every hour to gain urinary control.
- When starting to void, shut off stream for a few seconds, and then continue voiding; do this exercise until urinary control improves (which may take weeks).
- Avoid long automobile trips; prolonged sitting may increase tendency to bleed.

Medications
- Instruct patient on dosage, time of administration, purpose, and adverse effects.
- Avoid OTC drugs, especially anticholinergics and diuretics, unless approved by doctor.

Sexual functioning
- Instruct about absence of ejaculation fluid during sexual intercourse (fluid goes into bladder after ejaculation and is voided at next urination, which produces urine that appears milky).
- Allow 6 to 8 weeks before engaging in sexual intercourse.
- Encourage to seek psychological counseling if sexual functioning is problematic.

Critical thinking activities
1. Identify strategies for helping patients undergoing TURP and their families express concerns about sexual dysfunction.
2. List the most effective measures for ensuring compliance with daily performance of Kegel exercises after TURP.
3. Over the period of 1 year, determine the percent of TURP patients encountered in a general surgery unit who received yearly digital rectal examinations.
4. Develop a school-based teaching program to inform young males about the importance of early detection of prostate problems.
5. Describe one of the radiographic or endoscopic studies performed on the urinary system; explain one of the nursing responsibilities associated with the study.
6. Identify the defense mechanisms of the urinary tract, and describe the factors that alter these mechanisms.
7. Identify problems and concerns relevant to catheter care post-TURP.
8. Relate the clinical manifestations of BPH to the pathophysiologic processes that occur.

Suggested research topics
- Coping strategies for TURP
- Compliance with therapy
- Effectiveness of early detection programs

Urinary incontinence

DRG: 332 Mean LOS: 2.8 days

Urinary incontinence, the involuntary loss of urine, affects more than 12 million people in the United States. More women than men are incontinent. Though not a consequence of aging, incontinence affects about 26% of women between ages 30 and 59 and 15% to 30% of the noninstitutionalized population age 60 and older. Existing medical conditions and diseases, urinary or vaginal infections, surgical history, childbearing history, hormonal changes, sexual history, age, obesity, physical condition, and certain medications contribute to the risk and severity of incontinence. The condition results in physical, psychosocial, and economic costs to the individual and family.

Urinary incontinence is classified into these types:

- stress—occurs with increased intra-abdominal pressure and is characterized by the loss of 50 ml or less of urine
- urge—occurs when the "urge" to void is felt a few seconds to minutes before periodic leakage of urine; urge incontinence is frequent and varies in severity during psychologic stress
- overflow (paradoxical)—occurs when the pressure of urine in the overfull bladder overcomes sphincter control; characterized by small amounts of urine leakage frequently during day and night
- reflex—occurs when the detrusor contraction is stimulated by a full bladder, leaving a large residual of urine, and is characterized by involuntary but fairly predictable loss of a moderate to large amount of urine
- total—is an involuntary, unpredictable, and continuous loss of urine.

Certain types of urinary incontinence can be improved or corrected: Kegel exercises, for example, can strengthen pelvic floor muscles and may decrease incidence of stress incontinence. A urinary tract infection (UTI), which can cause frequency, urgency, and periods of incontinence, can be treated to decrease or eliminate the symptoms. And surgical repair can correct the underlying problem.

Subjective assessment findings

Health history
Stress incontinence: low estrogen and other conditions that predispose women to relaxed pelvis musculature, post-prostate surgery
Urge incontinence: cerebrovascular disease, brain tumor, Alzheimer's disease, bladder carcinoma, interstitial cystitis, spinal cord carcinoma, bladder outlet obstruction
Overflow incontinence: bladder outlet obstruction, benign prostatic hyperplasia, herniated disk, diabetic neuropathy, neurogenic bladder, postanesthesia and surgery (cystoscopy, hemorrhoidectomy, herniorrhaphy)
Reflex incontinence: spinal cord lesions (above S2)
Posttrauma or surgery (total incontinence): vesicovaginal or urethrovaginal fistula, hysterectomy, invasive cervical cancer, radiation therapy, prostatectomy (transurethral, perineal, or retropubic)

Medication history
Anesthesia, low-dose estrogen, numerous prescription and over-the-counter (OTC) drugs (diuretics, sedatives, hypnotics, antipsychotics, anticholinergics, and alpha-adrenergic blockers)

Functional health patterns
Activity-exercise: involuntary passage of urine during coughing, sneezing, heavy lifting, straining, laughing (stress incontinence)
Sleep-rest: interrupted sleep
Coping–stress tolerance: anxiety, emotional distress
Elimination: ineffective, involuntary passage of urine
Self-perception: depression, low self-esteem
Role-relationship: inability to perform activities of daily living (ADLs), isolation

Objective assessment findings

Physical findings
Gastrointestinal/Genitourinary: nausea before incontinence (reflex incontinence)
Integumentary: redness, rash, skin breakdown, diaphoresis and flushing before incontinence (reflex incontinence)
Neurologic: central nervous system disorders, conditions that interfere with spinal inhibitory pathways (urge incontinence), spinal cord lesions or trauma above S2 (reflex incontinence)

Diagnostic tests
Excretory urography, cystoscopy (including urethroscopy), urodynamic studies, catheterization for residual urine

Related nursing diagnoses
1 Impaired skin integrity
2 Risk for infection
3 Body image disturbance
4 Ineffective management of therapeutic regimen (community, family, or individual)
5 Social isolation
6 Altered urinary elimination

Expected outcomes
The following expected outcomes pertain to the patient or family. Numbers in parentheses refer to related nursing diagnoses above.
- Have patient's skin remain intact (1).
- Report signs and symptoms (S/S) of UTI, impairment of skin, and continued incontinence to doctor (1,2,4).
- Comply with medication regimen, exercise program, and bladder training program (2,4,6).
- State catheter care procedure (2,4).
- Express fears, feelings, concerns, and questions (3,4).
- Use techniques to control urine odor (3,5).
- Participate in ADLs at optimal level (4).
- Seek assistance from professionals and support groups (3,4,5).
- Assume increased responsibility for self-care (4).
- Demonstrate controlled urinary flow (6).

Potential complications
Acute urine retention

(Text continues on page 141.)

PLAN OF CARE	PREADMIT PHASE	INPATIENT CARE Day 1
DIAGNOSTIC TESTS	• Post-void residual • Urodynamic studies • Voiding cystourethrogram • Bladder ultrasound • Excretory urography • Cystoscopy • Bladder biopsy • Urine culture and sensitivity (C & S)	• Postvoid residual • Voiding diary • Urine C & S • Urodynamic studies • Catheterization for residual urine
MEDICATIONS	• Prescription • Over-the-counter	• Estrogen replacement • Anticholinergics • Parasympathomimetics • Sympathominetics • Alpha-adrenergic agonists • Imipramine • Calcium channel blockers • Antispasmodics • Antibiotics
PROCEDURES	*Based on cause:* • Behavioral techniques • Electrostimulation • Bladder training programs • Surgery	• Length of stay related to treatment or surgery: vesicourethral suspension, artificial urinary sphincter (stress incontinence); injection of urethral bulking agents (Teflon and collagen), augmentation, enterocystoplasty (urge incontinence); fistula repairs, genital deficit corrections, urinary diversion (total incontinence); surgery of bladder, pelvic area, and spinal cord (all types incontinence)
DIET	• Assess need for weight reduction.	• Assess need for weight reduction. • Maintain fluid intake (2½ qt [2.5 L]/day) unless contraindicated. • Avoid liquids past 7 or 8 p.m. to prevent nocturia.
ACTIVITY	• Assess exercise tolerance level and abilities to perform activities of daily living.	• Initiate bladder training programs.
ELIMINATION	• Take voiding history.	• Establish voiding schedule of every 2 hours; provide privacy. • Assess pain and comfort level prior to voiding schedule. • Assess for bladder distention.
HYGIENE	• Assess skin integrity.	• Keep perineal skin clean and dry. • Use moisture ointments on reddened areas.
PATIENT TEACHING	• Teach need for inpatient care.	• Teach and demonstrate skin care management. • Teach perineal muscle exercises (Kegel exercises) for stress incontinence. • Assist in establishing and maintaining voiding program. • Advise fluid intake of at least 2½ qt/day. Adjust intake so largest amounts are taken when patient feels continence will be successful. • Have patient avoid fluid intake past 7 or 8 p.m. to prevent nocturia. • Discuss effects of excess weight on bladder. • Teach and demonstrate activities that stimulate voiding (stroking inner thigh, anal stimulation, stroking vulva or glans penis) for reflex incontinence. • Teach self-catheterization and care of equipment (reflex and total incontinence). • Teach signs and symptoms of urinary tract infection.
DISCHARGE PLANNING	*Wound and skin consult:* • Determine if severe excoriation from urine is present.	*Social services:* • Discuss home care support groups.

Day 2

- Length of stay related to treatment of incontinence type and complications

- Same as Day 1

- Length of stay related to treatment or surgery

- Same as Day 1

- Same as Day 1

- Same as Day 1

- Same as Day 1

- Reinforce previous teaching.

Social services:
- Arrange for home equipment.

Day 3

- Same as previous day

- Same as Day 1

- Same as previous day

- Same as Day 1

- Same as Day 1

- Same as Day 1

- Same as Day 1

- Evaluate patient's performance of exercise program, voiding schedule management, and self-catheterization.

- Assess patient's and family's knowledge of home health and support groups.

(continued)

PLAN OF CARE	HOME CARE Visit 1	Visit 2	Visit 3
DIAGNOSTIC TESTS	• Urinalysis • Catheterization for residual urine if indicated	• Urine culture and sensitivity if indicated.	• Same as previous visit
MEDICATIONS	• Assess effectiveness of medications. • Assess compliance with drug therapy.	• Assess for positive and adverse effects of drug therapy.	• Same as previous visit
PROCEDURES	• Check vital signs. • Observe patient performing catheter care.	• Same as first visit	• Same as first visit
DIET	• Assess compliance with weight reduction diet. • Refer to nutrition consult if indicated. • Assess fluid intake.	• Same as first visit	• Same as first visit
ACTIVITY	• Assess exercise program (Kegel). • Assess patient's performance on activities of daily living (ADLs). • Assess bladder training program.	• Same as first visit	• Same as first visit
ELIMINATION	• Assess intake and output. • Assess catheter patency and leakage.	• Same as first visit	• Same as first visit
HYGIENE	• Assess skin integrity. • Assess catheter site. • Assess control of urine odor.	• Same as first visit	• Same as first visit
PATIENT TEACHING	• Teach signs and symptoms (S/S) of skin impairment, early action to take, and when to report to doctor. • Reinforce establishment and maintenance of voiding program. • Encourage patient to keep a voiding diary. • Discuss need to perform ADLs and resume self-care within capabilities. • Encourage performance of exercise program (Kegel) daily if appropriate. • Review techniques to control urine odor. • Teach catheter care if appropriate (site cleaning, check for patency, self-catheterization, storage and cleaning of equipment, catheter removal). • Discuss medications (name, dosage, purpose, time and route of administration, adverse effects).	• Teach definition and type of incontinence, urine retention, S/S of bladder distention, catheter function, and problem solving. • Reinforce need to evaluate episodes of incontinence for precipitating factors and to make changes in schedules and training as necessary. • Instruct patient to report continued incontinence.	• Reinforce and evaluate previous teaching sessions. • Stress need for regular follow-up care.
DISCHARGE PLANNING	• Assess home support and resource needs (for example, economic status to purchase medication and equipment). • Refer to appropriate agency or social services as indicated.	• Same as first visit	• Same as first visit

Patient teaching

Corrective measures
- Instruct patient to keep voiding diary and schedule.
- Instruct individuals with weakened pelvic muscles to perform appropriate exercises (Kegel exercises) daily.
- Explain importance of daily exercise and performance of ADLs at optimal level of function.
- Reinforce need for weight reduction if needed.
- Seek assistance from appropriate resources and support groups.
- Teach self-catheterization procedure.
- Reinforce need to evaluate episodes of incontinence for precipitating factors and make changes as necessary.
- Teach establishment and maintenance of a voiding program or schedule.
- Instruct to adjust fluid intake so that largest amounts are taken at time of day when patient feels attempts at continence will be successful.
- Discuss medications (name, dosage, purpose, time and route of administration, adverse effects).
- Discuss measures that control urine odor.

Signs and symptoms
- Teach S/S of UTI (fever, chills, dysuria, cloudy urine, foul-smelling urine, bladder spasms) and report immediately to health care provider.
- Instruct to avoid irritating fluids such as drinks with caffeine or alcohol.
- Keep perineal skin clean with mild soap and water and dry well.
- Teach early signs of skin impairment (redness, irritation, swelling, breakdown).
- Instruct to use skin barrier, protective spray, or sealant every 8 to 12 hours and after each episode of incontinence.
- Instruct to use absorbent products (briefs, shields, or underpants) if incontinence is frequent.
- Teach to keep certain plastic products from touching the skin.
- Teach proper application of external collection device.
- Teach care and storage of catheters and collection devices.
- Discuss the importance of maintaining fluid intake at $2\frac{1}{2}$ qt (2.5 L)/day unless contraindicated.
- Teach sterile technique of self-catheterization.

Activity
- Discuss the importance of exercise.
- Teach bladder training programs.

Medications
- Instruct patient on dosage, time of administration, purpose, and adverse effects.
- Avoid OTC drugs.
- Explain importance of drug use or avoidance in relationship to problem.

Nutrition
- Explain the importance of losing weight, if appropriate.
- Explain the importance of drinking enough fluids.
- Discuss the need to avoid drinking fluids late at night.

Lifestyle modifications
- Teach about establishing and maintaining a voiding schedule.
- Explain the importance of daily exercise and performing activities of daily living as tolerated.

Critical thinking activities

1. Discuss the therapeutic measures that are most effective in treating stress incontinence.
2. Identify the nursing interventions that effectively increase patient compliance with the bladder training program.
3. Describe the most reliable indicators for urinary catheterization in the incontinent individual.
4. Determine the effects of surgery or drugs used to treat the causes of urinary incontinence in a given patient situation.
5. Explain the process of evaluating an incontinent patient's level of emotional comfort.
6. List nursing interventions that improve body image and skin integrity when continence cannot be achieved.
7. Identify principles that apply to care of urethral, ureteral, suprapubic, and nephrostomy catheters.
8. Describe one of the imaging studies performed on the urinary system, and explain one of the nursing responsibilities associated with the study.
9. Develop a patient-teaching plan addressing collection of a clean-catch urine specimen.
10. Develop a patient-teaching plan addressing performance of Kegel exercises to control stress incontinence.

Suggested research activities

- Coping strategies for urinary incontinence
- Effectiveness of therapeutic measures for treating stress incontinence
- Compliance with therapy
- Effectiveness self catheterization
- Effectiveness of therapeutic measures for urge incontinence

PART 7

Musculoskeletal problems

Lower extremity amputation

Total hip replacement

Total knee replacement

Lower extremity amputation

DRG: 213 Mean LOS: 7 days

Amputation is the surgical removal of part of a limb because of trauma, disease, tumors, or congenital anomalies. A skin flap is generally constructed to facilitate healing and use of prosthetic equipment.

The stump is closed with sutures or staples unless massive infection was present before surgery, in which case a guillotine-like surgery is performed and the wound is left unsutured. Traction may be applied to prevent skin retraction and to allow healing.

Middle and older age-groups have the highest incidence of amputation because of advanced peripheral vascular disease, especially atherosclerosis and diabetes mellitus. Traumatic injury, such as crushing injuries from motor vehicle or industrial accidents, is the usual cause for amputation in a young adult. Men who engage in hazardous occupations are more apt to require amputation than other persons.

Subjective assessment findings

Health history
Diabetes, cerebrovascular accident, heart disease, peripheral vascular disease, inadequate tissue perfusion, trauma, malignant tumor, congenital deformities, osteomyelitis

Medication history
Use of analgesics, over-the-counter drugs, corticosteroids; cigarette smoking

Functional health patterns
Health perception–health management: circumstances related to inadequate tissue perfusion
Activity-exercise: decreased mobility, muscle spasms, activity restrictions
Cognitive-perceptual: phantom limb sensation
Role-relationship: changes in role responsibilities
Self-perception–self-concept: changes to body image, loss of self-worth, changes in perception of abilities, negative attitude toward self
Coping–stress tolerance: isolation, perceived powerlessness, dependency on others

Objective assessment findings

Physical findings
Cardiovascular: absent peripheral pulses, cold skin, severe cramping pain with exercise and relieved with rest
General: apprehension, guarding of affected limb
Integumentary: pallor, cyanosis, ulcerations, local infection, atrophy, thickened nails
Musculoskeletal: restricted function of affected limb
Neurologic: decreased sensation, pain, tingling or burning sensation

Diagnostic tests

Complete blood count (CBC), fasting blood sugar, prothrombin time/International Normalized Ratio (PT/INR), activated partial thromboplastin time (APTT), wound culture and sensitivity, arteriography, thermography, plethysmography, transcutaneous ultrasonic Doppler recordings, neurovascular physical examination

Related nursing diagnoses

1 Pain
2 Impaired physical mobility
3 Risk for trauma
4 Ineffective individual coping
5 Body image disturbance
6 Risk for impaired skin integrity
7 Activity intolerance
8 Ineffective management of therapeutic regimen (community, family, or individual)
9 Altered tissue perfusion
10 Risk for infection

Expected outcomes

The following expected outcomes pertain to the patient or family. Numbers in parentheses refer to related nursing diagnoses above.

- Use alternative pain relief measures (1).
- State that pain is controllable (1).
- Perform upper and lower extremity muscle strengthening exercises four times daily (2,8).
- Walk with walker and transfer from bed to walker independently (2,4,7,8).
- Understand phantom limb pain theory (1,4).
- Express feelings about impact of surgery (4,5).
- Identify and seek support systems (5,8).
- Exhibit well-approximated incision without drainage, redness, or edema (8,9,10).
- Participate in maintaining aseptic technique (8,10).
- Engage in prescribed physical and occupational therapy exercise and gait training programs (8).
- Participate in self-care (4,7,8).
- List signs and symptoms to report to doctor (8).
- Perform stump and incision care safely (3,6,8,9,10).
- Comply with home safety measures (3,8).
- Display no signs of joint contracture (2,4,7,8).
- Have no bleeding with PT, INR, APTT, and CBC within normal limits (8,9,10).
- Be free of infection with vital signs within normal limits (8,10).

Other possible nursing diagnoses

Constipation, self-care deficit (bathing/hygiene, feeding, dressing/grooming, or toileting)

Potential complications

Sepsis, negative nitrogen balance, hemorrhage, flexion contracture

Patient teaching

Stump conditioning and care

- Wrap residual limb with compression bandage to control edema and form a firm conical shape for prosthesis fitting.

(*Text continues on page 151.*)

CLINICAL PATHWAY

PLAN OF CARE	PREADMIT PHASE	INPATIENT CARE Day 1	Day 2
DIAGNOSTIC TESTS	• Doppler recordings • Complete blood count (CBC) • Fasting blood sugar (FBS) • Serum electrolytes (lytes) • Prothrombin time (PT) and International Normalized Ratio (INR) • Activated partial thromboplastin time (APTT) • Blood urea nitrogen • Arteriography • Thermography • Plethysmography • Neurovascular physical examination • Electrocardiogram	• CBC • FBS daily, if diabetic • Lytes • PT/INR • APTT • Accuchecks before meals (a.c.) and at bedtime (h.s.), if diabetic	• PT/INR • APTT • Hematocrit (Hct) • Hemoglobin (Hgb) • Accuchecks a.c. and h.s., if diabetic
MEDICATIONS	• Antibiotics	• Analgesics I.M., I.V., via patient-controlled analgesia pump, or epidural • I.V. antibiotics time 3-4 doses • Antiemetics • Antipyretics • Insulin if diabetic • Stool softener	• Oral (P.O.) analgesics • Antipyretics • Insulin if diabetic • Laxative, if no bowel movement (BM) in 3 days • Stool softener • Antispasmodic, anticonvulsant, or beta blocker for phantom limb pain
PROCEDURES	• Take psychosocial assessment. • Take system assessment.	• Check vital signs (VS) four times every hour then q 4 hr. • Assess stump dressing for drainage q 4 hr and as needed. • Assess for pain. • Check circulation q 4 hr and as needed. • Assess stump for bleeding. • Assess for compartment syndrome. • Elevate head of bed (HOB) no more than 30 degrees to maintain alignment. • Keep stump dressing clean and dry. • Prepare AV foot pump for unaffected leg. • Elevate stump for 24 hours (avoid use of pillow).	• Check VS every shift and as needed. • Assess stump dressing for drainage. • Assess for pain. • Check circulation every shift. • Assess stump for bleeding. • Assess skin around stump site for redness or breakdown. • Assess for compartment syndrome. • Turn from side to back to abdomen q 2 hr. • Prepare AV foot pump for unaffected leg. • Use sterile technique when changing stump dressing. • Do dressing change after first change by doctor; subsequent daily and as needed changes to be done by RN.
DIET	• Assess nutritional status.	• Give clear to full liquids as tolerated.	• Give full liquid to diet as tolerated (DAT). • Give diabetic or fat-restricted diet if diabetic.
ACTIVITY	• As tolerated	• Encourage bed rest. • Give complete care. • Turn q 2 hr with assistance and support stump (after 24 hr). • Provide overhead trapeze.	• Have patient get out of bed (OOB) in chair b.i.d. • Give partial bath. • Provide overhead trapeze. • Provide bedside commode (BSC). • Assist with active and passive ROM exercises to unaffected leg q 4 hr. • Adhere to physical therapy muscle strengthening program for UE and LE. • Assist with adduction and extension exercises to affected leg q 4 hr.

Day 3	Days 4 to 6	Day 7
• PT/INR • APTT • CBC • Lytes • Accuchecks a.c. and h.s., if diabetic	• PT/INR • APTT • Hct • Hgb • Accuchecks a.c. and h.s., if diabetic	• PT/INR • APTT • CBC • Accuchecks a.c. and h.s., if diabetic
• P.O. analgesics • Antipyretics • Insulin if diabetic • Stool softener • Antispasmodic, anticonvulsant, or beta blocker for phantom limb pain	• Same as previous day	• Same as previous day • Laxative, if no BM in 3 days
• Check VS 2 times every shift and as needed. • Assess for compartment syndrome. • Assess incision and surrounding area for signs and symptoms (S/S) of edema and infection every shift. • Observe for phantom limb pain. • Encourage self-care. • Remove JP or other wound drain. • Keep stump dressing clean and dry. • Change dressing and elastic bandage wrap b.i.d. • Praise patient for attempted or completed tasks. • Monitor AV foot pump for unaffected leg.	• Check VS every shift and as needed. • Assess for compartment syndrome. • Assess incision and surrounding area for S/S of edema and infection b.i.d. • Observe for phantom limb pain. • Apply firm fitting stump sock as needed. • Change dressing and elastic bandage wrap b.i.d. • Encourage self-care. • Praise patient for attempted or completed tasks. • Provide diversional activities.	• Check VS b.i.d. • Same as previous day
• Give DAT. • Encourage foods high in protein.	• Same as previous day	• Same as previous day
• Have patient stand at bedside. • Have patient lie prone t.i.d. for 20 to 30 minutes if tolerated. • Provide overhead trapeze. • Provide BSC. • Have patient perform self-care. • Assist with active and passive ROM exercises to unaffected leg q 4 hr. • Have patient adhere to physical therapy muscle strengthening program for UE and LE. • Assist with adduction and extension exercises to affected leg q 4 hr.	• Have patient walk to bathroom *PT consult:* • Discuss walker ambulation and gait training, and ROM and muscle strengthening exercises. • Have patient lie prone t.i.d. for 20 to 30 minutes if tolerated. • Provide overhead trapeze. • Provide BSC. • Have patient perform self-care. *OT consult:* • Discuss activities of daily living (ADLs) retraining if necessary.	• Have patient walk in hallway. • Have patient walk to bathroom. *PT consult:* • Have patient practice walker ambulation and gait training, and ROM and muscle strengthening exercises. • Have patient lie prone t.i.d. for 20 to 30 minutes if tolerated. • Have patient perform self-care. *OT consult:* • Assist with ADLs retraining if necessary.

(continued)

PLAN OF CARE	PREADMIT PHASE	INPATIENT CARE Day 1	Day 2
ELIMINATION	▪ Assess last BM. ▪ Assess voiding pattern.	▪ Measure intake and output. ▪ Assess Jackson-Pratt (JP) output or other wound drainage. ▪ Give catheter care.	▪ Assess BM. ▪ Assess urine output. ▪ Remove catheter; if no voiding in 8 hours, provide straight catheter.
HYGIENE	▪ Assess skin integrity. ▪ Assess for presence of open leg ulcers. ▪ Teach good hand-washing techniques after direct contact with affected extremity. ▪ Discuss skin preparation.	▪ Assess skin integrity.	▪ Same as Day 1
PATIENT TEACHING	▪ Explain operative procedure and need for rehabilitation. ▪ Explain types of prostheses available if appropriate. ▪ Give instruction for arteriovenous (AV) foot pump for unaffected leg.	▪ Teach use of overhead trapeze. ▪ Teach adduction and extension exercises ▪ Reinforce physical therapy muscle strengthening program for UE and LE. ▪ Teach proper elevation of stump and HOB. ▪ Teach active range-of-motion (ROM) exercises to unaffected leg. ▪ Teach medication usage.	▪ Reinforce previous teaching. ▪ Teach alternative methods of pain relief (imagery, relaxation, transcutaneous electrical nerve stimulation).
DISCHARGE PLANNING	*Physical therapy (PT)/Occupational therapy (OT) consult:* ▪ Evaluate upper and lower extremity (UE and LE) function. ▪ Evaluate for prosthesis. *Nutrition consult:* ▪ Discuss diet for diabetes, hyperlipidemia, or hypercholesterolemia if present.	*Social services consult:* *PT and OT consult:* ▪ Discuss need for skilled nursing facility, rehabilitation, home care, or nursing home. *Orthotic technician consult:* ▪ Discuss cast and prosthesis management (during operating room or later depending on healing).	*Social services consult:* ▪ Assess for home care needs, support systems, and economic status.

Day 3	Days 4 to 6	Day 7
• Assess BM. • Assess urine output.	• Same as previous day	• Same as previous day
• Use sterile technique when changing stump dressing.	• Same as previous day	• Same as previous day
• Teach dressing change procedure. • Reinforce transfer and walker activities per physical therapy. • Teach stump strengthening and conditioning (push against pillow and increase to firmer surface as tolerated).	• Teach stump wrap with compression bandage. • Reinforce walker ambulation and gait training per physical therapy. • Teach stump strengthening and conditioning (push against pillow and increase to firmer surface as tolerated).	• Same as previous day
Social Services consult: • Arrange for amputee support group member to visit while inpatient. • Make final arrangements for placement.	*PT consult:* • Discuss home care needs. • Assess patient's and family's understanding of home care and follow-up care. • Assess understanding of when to notify health care provider.	• Arrange for follow-up care visit with doctor.

(continued)

PLAN OF CARE	HOME CARE Visit 1	Visit 2	Visit 3
DIAGNOSTIC TESTS	• Serum electrolytes, complete blood count, prothrombin time and International Normalized Ratio, activated partial thromboplastin time	• As indicated	• As indicated
MEDICATIONS	• Assess analgesics, antispasmodics, need for stool softener. • Monitor insulin if diabetic.	• Same as first visit	• Same as first visit
PROCEDURES	• Check vital signs and perform physical assessment. • Assess stump incision site, patient's ability to perform incision care, safety needs in home environment, pain management, presence of contractures. • Assist with and reiterate postoperative conditioning exercises: sit-ups, trunk flexion, hopping in place. • Massage stump toward suture line as ordered. • Reapply compression wrap on postsurgical cast. • Assist with prosthesis management.	• Same as first visit	• Same as first visit
DIET	• Assess nutritional intake. • Encourage high-protein foods.	• Same as first visit	• Same as first visit
ACTIVITY	• Assess client performance of walker and crutch ambulation, muscle strengthening exercises and transfer techniques.	• Same as first visit	• Same as first visit
ELIMINATION	• Assess urine output and bowel movements (BMs).	• Assess urine output and BM.	• Assess urine output and BM.
HYGIENE	• Assess cleanliness of stump and wrap. • Teach patient and family hand-washing techniques.	• Assess cleanliness of stump and wrap and patient's ability to perform stump care.	• Assess cleanliness of stump and wrap.
PATIENT TEACHING	• Assess patient's comprehension of in-hospital teaching and ability to learn. • Teach environmental safety, nonpharmacologic pain relief measures, incision care, use of mirror to view all aspects of stump, application of compression ace bandage wraps, signs and symptoms to report to doctor. • Instruct to follow in-home physical therapy exercise program. • Reinforce correct use of walkers and crutches. • Instruct patient to wear low-heeled comfortable shoes. • Reinforce prosthesis application.	• Reinforce previous teaching. • Observe patient and family performing incision care, compression bandage wrap, muscle strengthening exercises, walker ambulation, and prosthetic application.	• Reinforce previous teaching.
DISCHARGE PLANNING	• Assess need for crutches, walker. • Consult social services, physical therapist, or psychological counselor if needed. • Assess access to phone communication with durable medical equipment company. • Assess availability of transportation for needed appointments. • Promote expression by patient and family about impact of surgery.	• Explain importance of follow-up care. • Assist with arrangements for follow-up visits. • Promote expression by patient and family about impact of surgery. • Consult psychological counselor if needed.	• Reinforce previous visits. • Promote expression by patient and family about impact of surgery. • Consult psychological counselor if needed.

- Apply air splint to stump to control edema.
- Perform strengthening exercises necessary for ambulation—hip flexion, abduction, adduction, and extension.
- Limit sitting with limb flexed to 30 minutes at a time.
- Perform residual limb-conditioning exercises to harden the residual limb (push limb against a soft pillow, then gradually push limb against harder surfaces).
- Massage limb as directed by physical therapist to soften scar, decrease tenderness, and improve vascularity.
- Cover limb with plastic material to protect incision in presence of incontinence.
- Wash healed residual limb with mild soap and water.
- Keep bedclothes off limb, and protect stump from injury.
- Inspect residual limb daily for potential and actual skin breakdown.
- Wrap limb at all times.
- Rewrap limb at least two to three times per day and as needed.
- Avoid soaking residual limb—soaking causes edema.

Signs and symptoms
- Temperature >101° F (38° C)
- Inflammation of incision
- Warmth and redness at the incision
- Unusual pain or tenderness at the incision
- Prolonged phantom limb pain, increasing edema of stump

Activity
- Perform strengthening exercises necessary for ambulation: hip flexion, abduction, adduction, and extension.
- Encourage prone position twice daily to stretch the flexor muscles and prevent flexion contracture of the hip (keep legs together in prone position to prevent abduction deformity).
- Engage in conditioning and balancing exercises, such as trunk flexion, sit-ups, hopping in place, and hopping with walker to maintain mobility.
- Perform range-of-motion exercises to affected leg four times daily.
- Gradually increase ambulation with assistive device.
- Practice quadriceps setting exercises, gluteal contraction exercises, and leg lift of affected extremity unless contraindicated.
- Practice ambulation with crutches or walker.
- Avoid long periods of chair sitting to prevent venous stasis.
- Encourage use of good walking shoes and maintain stump in normal position (relaxed and downward when ambulating with assistive device).

Safety
- Wear rubber-soled shoe.
- Use handrails with stairs and grab bars at tub and toilet.
- Use adequate lighting for safe movement.
- Keep flashlights near bed and chair.
- Remove throw rugs and unbacked carpets.
- Remove clutter from passageways and steps.
- Use easily accessible tables to store frequently used items.
- Use nonskid strips in tub.
- Bathe and shower only when someone is present to assist if needed.
- Raise height of chair and bed for easy transfer on and off each.

Phantom limb pain

- Explain phantom limb pain theory.
- Instruct patient in use of transcutaneous electrical nerve stimulation unit.
- Encourage increase in activity.
- Change position frequently.
- Engage in diversional activities.
- Teach and assist with alternative pain relief measures.
- Adhere to analgesic therapy as directed by doctor.

Coping

- Encourage and allow time for expression of feelings of loss and grief.
- Praise positive coping behaviors.
- Provide encouragement and praise for strengths observed.
- Encourage independence and self-care as much as possible.
- Encourage self-care of stump.
- Promote communication with family and significant others.
- Encourage socialization with another amputee.

Critical thinking activities

1. Describe the therapeutic measures most effective in treating phantom limb pain.
2. Discuss the nursing interventions that help a patient cope with the loss of a body part.
3. Describe the most reliable indicators for appropriate prosthesis fitting.
4. Identify nursing interventions and complications that would be different in the patient with an immediate prosthetic fitting.
5. Develop a teaching plan addressing the care of a prosthetic device.
6. Develop a plan of care addressing the complications of hemorrhage and infection postamputation.
7. Identify nursing interventions indicated for different prosthetic fitting techniques.
8. Identify nursing interventions related to stump care.
9. Develop a teaching plan addressing positioning and wrapping of the stump.

Suggested research topics

- Coping strategies for losing a body part
- Compliance with therapy
- Effectiveness of strategies for dealing with phantom limb pain

Total hip replacement

DRG: 211 Mean LOS: 5.6 days

Arthroplasty is the surgical reconstruction or replacement of a joint. It restores motion to the joint and function to the muscles, ligaments, and other soft tissue controlling the joint. Replacement arthroplasty is available for elbows, shoulders, knees, hips, ankles, feet, and the phalangeal joints of the fingers. Total hip replacement, which substitutes an artificial joint for a severely damaged one, is commonly used to treat patients with osteoarthritis, rheumatoid arthritis, and hip fractures. The procedure provides excellent pain relief and improved function. Inactive, older individuals usually receive implants that are "cemented" in place with polymethylmethacrylate, which bonds to bones. An active, young individual, however, usually gets a "cementless" version that facilitates biologic ingrowth of new bone tissue into the porous surface coating of the prosthesis.

A new surgical technique uses infrared sensors and a three-dimensional computerized image system to guide the surgeon. The system enables accurate positioning of the acetabular cup and takes into account patient-specific anatomy and range of motion, thereby improving the patient's chance for a speedy and complete recovery.

Subjective assessment findings

Health history
Recurring fractures, osteoarthritis, rheumatoid arthritis, failure of previous reconstructive surgery, congenital hip disease, joint instability, unremitting pain

Medication history
Use of analgesics and relief achieved

Functional health patterns
Health perception–health management: circumstances surrounding injury
Activity-exercise: loss of motion of affected part, muscle spasms
Cognitive-perceptual: pain in affected area, numbness, tingling, loss of sensation distal to joint

Objective assessment findings

Physical findings
Cardiovascular: reduced or absent pulse distal to affected joint, edema, hematoma
General: apprehension, guarding of affected joint, bleeding
Integumentary: skin lacerations, color changes, ecchymosis
Musculoskeletal: restricted function or loss of function of affected part, muscle weakness, shortening of leg, crepitation, local deformities
Neurologic: decreased sensation, paresthesia

Diagnostic tests
Complete blood count, electrocardiogram, serum electrolytes, arterial blood gases, prothrombin time/International Normalized Ratio, activated partial thromboplastin time, joint X-rays, bone scan, tomogram, computed tomography or magnetic resonance imaging scans

(Text continues on page 159.)

Total hip replacement

CLINICAL PATHWAY

PLAN OF CARE	PREADMIT PHASE	INPATIENT CARE Day 1	Day 2
DIAGNOSTIC TESTS	• White blood cell (WBC) count • Complete blood count • Arterial blood gases (ABGs) • Serum electrolytes (lytes) • Urinalysis (UA) • Prothrombin time and International Normalized Ratio (PT/INR) • Activated partial thromboplastin time (APTT) • Electrocardiogram • Joint X-rays • Bone scans	• PT/INR • APTT • Hematocrit (Hct) • Hemoglobin (Hgb) • ABGs • Lytes • Pulse oximetry q 4 hr. • Anterior and posterior (A & P) of hip	• PT/INR • APTT • Hct • Hgb • ABGs • Lytes • Pulse oximetry q 8 hr
MEDICATIONS	• I.V. antibiotics before operation • Analgesics	• I.V. fluids: rate based on intake and output, including oral intake • Analgesics (epidural or patient-controlled analgesia) • I.V. antibiotics • Stool softener • Antipyretics as needed • Aspirin (ASA), warfarin (Coumadin), enoxaparin, or heparin in evening of surgery if ordered	• Same as previous day • Laxative if no bowel movement (BM) in 3 days
PROCEDURES	• Take baseline vital signs (VS). • Initiate I.V. • Provide antiembolism (TED) stockings. • Teach turning, coughing, and deep breathing (TCDB) exercises. • Teach incentive spirometry (IS).	• Check VS q 15 minutes for 4 hours; q 30 minutes for 4 hours, q hour for 4 hours, q 4 hours for 24 hours, and as needed. • Give oxygen (O_2) as indicated to maintain arterial oxygen saturation (SaO_2) > 94%. • IS q hour for 10 hours. • Neurovascular assessment • Assess dressing, wound drain. • Assess calves for tenderness, redness, edema, heat, and pain q 4 hr. • Assess catheter or catheterize if unable to void. • Remove and replace TED stockings every shift; apply SCD • Apply abductor braces.	• Check VS q 4 hr. • Same as previous day
DIET	• Give nothing by mouth (NPO).	• NPO to clear liquids as tolerated	• Advance to diet as tolerated. • Encourage high-fiber, high-protein, high-vitamin C foods. • Encourage fluid intake of at least 2 to 3 qt (2 to 3 L)/day unless contraindicated.
ACTIVITY	• Encourage bed rest (BR).	• Provide overhead frame or trapeze on bed. • Have patient perform TCDB q 2 hr. • Use abductor pillow when supine and turning. • Assess pain level before and after turning. • Assess safety needs and maintain safety precautions. • Encourage BR. • Coordinate activity with physical therapy.	• Repeat Day 1 activities. • Have patient perform muscle strengthening exercises (gluteal and quadriceps sets, leg lifts, and plantar flexion) q 2 hr. • Have patient pivot to chair with 2 assists (2 people or 1 person and a stable object for patient to lean on) on affected side t.i.d. if tolerated.

Day 3	Day 4	Day 5	Day 6
• PT/INR • APTT • Hct • Hgb • WBC • Lytes • Pulse oximetry every day	• PT/INR • APTT	• PT/INR • APTT • Hct • Hgb	• PT/INR • APTT
• Saline or heparin lock I.V. if needed • P.O. analgesics • D/C antibiotics • Stool softener • ASA, Coumadin, enoxaparin, or heparin therapy if ordered	• D/C I.V. • Analgesics • Stool softener • ASA, Coumadin, enoxaparin, or heparin therapy if ordered	• Same as previous day	• Same as previous day
• Check VS q 4 hr. • IS every 2 hours. • Remove hemovac if drainage less than 30 ml during shift. • Change dressing and assess wound healing (doctor to perform first dressing change). • Abductor orthosis	• Check VS b.i.d. • Change dressing every day and as needed.	• Check VS b.i.d. • Assess wound healing. • Remove and replace every shift.	• Check VS every day. • Assess wound.
• Same as previous day	• Same as previous day	• Same as previous day	• Same as previous day
• Repeat Day 2 activities. • Have patient walk 10′ (3 m) with walker three or four times a day as tolerated. *Physical therapy consult:* • Discuss weight bearing and assistive devices.	• Repeat Day 2 activities. • Have patient walk 20′ to 30′ (6 to 9 m) q.i.d.	• Same as previous day	• Same as previous day

(continued)

PLAN OF CARE	PREADMIT PHASE	INPATIENT CARE	
		Day 1	Day 2
ELIMINATION	• Assess urine output. • Insert catheter if ordered.	• Measure intake and output (I & O). • Assess hemovac drainage.	• Measure I & O. • Assess hemovac drainage. • Discontinue (D/C) urinary catheter. • Assess BM.
HYGIENE	• Give preoperative skin preparation as ordered	• Give catheter care if ordered. • Give complete care. • Apply lotion to legs between TED stocking changes.	• Give partial care. • Apply lotion to legs between TED stocking changes.
PATIENT TEACHING	• Assess ability to learn. • Review postoperative care and need for early mobilization. • Review need for external device (I.V., hemovac, sequential compression device [SCD]) • Teach IS and TCDB. • Review pain management. • Teach safety precautions. • Teach use of abductor pillow when supine and turning.	• Review plan for early mobilization. • Teach TCDB. • Teach IS. • Inform about Hemovac, I.V. line, SCD, catheter, and pain management.	• Review need for early progressive exercise. • Reinforce hip precautions and safety measures for transfer, ambulation, and turning in bed.
DISCHARGE PLANNING	*Physical therapy (PT) consult:* • Assess need for home care, skilled nursing facility, or rehabilitation.	• Assess abilities to perform activities of daily living. *Social services consult:* • Assess knowledge of home care support groups. *Occupational therapy (OT) consult:* • Assess if needed.	• Same as Day 1

Day 3	Day 4	Day 5	Day 6
▪ Same as previous day	▪ Same as previous day	▪ Measure I & O. ▪ Assess BM.	▪ Assess BM.
▪ Give partial care. ▪ Apply lotion to legs between TED stocking changes. ▪ Leave incision open to air if no drainage. ▪ Keep wound site clean and dry	▪ Same as previous day	▪ Keep wound site clean and dry. ▪ Have patient perform self-care with assistance. ▪ Apply lotion to legs between TED stocking changes.	▪ Keep wound site clean and dry. ▪ Have patient perform self-care.
▪ Discuss importance of wound care, and demonstrate procedure. ▪ Evaluate previous teaching.	▪ Same as previous day	▪ Continue discharge teaching about wound care, diet, and activity. ▪ Review safety precautions for transfer and ambulation for home care. ▪ Allow patient to engage in wound care and evaluation. ▪ Evaluate understanding of teaching.	▪ Repeat Day 5 activities. ▪ Teach signs and symptoms of wound infection to report to doctor. ▪ Teach about medication (name, purpose, dose, frequency, route, dietary restrictions, and adverse effects. ▪ Discuss importance of follow-up care.
▪ Same as Day 1	*Social services consult:* ▪ Assess support and resource needs (for example, economic status to purchase equipment, medication, and supplies).	*Social services:* ▪ Complete referrals to home health, PT, and OT. ▪ Arrange for home health to visit while inpatient.	▪ Assess patient's and family's knowledge of home health, PT, and OT. ▪ Arrange for follow-up visit with doctor.

(continued)

PLAN OF CARE	HOME CARE Visit 1	Visit 2	Visit 3
DIAGNOSTIC TESTS	• Prothrombin time (PT)	• Complete blood count • PT	• PT
MEDICATIONS	• Assess use of analgesics for pain relief. • Assess compliance with therapeutic regimen.	• Same as first visit	• Same as first visit
PROCEDURES	• Check vital signs and perform physical assessment. • Assess incision site. • Perform incision care. • Assess safety needs in home environment.	• Same as first visit	• Same as first visit
DIET	• Assess food and fluid intake.	• Same as first visit	• Same as first visit
ACTIVITY	• Assess mobility status. • Assess patient walking at least 70′ (21 m) with assistive device. • Assess patient's performance of muscle strengthening exercises. • Assess transfer and ambulation techniques.	• Same as first visit	• Same as first visit
ELIMINATION	• Assess elimination patterns and need for laxatives.	• Same as first visit	• Same as first visit
HYGIENE	• Assess abilities to perform activities of daily living. • Make referral and arrange for home health aide.	• Same as first visit	• Assess progress toward goals; wean from home care visits.
PATIENT TEACHING	• Assess ability to learn and assess comprehension of previous in-hospital teaching. • Teach appropriate transfer and ambulation safety precautions. • Teach incisional care. • Teach importance of progressive ambulation. • Instruct to follow in-home physical therapy instruction and to increase exercise activities. • Teach position restrictions. • Teach signs and symptoms to report to doctor. • Teach home safety measures. • Teach nonpharmacologic pain relief measures.	• Reinforce previous teaching. • Observe patient and family performing incision care. • Observe patient using safety measures in transfer and ambulation. • Observe patient and family compliance to home safety measures.	• Reinforce previous teaching. • Assess understanding and compliance.
DISCHARGE PLANNING	• Consult physical therapist if needed. • Assess access to phone communication with durable medical equipment company. • Assess availability of appropriate assistive devices. • Consult social services if needed.	• Explain importance of follow-up care. • Assist with arrangements for follow-up visits: home health nurse has daily visits for 2 days, then one more visit during first week, two visits in second week, and then once a week for remainder until goals met.	• Assess patient's and family's understanding of importance of follow-up care.

Related nursing diagnoses

1 Risk for injury
2 Risk for infection
3 Impaired physical mobility
4 Altered peripheral tissue perfusion
5 Pain
6 Risk for impaired skin integrity
7 Activity intolerance
8 Ineffective management of therapeutic regimen (community, family, individual)

Expected outcomes

The following expected outcomes pertain to the patient or family. Numbers in parentheses refer to related nursing diagnoses above.

- Be independent in transfer, and verbalize safety measures (1,3).
- Comply with home safety measures (1,8).
- Exhibit no signs and symptoms (S/S) of infection and have stable vital signs (2).
- Have clean, dry wound with healing by first evaluation (2,4,6).
- Verbalize understanding of incision care (2,8).
- Perform safe incision care (2,8).
- Perform activities of daily living to patient's maximum level (3).
- Walk with assistive devices and gradually increase walking distance to 70′ (21 m) as directed by physical therapist (3,7,8).
- Perform muscle strengthening exercises (gluteal and quadriceps sets, leg lifts, and plantar flexion) daily (3,7,8).
- Be free of redness, edema, and pain in affected calf (4,6).
- Manage pain (5).
- Verbalize and demonstrate home care instructions (7,8).
- Void and defecate as before admission (8).
- Seek physical therapy consult as needed (8).
- Verbalize understanding of complications, S/S of infection, and when to call health care provider (1,2,8).

Other possible nursing diagnoses

Constipation, self-care deficit (bathing/hygiene, feeding, dressing/grooming, toileting)

Potential complications

Fat embolism, thrombophlebitis, pulmonary embolism, hemorrhage

Patient teaching

Preventing complications

- Wear antiembolism (TED) stockings until full activities are resumed.
- Avoid excessive hip adduction, flexion, and rotation.
- Avoid sitting on a low chair or toilet seat; get raised toilet seat.
- Keep knees apart; *do not* cross legs.
- Limit sitting to 30 minutes at a time.
- Do not turn affected leg inward.
- Do not bend affected hip more than a 90-degree angle (normal sitting position).
- Lie prone twice daily for 30 minutes.
- Check for calf edema, tenderness, local pain.

- Take prophylactic antibiotic if undergoing any procedure known to cause bacteremia (tooth extraction, manipulation of genitourinary tract).

Signs and symptoms
- Temperature above 101° F (38° C)
- Increased drainage from incision or change in drainage color; foul odor from drainage
- Warmth and redness at the incision site
- Unusual pain or tenderness at the incision site

Activity
- Perform quadriceps setting and range-of-motion exercises as directed.
- Do not participate in any activity placing undue or sudden stress on joint (jogging, jumping, lifting heavy loads, excessive bending and twisting); avoid becoming obese to prevent stress on joint.
- Use a stationary bicycle daily if possible with doctor's order.

Safety
- Use self-help and energy-saving devices (long-handled shoehorn, reacher, stocking donner, and so forth).
- Use handrails by toilet.
- Use bar-type stool for shower and kitchen work.
- Remove throw rugs.
- Remove clutter from passageways and steps.
- Use easily accessible tables to store frequently used items.
- Install railings on steps inside and outside home.
- Bathe and shower only when someone is present to assist if needed.
- Allow others to assist with household chores.
- Wear proper-fitting shoes with nonslip soles.
- When dressing, start with affected side first (the side of the operation).

Critical thinking activities
1. Discuss whether there are fewer implant complications among patients who had established exercise behaviors before hip replacement.
2. Discuss whether gender is a factor in success rates of hip replacements.
3. List the most common psychological ramifications of hip replacement.
4. Describe weight-bearing activities that can help rehabilitate the patient who has had a hip replacement.
5. Explain the purpose of TED stockings and list complications associated with TED stockings therapy.
6. Explain the rationale for using an abductor pillow when positioning a patient supine and when turning post hip replacement.
7. Describe the stages of wound healing.
8. Explain why 2 to 3 qt (2 to 3 L)/day of fluids is usually recommended after hip replacement.
9. List subjective and objective data that are essential for a safety needs assessment in relation to hip replacement.
10. Develop a teaching plan addressing wound care, activity and safety precautions for transfer, and ambulation for home care.

Suggested research topics
- Coping strategies for hip replacement
- Compliance with therapy
- Effectiveness of exercise and strength-building programs

Total knee replacement

DRG: 209 Mean LOS: 5.9 days

Arthroplasty is the surgical reconstruction or replacement of a joint. It restores motion to the joint and function to the muscles, ligaments, and other soft tissue controlling the joint. During total knee replacement, a part or all of the knee joint may be replaced with a metal and plastic device. The procedure is performed to relieve unremitting pain and joint instability from severe destructive deterioration caused by debilitating arthritis or traumatic degenerative bone disease.

During the procedure damaged tissues (bone, synovium, and cartilage) are removed and replaced by a metal implant. The prosthesis may be porous and coated with a material that allows bone to grow into the joint area, or it may be attached with an acrylic cement.

Subjective assessment findings

Health history
Osteoarthritis, rheumatoid arthritis, failure of previous reconstructive surgery, joint instability, unremitting pain, infection, trauma, obesity

Medication history
Short- or long-term use of analgesics and corticosteroids

Functional health patterns
Health perception–health management: circumstances surrounding injury
Activity-exercise: loss of motion of affected part, muscle spasms, decreased abilities to perform activities of daily living (ADLs)
Cognitive-perceptual: pain in affected area, numbness, tingling, loss of sensation distal to joint

Objective assessment findings

Physical findings
Cardiovascular: edema, hematoma
General: apprehension, guarding of affected joint, bleeding
Integumentary: skin lacerations, color changes, ecchymosis
Musculoskeletal: restricted function or loss of function of affected part, muscle weakness, shortening of leg, crepitation, local deformities, impaired gait
Neurologic: decreased sensation, paresthesia

Diagnostic tests
Complete blood count, electrocardiogram, serum electrolytes, arterial blood gases, prothrombin time and International Normalized Ratio, activated partial thromboplastin time, joint X-rays, bone scan, tomogram, computed tomography or magnetic resonance imaging scans, chest X-ray

Related nursing diagnoses
1 Risk for injury
2 Risk for infection

(Text continues on page 167.)

Total knee replacement — CLINICAL PATHWAY

PLAN OF CARE	PREADMIT PHASE	INPATIENT CARE Day 1	Day 2
DIAGNOSTIC TESTS	• Complete blood count • Blood gases • Serum electrolytes (lytes) • Prothrombin time (PT) and International Normalized Ratio (INR) • Joint X-rays • Bone scans • Electrocardiogram	• PT • Hematocrit (Hct) • Hemoglobin (Hgb) • Arterial blood gases (ABGs) • Lytes • Pulse oximetry q 4 hr • Anterior and posterior (A and P) X-ray of knee	• PT/INR • Activated partial thromboplastin time (APTT) • Hct • Hgb • Lytes • Pulse oximetry q 8 hr
MEDICATIONS	• Analgesics (patient-controlled analgesia [PCA], epidural, or I.M.) • I.V. antibiotics before operation	• Analgesics (PCA , epidural, or I.M.) • Stool softener • Antipyretics as needed • Acetylsalicylic acid (Aspirin [ASA]), warfarin (Coumadin), or enoxaparin if ordered • I.V. fluids.	• Analgesics by mouth (P.O.) • Laxative if no bowel movement (BM) in 3 days • Antipyretics as needed • ASA, Coumadin, or enoxaparin therapy if ordered • I.V. fluids; convert to intermittent device if P.O. fluids tolerated
PROCEDURES	• Check baseline vital signs (VS). • Access I.V. • Perform incentive spirometry (IS). • Perform turning, coughing, and deep breathing (TCDB) exercises. • Apply antiembolism (TED) stockings.	• Check VS q 15 minutes for 4 hours; q 30 minutes for 4 hours, q hour for 4 hours, q 4 hours for 24 hours, and as needed. • Maintain oxygen (O_2) as indicated to maintain oxygen saturation (O_2 sat) > 94%. • Encourage IS q 2 hr. • Do neurovascular assessment q 2 hr. • Assess dressing and Hemovac. • Assess calves for tenderness, redness, edema, heat, and pain q 4 hr. • Remove and replace TED stockings every shift. • Apply sequential compression device (SCD) or AV foot pump. • Perform catheter care. • Apply ice packs to affected knee.	• Check VS q 4 hr. • Maintain O_2 as indicated to O_2 sat > 94%. • Encourage IS q 2 hr. • Perform neurovascular, Hemovac, and dressing assessment q 4 hr and as needed. • Assess calves for tenderness, redness, edema, heat, and pain every shift. • Remove and replace TED stockings, SCD, or AV foot pump while in bed. • Provide catheter care.
DIET	• Give nothing by mouth (NPO).	• Give NPO to clear liquids as tolerated.	• Advance to full diet as tolerated (DAT). • Encourage fluid intake of at least 2 to 3 qt (2 to 3 L)/day unless contraindicated.
ACTIVITY	• Provide overhead frame or trapeze on bed.	• Encourage bed rest for 12 hours. • Have patient perform TCDB q 2 hr. • Assess pain level before and after movement. Encourage patient to put weight on the affected leg as tolerated. • Assess safety needs and maintain safety precautions. • Have patient pivot to chair with assistance. • Have patient perform frequent range of motion exercises with ankle and all toe joints. • Have patient perform muscle strengthening exercises: quadriceps sets, gluteal sets, plantar flexion, and leg lifts q 4 hr • Provide PT: Trapeze to bed, partial weight bearing, knee immobilizer (if ordered).	• Have patient perform muscle strengthening exercises (gluteal and quadriceps sets, leg lifts, and plantar flexion q 4 hr while awake) • Have patient pivot to chair with two assists, two to three times • Provide CPM if ordered. • Have patient practice partial weight bearing in room.

Day 3	Day 4	Day 5	Day 6
• PT/INR • APTT • Hct • Hgb • White blood cell count • Lytes • Pulse oximetry every day	• PT/INR • APTT	• PT/INR • APTT • Hct • Hgb	• PT/INR • APTT
• Analgesics • Stool softener • ASA, Coumadin or enoxaparin if ordered • Intermittent I.V. device if needed	• Analgesics • Stool softener • ASA, Coumadin or enoxaparin if ordered • D/C I.V. device.	• Analgesics • Stool softener • Coumadin or enoxaparin therapy if ordered • Laxative if no BM in 3 days	• Analgesics • Stool softener • Coumadin or enoxaparin if ordered
• Repeat Day 2 procedures. • Remove Hemovac as ordered if drainage less than 30 ml per shift. • Change dressing and assess wound healing (doctor to change first dressing; RN to change subsequent dressings).	• Check VS b.i.d. • Assess wound healing. • Assess calves for tenderness, redness, edema, heat, pain every shift. • Remove and replace TED stockings every shift. • Apply SCD or AV foot pump while in bed. • Change dressing every day and as needed.	• Check VS every shift. • Assess wound healing • Remove and replace TED stockings every shift. • Change dressing every day and as needed.	• Check VS every shift. • Assess wound healing. • Change dressing every day. • Remove dressing.
• Give DAT. • Encourage foods high in fiber, protein, vitamin C, iron, and protein.	• Same as previous day	• Same as previous day	• Same as previous day
• Repeat Day 2 activities. *PT consult:* • Discuss gait training with assistive device.	• Have patient walk 20' to 30' (6 to 9 m) q.i.d. *PT consult:* • Review weight bearing and assistive devices. • Provide CPM if ordered. • Continue progressive gait training. • Have patient continue muscle strengthening exercises.	• Have patient continue muscle strengthening exercises. • Continue progressive gait training. • Have patient walk 30' to 50' (9 to 15 m) q.i.d. *PT consult:* • Review weight bearing, assistive devices, and stair training. • Continue CPM if ordered.	• Have patient continue muscle strengthening exercises. • Have patient walk 50' to 70' (15 to 21 m) q.i.d. *PT consult:* • Review weight bearing, assistive devices, and stair training.

(continued)

PLAN OF CARE	PREADMIT PHASE	INPATIENT CARE Day 1	Day 2
ELIMINATION	• Assess urine output. • Provide catheter if ordered.	• Measure intake and output (I & O). • Assess hemovac drainage.	• Measure I & O. • Assess hemovac drainage. • Assess BM. • Discontinue (D/C) catheter (if present); if no void in 8 hours, provide straight catheter as needed.
HYGIENE	• Perform preoperative skin preparation as ordered.	• Assess dressing site for dryness. • Provide complete care. • Apply lotion to legs as part of TED stockings changes.	• Assess dressing site for dryness. • Have patient perform self-care with assistance. • Apply lotion to legs as part of TEDS changes.
PATIENT TEACHING	• Review postoperative care and need for early mobilization. • Review need for external devices (I.V., Hemovac) • Teach IS and TCDB. • Review pain management: epidural or PCA pump. • Teach continuous passive motion (CPM) machine if ordered and arteriovenous (AV) foot pump. • Review safety precautions.	• Review plan for early mobilization. • Teach about TCDB. • Teach IS. • Inform about Hemovac, I.V., catheter, and pain management. • Teach muscle strengthening exercises and signs and symptoms (S/S) of deep vein thrombosis.	• Review need for early progressive exercise. • Reinforce knee precautions and safety measures for transfer, ambulation, and turning in bed. • Evaluate understanding of teaching. • Discuss physical therapy for gait training and assistive devices.
DISCHARGE PLANNING	• Assess need for home care (need for home health, skilled nursing facility, or rehabilitation). • Consult physical therapy (PT) and occupational therapy (OT).	• Assess abilities to perform activities of daily living. *Social services consult:* • Provide information about home care support groups. *PT consult:* • Discuss collaborative care. *OT consult:* • Determine if needed for collaborative care.	*Social services:* *PT:* *OT:* • Assess needs.

Day 3	Day 4	Day 5	Day 6
• Measure I & O. • Assess hemovac drainage.	• Measure I & O.	• Measure I & O. • Assess BM.	• Assess urine output. • Assess BM.
• Keep wound site clean and dry • Have patient perform self-care with assistance. • Apply lotion to legs between TED stockings changes.	• Keep wound site clean and dry. • Have patient take a shower. • Apply lotion to legs between TED stockings changes.	• Keep wound site clean and dry. • Have patient perform self-care with assistance. • Apply lotion to legs as part of TED stockings changes.	• Keep wound site clean and dry. • Have patient perform self-care.
• Discuss importance of wound care and demonstrate procedure for changing dressing if needed. • Repeat Day 2 activities.	• Repeat Day 3 teaching.	• Continue teaching about wound care, diet, and activity. • Review safety precautions for transfer and ambulation for home care. • Teach safe use of immobilizer (if ordered), elastic bandage rewrap procedure, and ice pack application to knee for pain, swelling, or stiffness. • Allow patient to engage in wound care and evaluation. • Evaluate understanding of teaching.	• Repeat Day 5 activities. • Teach S/S of wound infection to report to doctor. • Teach about medications: name, purpose, dose, frequency, route, dietary restrictions, and adverse effects. • Discuss importance of follow-up care.
Social services: *PT:* *OT:* • Assess needs.	*Social services:* • Assess support and resource needs (for example, economic status to purchase equipment, medication, and supplies).	*Social services:* • Complete referrals to home health, PT, and OT. • Arrange for home health to visit while inpatient.	• Assess patient's and family's knowledge about home health, PT, and OT. • Arrange for follow-up visit with doctor.

(continued)

PLAN OF CARE	HOME CARE Visit 1	Visit 2	Visit 3
DIAGNOSTIC TESTS	• Prothrombin time and International Normalized Ratio (PT and INR)	• PT and INR • Complete blood count	• PT and INR
MEDICATIONS	• Assess use of analgesics for pain relief. • Assess compliance with therapeutic regimen.	• Same as first visit	• Same as first visit
PROCEDURES	• Check vital signs and physical assessment. • Assess incision site for drainage, and condition of surrounding tissue. • Assess incision care. • Assess safety needs in home environment. • Assess affected leg for color, motion, and sensation.	• Same as first visit	• Same as first visit
DIET	• Assess food and fluid intake.	• Same as first visit	• Same as first visit
ACTIVITY	• Assess mobility status. • Assess patient walking at least 70' (21 m) with assistive device. • Assess patient's performance of muscle strengthening exercises. • Assess transfer and ambulation techniques.	• Same as first visit	• Same as first visit
ELIMINATION	• Assess elimination patterns and need for laxatives.	• Same as first visit	• Same as first visit
HYGIENE	• Assess ability to perform activities of daily living.	• Same as first visit	• Same as first visit
PATIENT TEACHING	• Evaluate comprehension of previous teaching. • Teach appropriate transfer and ambulation safety precautions. • Teach incision care. • Teach importance of progressive ambulation. • Instruct to follow in-home physical therapy. • Instruct to increase exercise activities. • Teach safe immobilizer application (if ordered). • Teach elastic bandage rewraps. • Teach safe use of ice packs to knee every 20 to 30 minutes for swelling, pain, or stiffness. • Teach signs and symptoms (S/S) to report to doctor. • Teach home safety measures. • Teach nonpharmacologic pain relief measures and medication instruction. • Teach S/S of deep vein thrombosis.	• Reinforce previous teaching. • Observe patient and family performing incision care. • Observe patient using safety measures in transfer and ambulation. • Observe patient and family compliance with home safety measures. • Observe patient and family performing application of immobilizer (if ordered), elastic bandage rewrap, and ice pack. • Reevaluate safety in home.	• Reinforce previous teaching.
DISCHARGE PLANNING	• Consult physical therapy if needed. • Assess access to phone communication with durable medical equipment company. • Assess availability of appropriate assistive devices. • Consult social services if needed.	• Explain importance of follow-up care. • Assist with arrangements for follow-up visits.	• Assess patient's and family's understanding of importance of follow-up care.

3 Impaired physical mobility
4 Altered peripheral tissue perfusion
5 Pain
6 Risk for impaired skin integrity
7 Activity intolerance
8 Ineffective management of therapeutic regimen (community, family, or individual)

Expected outcomes

The following expected outcomes pertain to the patient or family. Numbers in parentheses refer to related nursing diagnoses above.

- Comply with home safety measures (1,3,8).
- Use immobilizers (if ordered), ice packs, and elastic bandages safely (1,3,8).
- Exhibit no signs or symptoms (S/S) of infection (2,8).
- Have a clean, dry wound with healing by first evaluation (2,4,6).
- Drink six to eight glasses of fluid a day (2).
- Be independent in transfer (3,7).
- Walk with assistive devices and increase walking distance gradually to at least 70′ (21 m) four times daily as directed by physical therapy (PT) (3,7,8).
- Perform muscle strengthening exercises (gluteal and quadriceps sets, leg lifts, and plantar flexion) daily (3,8).
- Be free of redness, edema, and pain in affected calf (2,4,6).
- Manage pain (5).
- Perform activities of daily living to patient's maximum level (3,7).
- Perform safe incision care (2,8).
- Void and defecate as before admission (8).
- Verbalize or demonstrate home care instructions (7,8).
- Seek PT consult as needed (8).
- Verbalize S/S of infection and deep vein thrombosis and when to notify health care provider (1,2,8).

Other possible nursing diagnoses

Constipation, self-care deficit (bathing/hygiene, feeding, dressing/grooming, toileting)

Potential complications

Fat embolism, thrombophlebitis, pulmonary embolism, hemorrhage, disarticulation of prosthesis, pneumonia, neurovascular damage in the extremity, osteomyelitis

Patient teaching

Preventing complications

- Wear antiembolism stockings until full activities are resumed.
- Avoid sitting on a low chair or toilet seat; use a raised toilet seat.
- Limit sitting to 30 minutes at a time.
- Check for calf edema, tenderness, and local pain.
- Use knee immobilizer as directed.
- Apply elastic bandage wrap to knee as directed.
- Take prophylactic antibiotic if undergoing any procedure known to cause bacteremia (tooth extraction, manipulation of genitourinary tract).

Signs and symptoms
- Temperature >101° F (38° C)
- Increased drainage from incision or change in drainage color
- Warmth and redness at the incision site
- Unusual pain or tenderness at the incision site

Activity
- Perform quadriceps sets, gluteal sets, plantar flexion, straight leg lifts, and progressive range-of-motion exercises daily.
- Do not participate in any activity placing undue or sudden stress on joint (jogging, jumping, lifting heavy loads, excessive bending and twisting); avoid becoming to prevent stress on joint.
- Use a stationary bicycle daily if possible.

Safety
- Use self-help and energy-saving devices.
- Use handrails by toilet.
- Use bar-type stool for shower and kitchen work.
- Remove throw rugs.
- Remove clutter from passageways and steps.
- Use easily accessible tables to store frequently used items.
- Install railings on steps inside and outside home.
- Bathe and shower only when someone is present to assist if needed.
- Allow others to assist with household chores.
- When dressing, start with the side that was operated on.

Exercise
- Perform exercises as specified by doctor or PT.
- Follow instructions as to how long to hold any movement.
- Follow instructions as to how many times a day to do the exercise.
- Follow instructions as to how many times to repeat the exercise at each session.
- Follow instructions as to how long to rest between sessions.

Critical thinking activities
1. Compare the differences in success rates of total knee replacements to those of total hip replacements among the elderly population.
2. Determine whether more men than women require total knee replacement. Discuss the reasons for any difference.
3. Identify nursing measures that help the patient comply with a daily exercise program.
4. Develop a teaching plan addressing the purpose and procedure of arthroscopy.
5. Identify nursing interventions associated with a sequential compression device or arteriovenous foot pump.
6. List the effects of heparin therapy and complications related to it.
7. Develop a teaching plan addressing muscle strengthening exercises such as quadriceps sets, gluteal sets, planter flexion, and leg lifts.
8. Identify safety measures for transfer, ambulation, and turning in bed.
9. Describe a progressive gait training program.
10. Explain why a diet high in vitamin C and iron is recommended after knee replacement.

Suggested research topics
- Coping strategies for having a knee replaced
- Compliance with therapy
- Success rates for knee replacement surgery

PART 8

Neurologic problems

Cerebrovascular accident

Lumbar laminectomy

Parkinson's disease

Cerebrovascular accident

DRG: 014 Mean LOS: 5.5 days

A cerebrovascular accident (CVA), also known as a stroke or brain attack, is the onset of neurologic dysfunction resulting from disruption of the blood supply to the brain. CVAs are classified according to pathophysiology: thrombotic (blood clot within a blood vessel of the brain or carotids producing stenosis), embolic (cerebral embolism), or hemorrhagic (rupture of a cerebral vessel with bleeding or pressure into the brain).

Symptoms of CVAs depend on the location and size of the lesion and will vary in intensity. In its mildest form, a CVA is so minimal it may go almost unnoticed. In its most severe state, hemiplegia, coma, and death result.

CVAs are the third leading cause of death in the United States. The highest incidence of CVA is among individuals older than age 65. They also occur in a 3 to 10 ratio in individuals younger than age 65, tend to run in families, and are more frequent in women. The incidence is greater in blacks than whites, possibly because of the greater incidence of hypertension in blacks.

Subjective assessment findings

Health history
Hypertension, previous stroke, transient ischemic attacks, aneurysm, cardiac disease, arrhythmias (particularly atrial fibrillation), heart failure, valvular disease, infective endocarditis, alcohol abuse, smoking, hyperlipidemia, diabetes, gout, past myocardial infarction, carotid endarterectomy

Medication history
Use of oral contraceptives, use of and compliance with antihypertensive and anticoagulant agents

Functional health patterns
Health perception–health management: positive family history, easy fatigability
Nutritional-metabolic: anorexia, nausea, vomiting, dysphagia, disturbances in taste and smell
Elimination: change in bladder and bowel patterns
Cognitive-perceptual: loss of memory; alteration in speech, language, problem solving; pain; headache; visual disturbances

Objective assessment findings

Physical findings
Cardiovascular: hypertension, tachycardia, carotid bruit
Gastrointestinal: loss of gag reflex, bowel incontinence, decreased or absent bowel sounds, dysphagia
General: emotional lability, lethargy, apathy or combativeness, fever
Neurologic: contralateral motor and sensory deficits, including weakness, paresis, paralysis, anesthesia, unequal pupils, unequal hand grasps, akinesia, aphasia (expressive, receptive, global), agnosias, apraxia, visual deficits, perceptual or spatial disturbances, altered level of consciousness (drowsiness to deep coma), positive Babinski sign, decreased followed by increased deep tendon reflexes, flaccidity followed by spasticity, amnesia, ataxia, personality change, nuchal rigidity, seizures

Respiratory: loss of cough reflex, labored or irregular respirations, tachypnea, rhonchi, airway occlusion, apnea
bowel sounds, dysphagia
Urinary: incontinence or retention

Diagnostic tests

Computed tomography scan, magnetic resonance imaging, brain scan, positron emission tomography scan, B-mode ultrasound, skull X-ray, electrocardiogram, electroencephalogram, echoencephalography, Doppler ultrasonography, cerebral angiography, lumbar puncture

Related nursing diagnoses

1 Impaired physical mobility
2 Risk for injury
3 Impaired verbal communication
4 Self-care deficit (bathing/hygiene, feeding, dressing/grooming, or toileting)
5 Sensory/perceptual alteration (visual, auditory, kinesthetic, gustatory, tactile, or olfactory)
6 Altered urinary elimination
7 Constipation
8 Altered nutrition: less than body requirements
9 Impaired swallowing
10 Ineffective breathing pattern
11 Self-esteem disturbance
12 Ineffective management of therapeutic regimen (community, family, or individual)

Expected outcomes

The following expected outcomes pertain to the patient or family. Numbers in parentheses refer to related nursing diagnoses above.
- Exhibit a stable neurologic exam (1,2,5,9,10).
- Remain free of injury (1,2).
- Acquire increasing independence in self-care (1,4).
- Obtain optimum mobility (exercises extremities, remains free of contractures, attains sitting balance, transfers to wheelchair, ambulates with assistive devices or with reciprocal pattern) (1,4,12).
- List signs and symptoms (S/S) to report to doctor (2,12).
- State risk factors for stroke (2,12).
- Demonstrate home safety measures (2,12).
- Adapt home environment for accessibility (2,12).
- Effectively communicate needs to others (3,5).
- Compensate for sensory deficits (achieves increasing ability in self-care, feeds self, remembers to look at feet occasionally) (3,4,5).
- Attain or maintain bladder and bowel control and elimination (6,7).
- Tolerate diet without difficulty swallowing (8,9).
- Have stable vital signs, neurovital signs, and oxygen saturation (10).
- Demonstrate patent airway (10).
- Exhibit clear breath sounds to auscultation and remain free of respiratory distress (10).
- Verbalize feelings related to impact of CVA (11).
- Recognize need for resource or support groups (11,12).
- Demonstrate coping strategies with changes in lifestyle (11,12).
- Demonstrate a realistic perception of deficits (12).
- Verbalize or demonstrate home care interventions or need to transfer to rehabilitation or long-term care facility (12).

(Text continues on page 177.)

PLAN OF CARE	PREADMIT PHASE	INPATIENT CARE Day 1	Day 2
DIAGNOSTIC TESTS	• Complete blood count (CBC) • Prothrombin time (PT)/ International Normalized Ratio (INR) • Activated partial thromboplastin time (APTT) • Computed tomography (CT) scan of head • Magnetic resonance imaging • Electroencephalogram • Electrocardiogram (ECG) • Consider angioplasty	• CBC • PT/INR • APTT • Serum chemistries • Arterial blood gases (ABGs) • Lipid profile • Pulse oximetry q 4 hr and as needed • Urinalysis • Chest X-ray • CT scan of head (if neurologic examination shows worsening of condition) • Echocardiography and carotid Doppler • ECG	• CBC • PT/INR • APTT • Serum albumin • Pulse oximetry q 8 hr and as needed • Serum albumin • Cerebral arteriogram
MEDICATIONS	• Antihypertensives: angiotensin-converting enzyme (ACE) inhibitors, beta blockers, calcium channel blockers • Anticoagulants: heparin or enoxaparin • Diuretics: furosemide (Lasix, bumetanide (Bumex), mannitol • Antiplatelets: aspirin, clopidogrel • Antilipidemia agents • Consider thrombolytic: alteplase, tissue plasminogen activator (tPA)	• Antihypertensives: ACE inhibitors, beta blockers, calcium channel blockers • Anticoagulants: heparin or enoxaparin • Diuretics: Lasix, Bumex, mannitol • Analgesics • Anticonvulsants: clonazepam, phenytoin • Stool softeners • I.V. 0.9% sodium chloride or 0.45% sodium chloride solution at 80 ml/hr or I.V. intermittent device	• Same as Day 1
PROCEDURES	• Establish I.V. • Obtain baseline physical and neurologic assessment.	• Check vital signs (VS) q 4 hr and as needed. • Give oxygen (O_2) therapy to maintain O_2 saturation (O_2 sat) at > 95%. • Check neurovital signs and mental status every 1 to 2 hours until stable, then every 2 to 4 hours and as needed. • Assess for presence of visual field deficit, cognitive and language deficit, cranial nerve deficit, changes in level of consciousness (LOC), aspiration, and paralytic ileus. • Assess for changes in heart sounds and rhythm. • Assess for bleeding and for signs of increasing intracranial pressure (ICP). *Neurology consult:* • Apply antiembolism (TED) stockings. • Take seizure precautions. • Protect patient from injury. • Suction as needed and maintain airway; tracheostomy if needed. • Develop communication system.	• Check VS q 4 hr and as needed. • Give O_2 therapy to maintain O_2 sat > 95%. • Check neurovital signs and mental status q 4 hr and as needed. • Assess swallowing and gag reflex. • Assess for presence of visual field deficit, cognitive and language deficit, cranial nerve deficit, changes in LOC, aspiration, and paralytic ileus. • Assess for changes in heart sounds and rhythm. • Assess for bleeding and for signs of increasing ICP. • Apply TED stockings. • Take seizure precautions. • Protect patient from injury. • Suction as needed. • Maintain airway.

CLINICAL PATHWAY ■ Cerebrovascular accident

Day 3	Day 4	Day 5
- CBC - PT/INR - APTT - Serum albumin - Pulse oximetry q 12 hr and as needed	- CBC - PT/INR - APTT - Serum albumin - Pulse oximetry	- Same as previous day
- Antihypertensives - Anticoagulants: heparin or enoxaparin; start warfarin (Coumadin) - Diuretics - Analgesics - Anticonvulsants - Stool softeners - Saline or heparin lock I.V.	- Same as previous day	- Same as previous day
- Check VS q 4 hr and as needed. - Discontinue (D/C) O_2 therapy if O_2 sat > 95% on room air. - Check neurovital signs and mental status q 4 hr and as needed. - Assess systems every shift. - Apply TED stockings. - Take seizure precautions. - Protect patient from injury. - Suction as needed. - Maintain airway.	- Same as previous day	- Check VS q 4 hr. - Assess neurovascular and respiratory status every shift. - Apply TED stockings. - Prevent injury and falls.

(continued)

PLAN OF CARE	PREADMIT PHASE	INPATIENT CARE Day 1	Day 2
DIET	• Obtain baseline nutritional and hydration needs.	• Give nothing by mouth (NPO). • Request nutrition consult. • Request speech therapy and dysphagia consult.	• Thicken liquids if swallowing reflex is intact. • Assist with medications. • Keep head elevated and tilt head slightly forward when eating. • Teach patient to eat small, frequent meals, and supplement feedings if indicated. • Teach patient to avoid foods that may cause choking (mashed potatoes, large pieces of meat, soft breads). • Assess need for total parenteral nutrition and enteral feeds for patients who are NPO.
ACTIVITY	• Assess abilities to perform activities of daily living (ADLs).	• Encourage bed rest with head of bed elevated > 30 degrees. • Turn and position q 2 hr. *Physical therapy consult: Occupational therapy consult:* • Assess rehabilitation needs. • Use splints and orthotics to prevent footdrop and contractures. • Have patient perform range-of-motion (ROM) exercises to extremities. • Assess safety needs and provide appropriate measures.	• Have patient get up in chair b.i.d. if tolerated. • Turn and position patient q 2 hr. • Have patient perform ROM to extremities. • Have patient begin walking. • Assess safety needs and provide appropriate measures. • Praise activities and tasks accomplished.
ELIMINATION	• Take baseline assessment of urine and bowel patterns of elimination. • Insert indwelling urinary catheter if needed.	• Measure intake and output (I & O). • Assess bowel elimination and urinary voidings. • Assess bowel sounds. • Observe for presence of constipation and paralytic ileus.	• Measure I & O. • Assess bowel elimination and urinary voiding. • Assess bowel sounds. • Observe for presence of constipation and paralytic ileus.
HYGIENE	• Take baseline integumentary assessment.	• Keep skin clean and dry. • Protect skin from breakdown. • Give complete care. • Provide oral hygiene q.i.d.	• Keep skin clear and dry. • Protect skin from breakdown. • Encourage as much self-care as possible. • Provide or assist with oral hygiene before and after meals and at bedtime.
PATIENT TEACHING	• Teach need for in-patient treatment.	• Orient patient to environment. • Prepare for diagnostic tests. • Give brief, simple instructions related to care. • Include family in care as appropriate.	• Reorient patient to environment. • Educate about diagnosis. • Begin teaching related to ADL training. • Evaluate understanding of teaching. • Instruct in use of assistive devices for communication, eating, and walking. • Teach transfer technique.
DISCHARGE PLANNING	*Social services consult: Ophthalmology consult:* • Assess visual changes. *Psychiatric consult:* • Assess if needed	*Social services:* • Assess need for home care (placement, economic status, support systems, skilled nursing unit). • Refer to support groups.	*Social services:* • Identify placement for discharge.

Day 3	Day 4	Day 5
• Advance diet as tolerated (DAT). • Assist with meals. • Keep head elevated and tilt head slightly forward when eating.	• Advance DAT. • Assist with meals. • Keep head elevated and tilt head slightly forward when eating. *GI consult:* • Consider percutaneous endoscopic gastrostomy (PEG) tube if necessary.	• Give DAT. • Assist with meals as needed.
• Have patient get up in chair b.i.d. if tolerated. • Have patient begin walking. • Turn and position patient q 2 hr. • Have patient perform ROM to extremities. • Assess safety needs and provide appropriate measures. • Praise activities and tasks accomplished.	• Have patient get up in chair t.i.d. • Have patient walk with physical therapist b.i.d. • Turn and position patient q 2 hr. • Have patient perform ROM to extremities. • Assess safety needs and provide appropriate measures. • Praise activities and tasks accomplished.	• Have patient get up in chair t.i.d. and as needed. • Have patient walk with physical therapist t.i.d. • Turn and position patient q 2 hr. • Have patient perform ROM to extremities. • Assess safety needs and provide appropriate measures.
• Measure I & O. • Assess bowel elimination and urinary voiding. • Assess bowel sounds. • Observe for presence of constipation and paralytic ileus. • Begin bladder training.	• Measure I & O. • Assess bowel elimination and urinary voiding. • Assess bowel sounds. • Observe for presence of constipation and paralytic ileus. • D/C indwelling urinary catheter. • Continue bladder training.	• Assess bowel and urine elimination. • Continue bladder training.
• Same as previous day	• Same as previous day	• Encourage as much self-care as possible.
• Repeat previous teaching. • Teach lifestyle modification (diet, exercise, smoking cessation • Teach importance of blood pressure monitoring.	• Repeat previous teaching. • Teach about medications: name, route, dosage, time, action, adverse effects. • Explain safety precautions related to anticoagulant therapy. • Teach PEG site care and feedings if applicable.	• Reinforce previous teaching. • Give specific verbal and written discharge instructions. • Teach importance of follow-up care.
• Begin referrals to rehabilitation or long-term care, or ensure that home has assistive devices. *Physical therapy consult:* • Teach use of home assistive devices to patient and family. • Evaluate patient's and family's knowledge related to resource support needs.	• Same as previous day • Begin arrangements for follow-up visits with doctor.	• Finalize plans for home care.

(continued)

PLAN OF CARE	HOME CARE Visit 1	Visit 2	Visit 3
DIAGNOSTIC TESTS	▪ Oxygen saturation ▪ Prothrombin time (PT)	▪ PT	▪ PT
MEDICATIONS	▪ Assess compliance with drug therapy. ▪ Assess effectiveness of drugs. ▪ Assess for adverse effects of drugs.	▪ Same as first visit	▪ Same as first visit
PROCEDURES	▪ Check vital signs and perform neurologic assessment. ▪ Assess lung and heart sounds. ▪ Assess for signs and symptoms (S/S) of cerebrovascular accident (CVA): bleeding, headache, edema, increased or new blurred vision, weakness, immobility, slurred speech. ▪ Assess for S/S of seizure activity.	▪ Same as first visit	▪ Same as first visit
DIET	▪ Assess nutritional and fluid intake. ▪ Teach patient to eat small, frequent, and supplemental feedings if indicated. ▪ Teach patient to avoid foods that may cause choking (mashed potatoes, large pieces of meat, soft breads).	▪ Same as previous visit	▪ Same as previous visit
ACTIVITY	▪ Assess mobility and ability to perform activities of daily living. ▪ Assess safe and appropriate use of assistive devices. ▪ Consult physical therapist if needed. ▪ Encourage patient to plan rest periods daily. ▪ Encourage range-of-motion (ROM) exercises to extremities and regular daily exercise.	▪ Same as first visit ▪ Assess compliance to rest periods.	▪ Same as first visit
ELIMINATION	▪ Assess urinary and bowel elimination. ▪ Reinforce bladder training program.	▪ Same as first visit	▪ Same as first visit
HYGIENE	▪ Assess skin integrity. ▪ Assess oral cavity. ▪ Encourage frequent oral hygiene.	▪ Same as first visit	▪ Same as first visit
PATIENT TEACHING	▪ Teach S/S of CVA. ▪ Teach S/S to report to doctor. ▪ Teach safety precautions related to anticoagulant therapy. ▪ Teach patient and family ways of adapting the home for accessibility. ▪ Reinforce physical therapy training related to use of wheelchair, crutches, or walker. ▪ Teach family and caregiver proper body mechanics and how to protect their back when assisting patient. ▪ Teach safety measures to prevent falls. ▪ Encourage speech exercises daily. ▪ Teach family to engage in communication with patient as much as possible. ▪ Teach family, if needed, to develop competency in the following: home ventilation, suctioning, positioning techniques, parenteral or enteral home nutrition, tracheostomy care.	▪ Reinforce previous teaching. ▪ Teach definitions and S/S of CVA. ▪ Teach risk factors (high blood pressure, blood clot in neck vessels or brain, high cholesterol, atherosclerosis, excessive stress in presence of these listed risk factors, tobacco use in presence of these listed risk factors). ▪ Teach importance of follow-up care. ▪ Teach need to consult occupational therapy, physical therapy, speech therapy (ST), social services, and psychological counseling as needed. ▪ Evaluate understanding of teaching.	▪ Reinforce previous teaching. ▪ Evaluate understanding of teaching.

PLAN OF CARE	HOME CARE Visit 1	Visit 2	Visit 3
DISCHARGE PLANNING	• Assess availability of pertinent phone numbers (pharmacy, durable medical equipment, occupational therapy, physical therapy, ST, social services). • Assess resource and support needs. • Consult psychological counselor if needed. • Discuss importance of follow-up care. • Assess need for modifications in the home environment, and refer to social services if needed.	• Assess resource and support needs. • Evaluate patient and family understanding of follow-up care. • Evaluate patient and family seeking appropriate support groups. • Assess resource and support needs. • Consult psychological counselor if needed. • Discuss importance of follow up care. • Assess need for modifications in the home environment, and refer to social services if needed.	• Same as previous visit. • Plan for more visits if necessary. • Encourage continued visits from occupational therapy, physical therapy, ST, social services, and psychological counselor if needed.

Other possible nursing diagnoses

Ineffective airway clearance

Potential complications

Seizures, increased intracranial pressure

Patient teaching

Optimal functioning capacity

- Explain disease, its causes, symptoms, and various treatment methods.
- Explain importance of daily exercise within functional abilities (stretching, range-of-motion, and breathing and speech exercises, and ambulating with assistive device).
- Explain importance of maintaining constancy of the environment without too many distractions.
- Explain importance of ongoing outpatient care.
- Discuss adhering to medication therapy as directed by doctor.
- Explain the need for family members to avoid doing things for the patient that he can do for himself.

- Discuss using assistive devices to help perform activities of daily living and transfer activities (bed to chair, chair to toilet, and so forth); modify and adapt devices to encourage independence.
- Teach the importance of taking planned rest periods daily.
- Comply with physical, occupational, and speech therapy programs and seek assistance as needed.
- Teach patient and family members to seek community resource and support services.
- Teach bladder training program if necessary.
- Reinforce speech therapy communication program by encouraging communication measures and use of adaptive communication devices.

Medications
- Discuss name, purpose, dosage, schedule, route of administration, and adverse effects.
- Explain safety precautions related to anticoagulant therapy (do not use a straight razor, check for bright red or black stools, avoid foods high in vitamin K, take right amount of medication at same time every day, notify doctor about any S/S of bleeding, hold direct pressure for extended period if bleeding occurs).
- Caution to prevent falls.

Nutrition
- Drink at least 2 to 3 qt (2 to 3 L)/day unless contraindicated.
- Encourage frequent, small feedings if indicated.
- Instruct patient to swallow slowly and take small bites of food.
- Use blender for thick foods if patient has difficulty with swallowing; use a thickening agent for thin liquids.
- Teach patient to turn head to compensate for visual field deficits while feeding self.
- Use adaptive dinnerware and utensils for self-feeding.
- Avoid foods high in vitamin K.
- Avoid foods such as soft breads, mashed potatoes, semicooked vegetables, and large pieces of meat that may cause choking if patient has difficulty with swallowing.

Safety
- Wear rubber-soled shoes.
- Use handrails by the toilet and tub or shower, and put safety rails on bed.
- Remove throw rugs and unbacked carpets.
- Remove clutter from passageways and steps.
- Use nonskid strips in tub.
- Bathe and shower only when someone is present to assist if needed.
- Use assistance as needed to go up and down stairs.
- Use an elevated toilet seat.

Coping
- Encourage and allow time for expression of feelings about impact of disease.
- Praise positive coping behaviors.
- Provide encouragement and praise for strengths observed.
- Encourage independence and self-care as much as possible.
- Set realistic goals and make the best of what remains.
- Promote communication with family and significant others.
- Encourage socialization.
- Discuss need for family to show security, love, and need for patient.
- Discuss need for family to have patience with and understanding of patient's disabilities.
- Explain to family to expect some emotional lability and some degree of brain damage in severe CVA (episodes of inappropriate laughing, crying, and temper outbursts).
- During emotional periods as described above, instruct family to change the subject or ask patient to perform some motor activity, and reassure the patient that this will gradually subside.

Signs and symptoms
- New or increased weakness
- New or increased slurred speech
- New or increased immobility
- Severe headaches
- Unpleasant adverse effects from medications (for example, bleeding from warfarin use)
- Edema of feet and ankles

Critical thinking activities
1. Discuss the quality of life for persons with functional disabilities after CVA.
2. Identify and describe effective strategies to improve patient compliance with medication therapy.
3. Design an educational program for effectively reducing stress for caregivers of CVA patients.
4. Discuss the effectiveness of a supportive educational nursing intervention in helping the patient make decisions regarding self-care goals.
5. Detail the cost-effectiveness of preventive testing or teaching of high-risk individuals as a means of reducing the occurrence or severity of a CVA.
6. Describe which patients have benefited most from angioplasty procedures.
7. Develop a teaching plan that addresses teaching family members who are assuming the care of the patient at home.
8. Identify additional problems and demands on caregivers that occur when an elderly patient suffers from strokes.
9. Describe the goals of rehabilitative management of the stroke patient.
10. Identify community resources that can provide respite for caregivers.

Suggested research activities
- Coping strategies for CVA
- Compliance with therapy
- Effectiveness of preventive testing programs
- Effectiveness of angioplasty procedures

Lumbar laminectomy

DRG: 214 Mean LOS 4.9 days

Often performed to treat a herniated disk or spinal stenosis, laminectomy is the removal of the lamina (arch of bone covering the spinal cord) to expose the neural elements in the spinal canal. The process allows for inspection of the canal as well as identification and removal of pathology and compression from the cord and roots. The goal of lumbar laminectomy is to relieve pressure on nerve roots and eliminate or relieve pain or weakness, that is caused by a progressive neurologic deficit (muscle weakness and atrophy, loss of sensory and motor function, loss of sphincter control).

A common cause of low back pain is herniation of the nucleus pulposus in the lumbar region, an area of the back that is vulnerable to injury because it is flexible, contains numerous nerve roots, carries most of the body's weight, and has poor biomechanics. Factors associated with lumbar injury and pain include jobs that require repetitive heavy lifting, vibration (jackhammer operator), and extended periods of driving.

Other causes of low back pain include spinal cord compression from a fracture, dislocation, stenosis, hematoma, abscess, or spinal nerve surgery.

Low back pain affects millions of Americans yearly. It is the single most common cause of lost working hours and represents one of the most costly health problems in our country today.

Subjective assessment findings

Health history
Acute or chronic lumbosacral strain, osteoarthritis, degenerative disk disease, obesity, occupational risk factors, previous back surgeries, epidural injections

Medication history
Use of analgesics, muscle relaxants, nonsteroidal anti-inflammatory drugs, corticosteroids, and over-the-counter remedies

Functional health patterns
Activity-exercise: muscle spasms, poor posture, activity restrictions, missed work days
Cognitive-perceptual: pain in back, buttocks, or leg associated with walking, straining, turning, coughing, and leg raising; numbness or tingling of legs, feet, or toes

Objective assessment findings

Physical findings
General: guarding
Musculoskeletal: tense, tight paravertebral muscles on palpation; decreased range of motion of spine
Neurologic: depressed or absent Achilles tendon reflex

Diagnostic tests
Myelogram, computed tomography scan, electromyography, magnetic resonance imaging, hematocrit, hemoglobin, lumbar spine X-rays, complete blood count with differential, electrolytes,

blood type and screen, prothrombin time, International Normalized Ratio, activated partial thromboplastin time, urinalysis

Related nursing diagnoses

1 Impaired physical mobility
2 Risk for infection
3 Pain
4 Body image disturbance
5 Ineffective management of therapeutic regimen (community, family, or individual)
6 Ineffective individual coping
7 Constipation
8 Risk for injury

Expected outcomes

The following expected outcomes pertain to the patient or family. Numbers in parentheses refer to related nursing diagnoses above.

- Be fully ambulatory (1).
- Comply with activity restrictions (1).
- Ambulate independently daily, increasing distance (1,5).
- Have intact neurovascular status in lower extremities (1,3,4,8).
- Be afebrile (2).
- Have clean, dry wound, healing by first evaluation (2).
- Perform wound care safely (2,8).
- Manage pain (3).
- Tolerate usual diet (5,7).
- Express concerns and feelings related to stressors of surgery and condition (5,6).
- List signs and symptoms to report to doctor (2,5).
- Perform neurovascular status monitoring daily (5).
- Perform muscle strengthening exercises daily (5).
- Seek appropriate support groups (5,6).
- Engage in self-care (5,6).
- Have established urine and bowel elimination patterns as before surgery (7).

Other possible nursing diagnoses

Altered role performance

Potential complications

Paralysis, unrelieved acute pain, altered bowel or bladder function

Patient teaching

Preventing recurrence

- Establish a regular period of walking, increasing the distance as tolerated.
- Reduce or restrict activities that precipitate or aggravate discomfort.
- Avoid repetitive heavy lifting and activities that produce flexion strain on the spine (stair climbing, extended automobile riding or driving, bending, sudden twisting of the back).
- Allow scheduled rest periods.
- Wear a proper fitting low back brace or corset.
- Keep follow-up appointments with doctor as directed.

(Text continues on page 187.)

CLINICAL PATHWAY	PLAN OF CARE	PREADMIT PHASE	INPATIENT CARE Day 1	Day 2
Lumbar laminectomy	DIAGNOSTIC TESTS	• Complete blood count (CBC) • Serum electrolytes (lytes) • Prothrombin time/International Normalized Ratio • Activated partial thromboplastin time • Type and screen • Urinalysis • Chest X-ray • Myelogram • Computed tomography scan • Magnetic resonance imaging • Electrocardiogram	• Hemoglobin • Hematocrit • Pulse oximetry	• Pulse oximetry
	MEDICATIONS	• Take medication history • Discontinue (D/C) aspirin (ASA) and nonsteroidal anti-inflammatory drugs 24 hours before surgery, and warfarin (Coumadin) 5 to 7 days before surgery.	• Analgesics as ordered (patient-controlled analgesia/I.M.) • I.V. antibiotics • I.V. fluids if not tolerating fluids by mouth (P.O.) • Stool softener • Antiemetic for postoperative nausea and vomiting	• Analgesics as ordered (wean to P.O.) • I.V. antibiotics • Heparin or saline lock I.V. device • Stool softener • Laxative if no bowel movement (BM) in 3 days
	PROCEDURES	• Apply thigh-high antiembolism (TED) stockings or compression boots. • Take baseline vital signs (VS). • Discuss need for early ambulation.	• Check VS and perform neurovascular and wound assessment every 15 minutes for 4 hours, every 30 minutes for 4 hours, every hour for 4 hours, and then q 4 hr and as needed. • Assess neurologic, respiratory, urinary, musculoskeletal, and GI status q 4 to 8 hr. • Assess wound drainage q 2 to 4 hr. • Have patient perform IS q 2 hr. • Remove and replace TED stockings or compression boots every shift.	• Check VS and perform neurovascular and wound assessment q 4 hr and as needed. • Assess neurologic, respiratory, urinary, musculoskeletal, and GI status q 4 to 8 hr. • Assess wound drainage q 2 to 4 hr. • Incentive spirometry q 2 hr. • Remove and replace TED stockings or compression boots every shift. • Assess straight catheter q 8 hr and as needed. • Change dressing b.i.d.; first change by doctor, subsequent changes by RN. • Provide wound care.
	DIET	• Assess nutritional status.	• Keep nothing by mouth for 4 hours. • Progress to ice chips, then clear liquid, and advance as tolerated.	• Give diet as tolerated (DAT).
	ACTIVITY	• Assess limitations. • Assess ability to perform activities of daily living (ADLs).	• Encourage bed rest. • Have patient get out of bed to chair in afternoon with assistance. • Have patient stand to void. • Have patient turn, cough, and deep breathe (TCDB) q 2 hr and as needed (log roll). • Place "Log Roll Only" sign at bedside. • Have patient perform passive and active range of motion to all extremities three to four times daily.	• Have patient TCDB q 2 hr and as needed (log roll). • Have patient walk with assistance in room q.i.d. • Encourage participation in ADLs as tolerated.

Day 3	Day 4
▪ CBC ▪ Lytes if indicated	▪ Same as previous day
▪ Analgesics as ordered ▪ I.V. antibiotics ▪ Stool softener ▪ Laxative if no BM in 3 days	▪ Analgesics as ordered ▪ D/C I.V. ▪ Stool softener ▪ Laxative if no BM in 3 days
▪ Check vital signs q 4 hr and as needed. ▪ Assess neurologic, respiratory, urinary, musculoskeletal, and GI status every 4 to 8 hours. ▪ Assess wound drainage q 4 hr. ▪ Have patient use IS until fully ambulatory. ▪ Remove and replace TED stockings or compression boots every shift ▪ Remove Hemovac or Jackson-Pratt drain. ▪ Change dressing b.i.d. ▪ Provide wound care.	▪ Check VS q 4 hr. ▪ Assess neurologic, respiratory, urinary, musculoskeletal, and GI status every shift. ▪ Assess wound drainage q 4 hr. ▪ Have patient use IS until fully ambulatory. ▪ Remove and replace TED stockings or compression boots every shift. ▪ Change dressing b.i.d. ▪ Provide wound care.
▪ Give DAT.	▪ Give DAT.
▪ Have patient walk q.i.d. with assistance. ▪ Increase walking distance each time. ▪ Encourage participation in ADLs as tolerated.	▪ Have patient walk ad lib. ▪ Encourage participation in ADLs as tolerated.

(continued)

PLAN OF CARE	PREADMIT PHASE	INPATIENT CARE *Day 1*	*Day 2*
ELIMINATION	• Assess elimination patterns. • Explain need for catheter after surgery.	• Measure intake and output (I & O). • Initiate straight catheter q 8 hr and as needed.	• Measure I & O. • Continue straight catheter q 8 hr and as needed.
HYGIENE	• Prepare skin.	• Assist with ADLs as needed.	• Same as Day 1.
PATIENT TEACHING	• Review postoperative plan of care with patient and family. • Discuss pain management. • Teach good body alignment. • Teach incentive spirometry (IS). • Teach turning (log roll) and transfer bed to chair to stand. • Teach about tubes and drainage systems. • Include family in teaching.	• Teach transfer technique.	• Reinforce teaching. • Evaluate understanding of teaching. • Discuss importance of early walking. • Teach movement restrictions (no twist, flex, hyperextend, pull on rails). • Include family in training. • Teach muscle strengthening exercises.
DISCHARGE PLANNING	• Identify need for home care. *Social services consult:* • Discuss work restrictions and time off. • Consult physical therapy and rehabilitation if preexisting physical deficit.	*Social services consult:* • Assess home care, support groups, economic status, and work situation.	*Social services:* • Assess home support and resource needs. • Prescription for elevated toilet seat.

Day 3

- Measure I & O.

- Assist with ADLs as needed.
- May shower with waterproof dressing.

- Reinforce previous teaching.
- Teach signs and symptoms of infection, increased pain, neurovascular changes, and difficulty with walking to report to doctor.
- Teach pharmacologic drug therapy for pain management.
- Teach activity restriction (stair climbing, automobile, riding, bending, heavy lifting, sitting for prolonged periods of time, twisting of back).
- Teach muscle strengthening exercises.

- Refer to appropriate agency.

Day 4

- Measure I & O if indicated.

- Assist with ADLs as needed.

- Reinforce previous teaching.
- Discuss importance of follow-up care.
- Evaluate understanding of teaching.

- Assess patient's and family's knowledge of home health and support groups.

(continued)

PLAN OF CARE	HOME CARE		
	Visit 1	*Visit 2*	*Visit 3*
DIAGNOSTIC TESTS	▪ Hematocrit, hemoglobin if indicated	▪ Same as first visit	▪ Same as first visit
MEDICATIONS	▪ Assess compliance with drug regimen. ▪ Assess effectiveness of medications.	▪ Same as first visit	▪ Same as first visit
PROCEDURES	▪ Check vital signs (VS). ▪ Evaluate neurovascular status to lower extremities. ▪ Assess incision site. ▪ Teach nonpharmacologic pain therapy.	▪ Same as first visit	▪ Same as first visit
DIET	▪ Assess fluid and nutritional intake. ▪ Encourage fluid intake to 2 to 3 qt (2 to 3 L)/ day if tolerated.	▪ Same as first visit	▪ Same as first visit
ACTIVITY	▪ Assess ambulatory status. ▪ Assess compliance with activity restrictions. ▪ Assess participation in self-care.	▪ Same as first visit	▪ Same as first visit
ELIMINATION	▪ Assess urine output. ▪ Assess presence of constipation.	▪ Same as first visit	▪ Same as first visit
HYGIENE	▪ Assess cleanliness of wound. ▪ Teach hand-washing techniques.	▪ Same as first visit	▪ Same as first visit
PATIENT TEACHING	▪ Teach signs and symptoms (S/S) of infection. ▪ Teach S/S to report to doctor (temperature > 101° F (37.3° C), redness and increased drainage at wound, difficulty in walking, increased pain, neurovascular changes). ▪ Teach neurovascular status monitoring. ▪ Teach activity restrictions.	▪ Teach muscle strengthening exercises. ▪ Reinforce previous teaching. ▪ Observe patient and family performing incision care. ▪ Observe patient ambulating and performing muscle strengthening exercises and neurovascular status monitoring.	▪ Reinforce previous teaching. ▪ Evaluate understanding of teaching.
DISCHARGE PLANNING	▪ Assess level of anxiety. ▪ Refer to psychological counselor if needed. ▪ Consult physical therapy if needed. ▪ Discuss importance of follow-up care. ▪ Refer to appropriate agency for social services and resource needs.	▪ Assess home and support resource needs.	▪ Same as previous visit

- Engage in daily exercises that strengthen the abdominal muscles and the erector muscles of the spine, as directed by physical therapist or doctor.
- Maintain appropriate body weight.
- Sleep on firm mattress in a supine position with small 10″ (25.4 cm) pillow lifting knees or in a side-lying position with knees and hips flexed and pillow between knees; avoid prone position.
- Enroll in the program called "Back School" aimed at preventing back injury.
- Maintain proper posture and body alignment when standing, lying, or sitting.
- Use proper body mechanics when reaching, lifting, or bending.
- Use a lumbar roll or pillow when sitting.
- Sit in chairs with knees higher than hips and support arms on chair or knees.
- Avoid chilling during and after exercising.
- If you become tired or experience low back pain, go to bed immediately.

Signs and symptoms
- Pain that is different from pain before surgery
- Any increase in pain in the back or legs
- Any increase in swelling or redness around the incision
- Any cloudy or foul-smelling drainage from the incision
- Any new development of numbness, tingling, or decreased sensation of foot, leg, or toes
- Any increase in body temperature > 100°F (37.8° C).

Medications
- Instruct patient on dosage, time of administration, purpose, and adverse effects.
- Avoid over-the-counter remedies unless recommended by doctor.

Coping
- See appropriate resources to assist with pain relief.
- Comply with a daily walking and exercise program.

Nutrition
- Explain importance of maintaining a well-balanced diet.
- Explain importance of drinking 2 to 3 qt (2 to 3 L)/day.

Critical thinking activities
1. Identify and discuss strategies that assist postlaminectomy patients and families to express concerns about loss of work and wages.
2. Identify and discuss the most effective measures for ensuring compliance with daily postlaminectomy exercise regimens.
3. Discuss whether decreasing the physical demands of a job by altering the environment reduces back stress.
4. Define and discuss the best measures for helping patients manage chronic back pain.
5. List the differences between acute and chronic low back pain.
6. Explain the significance of abnormal neurologic signs postlaminectomy.
7. Develop a teaching plan including exercises that strengthen back muscles.

Suggested research topics
- Coping strategies for laminectomy and low back pain
- Compliance with therapy
- Effectiveness of exercise regimens

Parkinson's disease

DRG: 012 Mean LOS: 5.4 days

Parkinson's disease is a progressive, degenerative disease of the brain's dopamine neuronal system and is most commonly idiopathic in nature. The primary neurohumoral defect is deficiency of dopamine in the striatum of the basal ganglia, which affects the brain centers responsible for movement. The disease is characterized by bradykinesia (slowness of movement), tremor, and muscle stiffness or rigidity. Its onset is gradual and insidious, with slow progression and a prolonged course.

No specific diagnostic test confirms Parkinson's disease, and diagnosis is made solely on physical examination, history, and exclusion of other diseases. A firm diagnosis is made when two of the three characteristic signs (bradykinesia, tremor, and rigidity) are present. Ultimately, a confirming diagnosis is made when the individual exhibits a positive response to antiparkinsonian drugs.

Symptoms usually first appear in persons older than age 50, with age 65 being the average age of onset. Approximately 500,000 persons in the United States have Parkinson's disease. The disease shows no cultural, gender, or socioeconomic preferences but rarely occurs in African-Americans.

There is no known cure, although a surgical treatment, pallidotomy, which produces lesions in the globus pallidus (a part of the extrapyramidal brain nuclei) , has been demonstrated to slow the progression of symptoms in some patients who do not respond to drug therapy. Pallidotomy destroys the ventrolateral nucleus of the thalamus to prevent involuntary movement. Deterioration progresses for an average of 10 years, at which time death usually results from aspiration pneumonia or another infection.

Subjective assessment findings

Health history
Central nervous system trauma, cerebrovascular disorders, syphilis, exposure to metals and carbon monoxide, encephalitis

Medication history
Use of central nervous system drugs, especially haloperidol (Haldol) and phenothiazines; reserpine, methyldopa

Functional health patterns
Health perception–health management: fatigue
Nutritional-metabolic: excessive salivation, dysphagia, excessive sweating, weight loss
Elimination: constipation
Activity-exercise: difficulty in initiating movements, frequent falls, loss of dexterity, micrographia
Cognitive-perceptual: diffuse pain in legs, shoulders, neck, back, and hips; muscle soreness and cramping
Self-perception–self-concept: depression, mood swings

Objective assessment findings

Physical findings
General: blank (masked) face, slow and monotonous speech, infrequent blinking
Cardiovascular: postural hypotension
Gastrointestinal: drooling
Integumentary: seborrhea
Musculoskeletal: cogwheel rigidity, dysarthria, bradykinesia, contractures, stooped posture
Neurologic: tremor at rest, first in hands (pill-rolling) and later in legs, arms, face, and tongue; aggravation of tremor with anxiety and absence in sleep; shuffling gait; poor coordination; subtle dementia

Diagnostic tests
Complete blood count, cerebrospinal fluid analysis, computed tomography scan, electroencephalogram, skull X-rays, cineradiographic study of swallowing

Related nursing diagnoses
1 Impaired physical mobility
2 Self-care deficit (bathing/hygiene, feeding, dressing/grooming, or toileting)
3 Ineffective management of therapeutic regimen (community, family, or individual)
4 Impaired verbal communication
5 Impaired social interaction
6 Constipation
7 Altered nutrition: less than body requirements
8 Sleep pattern disturbance

Expected outcomes
The following expected outcomes pertain to the patient or family. Numbers in parentheses refer to related nursing diagnoses above.
- Ambulate safely at maximum functioning (1).
- Perform daily strengthening exercises (1,3).
- Have daily physical needs met (2).
- Engage in optimal self-care (2).
- Comply with medication therapy (3).
- Express understanding of disease process (3).
- Express feelings about impact of disease (3,5,8).
- Develop effective methods of communication (4,5).
- Engage in diversional activities (5).
- Maintain a regular bowel and urine elimination pattern (6,).
- Maintain satisfactory body weight (7).
- Verbalize feelings of being rested (8).

Other possible nursing diagnoses
Impaired skin integrity, altered role performance

Potential complications
Aspiration pneumonia

(Text continues on page 192.)

■ Parkinson's disease

CLINICAL PATHWAY

PLAN OF CARE	PREADMIT PHASE	INPATIENT CARE *Day 1*
DIAGNOSTIC TESTS	• Medical history and physical exam	• Blood urea nitrogen, white blood cell count, hematocrit, hemoglobin • Electroencephalogram, computed tomography scan, magnetic resonance imaging
MEDICATIONS	• Rule out adverse effects of phe-nothiazines, reserpine, benzodi-azepines, and haloperidol.	• Dopaminergic, anticholinergic, antihistamine, monoamine oxidase-B inhibitor • Stool softener • Assess for positive response to antiparkinsonian medications.
PROCEDURES	• *Physical therapy (PT) consult* • *Occupational therapy (OT) consult* • *Speech therapy (ST) consult* • *Neurosurgery consult if possible pallidotomy candidate*	• Take vital signs. • Assess lung sounds, risk of falling, ability to communicate verbally, difficulty in swallowing, functional disability related to self-care needs. • Institute safety measures.
DIET	• Take weight history. *Nutrition consult:* • Assess needs for a soft, high-bulk diet.	• Avoid foods that contain pyridoxine hydrochloride (vitamin B₆). • Give frequent small feedings if needed. • Use bibs and straws as indicated. • Maintain fluid intake to 2 to 3 qt (2 to 3 L)/day unless contraindicated. • Give supplemental high-calorie fluids (eggnog, milk shake).
ACTIVITY	• Assess ability to perform activities of daily living (ADLs).	• Assess level of disability. • Encourage ambulation to tolerance. • Have patient perform range-of-motion q 4 hr. • Assist with turning every 2 to 4 hours if unable to move self. *PT consult:* • Review gait retraining, massage, and muscle stretching exercises. • Maintain planned rest periods. *OT consult:* • Will be indicated by amount of tremors present. • Encourage diversional activities to decrease attention on symptoms (reading, TV, radio, hobbies, painting).
ELIMINATION	• Assess bladder control.	• Institute bladder control program as indicated. • Assess bowel elimination.
HYGIENE	• Assess abilities to perform ADLs.	• Provide or assist with general hygiene; encourage self-care. • Provide oral hygiene every 4 to 6 hours and as needed.
PATIENT TEACHING	• Teach need for medication therapy.	• Reinforce doctor's explanation of disease and its causes, signs and symptoms, and treatments. • Discuss importance of verbalization about loss of body function, self-esteem, and sexuality. • Explain need for psychologic support and socialization. • Explain to family the need to encourage self-care and independence. • Teach importance of daily exercise and ambulation to delay progression of disease. • Teach patient to perform any physical task that is difficult 5 to 10 times a day. • Teach pressure ulcer prevention. • Discuss importance of on-going follow-up care with doctor and PT. • Discuss medications: name, dosage, frequency, purpose, and adverse effects. • Teach patient to avoid over-the-counter drugs without doctor approval. • Teach home safety measures (clearing walkways and use of hand rails). • Evaluate understanding of teaching.
DISCHARGE PLANNING	• *Social services consult*	*Social services:* • Assess resources and support needs. • Refer to OT, PT, ST, or home care as indicated. • Discuss availability of resources, such as the American Parkinson's Disease Association.

Days 2 to 5	HOME CARE Visit 1	Visit 2	Visit 3
▪ As indicated	▪ Blood urea nitrogen ▪ Hematocrit ▪ Hemoglobin	▪ Same as first visit	▪ Same as first visit
▪ Same as Day 1	▪ Assess compliance with medication therapy. ▪ Monitor effectiveness of medications.	▪ Same as first visit	▪ Same as first visit
▪ Same as Day 1	▪ Check vital signs and lung sounds. ▪ Evaluate level of consciousness, orientation, neurologic status, home safety.	▪ Same as first visit	▪ Same as first visit
▪ Same as Day 1	▪ Assess nutritional and fluid intake. ▪ Weigh patient. ▪ Observe ability to swallow.	▪ Same as first visit	▪ Same as first visit
▪ Same as Day 1	▪ Monitor disabilities related to activities of daily living (ADLs). ▪ Assess compliance with physical therapy (PT), occupational therapy (OT), and speech therapy (ST) programs. ▪ Evaluate patient performance of stretching and range-of-motion (ROM) exercises and ambulation.	▪ Same as first visit	▪ Same as first visit
▪ Same as Day 1	▪ Assess urinary and bowel elimination patterns, and evaluate urinary control.	▪ Same as first visit	▪ Same as first visit
▪ Same as Day 1	▪ Evaluate degree of self-care. ▪ Encourage frequent oral hygiene.	▪ Same as first visit	▪ Same as first visit
▪ Reinforce previous teaching. ▪ Evaluate understanding of teaching.	▪ Teach medications: names, dosage, purpose, route, time, adverse effects. ▪ Teach definition and causes of Parkinson's disease. ▪ Discuss signs and symptoms (S/S) of Parkinson's disease (tremors, rigid movement, unstable posture) and progressive Parkinson's disease (expressionless face, drooling, infrequent blinking, rapid rolling movement of fingers, tremors at rest, soft and expressionless voice). ▪ Teach home safety. ▪ Evaluate understanding of instruction.	▪ Reinforce previous teaching. ▪ Instruct proper feeding. ▪ Reinforce PT, OT, and ST teaching about stretching, strengthening, ROM exercises; speech pattern exercises; daily routine skills and safety with ADLs; and proper use of adequate equipment. ▪ Evaluate understanding of teaching.	▪ Reinforce previous teaching. ▪ Evaluate understanding of teaching.
▪ Evaluate knowledge of home care visits and follow-up care.	▪ Assess accessibility to pertinent phone numbers for durable equipment, pharmacy, PT, OT, ST, and doctor. ▪ Assess resource and support needs. ▪ Refer to social services or psychological counselor if indicated. ▪ Discuss importance of follow-up care.	▪ Same as first visit	▪ Same as first visit

(continued)

Patient teaching

Optimal functioning
- Explain the disease, its causes, symptoms, and treatment.
- Explain that behavioral changes may be part of the disease process or caused by medications.
- Explain importance of daily exercise to delay progression of disease (stretching, range-of-motion, breathing, and facial muscle exercises; ambulating with long strides).
- Explain importance of performing any physical task that is difficult 5 to 10 times per day.
- Explain importance of ongoing outpatient care.
- Teach postural exercises and walking techniques to offset shuffling gait and tendency to lean forward (use a broad-based gait—keep feet wide apart, increase width of walking stride, swing arms when walking, raise the feet while walking, use a heel-toe, heel-toe gait).
- Instruct patient to take warm baths and massages to relax muscles and relieve painful muscle spasms that accompany rigidity.
- Use assistive devices to perform activities of daily living.
- Take planned rest periods daily.
- Seek help from physical therapy, occupational therapy, and speech therapy as needed.
- Seek resources and support from groups such as the American Parkinson's Disease Association.

Medications
- Instruct patient on name, purpose, dosage, route of administration, time, and adverse effects.
- Explain need to avoid taking over-the-counter medications without doctor approval.
- Avoid foods high in vitamin B_6 (reverses effects of levodopa).
- Limit high-protein foods, which may block effects of drugs.
- Periodically assess blood urea nitrogen, hematocrit, and white blood cell count because of levodopa treatment, which can cause hemolytic anemia, leukopenia, and agranulocytosis.

Nutrition
- Teach need for soft diet with progression to diet as tolerated.
- Drink fluid to at least 2 to 3 qt (2 to 3 L)/day unless contraindicated.
- Add supplemental high-calorie foods to daily diet (milk shakes, malts, eggnog).
- Encourage frequent, small feedings if indicated.
- Use bibs and straws for excessive drooling.
- Weigh patient daily.
- Instruct patient to swallow slowly and take small bites of food.
- Use blender for thick foods.
- Use braces for severe tremors occurring during meals.

Safety
- Wear rubber-soled shoes.
- Use handrails with stairs and grab bars at tub and toilet.
- Remove throw rugs and unbacked carpets.
- Remove clutter from passageways and steps.
- Use nonskid strips in tub.
- Bathe and shower only when someone is present to assist if needed.
- Remain within hearing distance within the home setting.

Coping
- Encourage and allow time for expression of feelings about impact of disease.
- Praise positive coping behaviors.
- Provide encouragement and praise for strengths observed.
- Encourage independence and self-care as much as possible.

- Encourage participation in activities that decrease attention on symptoms (reading, watching TV, listening to radio, engaging in hobbies, painting).
- Promote communication with family and significant others.
- Encourage socialization.
- Explain that the physical disability is not related to intelligence.
- Discuss need for family to show security, love, and need for patient.
- Discuss need for family to have patience with and understanding of patient's slowness and clumsiness.
- Encourage patient to dress daily (clothes with zippers instead of buttons and shoes without laces or small buckles).

Critical thinking activities

1. Describe the quality of life for persons with Parkinson's disease.
2. Identify effective ways to assist the patient with Parkinson's disease maintain positive self-esteem.
3. Discuss how exercise programs help patients with Parkinson's disease improve their self-concept.
4. List symptoms of Parkinson's disease and classify these as related to tremor, rigidity, or bradykinesia.
5. Identify complications that may result from rigidity and bradykinesia.
6. Identify whether antiparkinsonian drugs are dopaminergic or anticholinergic.
7. Relate the loss of dopamine in the corpus striatum to the clinical manifestations seen in the patient with Parkinson's disease.
8. Identify specific nursing interventions for adjusting to the illness, avoiding precipitating factors, and preventing complications.
9. Compare the effects of drugs that block dopamine receptors, such as phenothiazines, with the symptoms of Parkinson's disease.
10. Identify nursing diagnoses that are supported by the clinical manifestations characteristic of Parkinson's disease.

Suggested research topics

- Coping strategies for Parkinson's disease
- Compliance with therapy
- Effectiveness of exercise programs

PART 9

Bowel elimination problems

Colostomy

Ileostomy

Colostomy

DRG: 148 Mean LOS 11.2 days

A colostomy is the surgical creation of an opening, or stoma, between the colon and the abdominal wall. Colostomies can be either temporary or permanent; the consistency of the stool draining from the ostomy depends on the placement of the ostomy. For example, the drainage from a sigmoid colostomy is solid stool, and the drainage from an ascending colostomy is usually liquid. Colostomies are performed to treat cancer of the colon or rectum, inflammatory bowel disease, familial polyposis, and diverticulitis. They are also created to treat abdominal trauma and mechanical obstruction of the bowel.

For most patients, the colostomy will begin to function within several days to 1 week postoperatively. Before discharge from the hospital, the nurse must begin to teach the patient and family about colostomy care, which includes care of the peristomal skin; inspection of the stoma; application, drainage, and removal of the drainage pouch; and irrigation of the colostomy. Colostomy care is continued by the home care nurse after the patient has been discharged from the hospital.

Complications associated with colostomies include prolapse of the stoma, perforation of the colon (during improper irrigation), retraction of the stoma into the abdomen, fecal impaction, and irritation of the peristomal skin. Surgical repair may be necessary to manage these complications.

Subjective assessment findings

Health history
Bowel elimination patterns (frequency of diarrhea and constipation), episodes of abdominal or rectal cramping, blood in stool (melena), colonic impactions, personal or family history of colon polyps or cancer, recent trauma to the abdomen, inflammatory bowel disease, dietary intake of fiber, allergies (for consideration of colostomy products)

Medication history
Prescription and over-the-counter (OTC) cathartics, enemas, laxatives, antidiarrheals

Functional health patterns
Nutritional-metabolic: anorexia, abdominal fullness, unexplained loss of > 10% of body weight, nausea with vomiting after eating
Elimination: frequent diarrhea or constipation; thin, ribbonlike stool; sensation of rectal pressure or cramping; blood in stool
Cognitive-perceptual: pain experienced with defecation, fear, anxiety

Objective assessment findings

Physical findings
Elimination: color, odor, and consistency of stool;, presence of blood, mucus, or pus in stool; location, duration, and frequency of rectal pain
Gastrointestinal: abdominal distension, abdominal masses, hyperactive or hypoactive bowel sounds
Integumentary: pallor, poor skin turgor, skin infections, skin disruption in rectal area

Diagnostic tests

Digital rectal examination, stool guaiac test, urinalysis, chest X-ray, electrocardiogram, carcinoembryonic antigen, colon X-rays, ultrasound and computed tomography of the abdomen, flexible sigmoidoscopy, colonoscopy, barium enema, complete blood count with differential, electrolytes, blood chemistries, coagulation profile, blood urea nitrogen and creatinine, liver function tests, amylase

Related nursing diagnoses

1 Body image disturbance
2 Pain
3 Constipation or diarrhea
4 Risk for infection
5 Risk for injury
6 Ineffective management of therapeutic regimen (community, family, or individual)
7 Altered nutrition: less than body requirements
8 Risk for impaired skin integrity

Expected outcomes

The following expected outcomes pertain to the patient or family. Numbers in parentheses refer to related nursing diagnoses above.

- Have concerns such as sexuality, body image, and reproductive issues addressed to their satisfaction (1).
- Have pain controlled to patient's satisfaction (2).
- Have bowel elimination regulated before discharge, (that is, no diarrhea or constipation will be present) (3,6).
- Maintain peristomal skin without signs of infection or irritation (4,5,8).
- Have abdominal and perineal incisions that are clean and free of infection before discharge (4,5).
- Have a moist, brick red stoma on discharge (5,8).
- Be knowledgeable about community support services and resources related to ostomy care before discharge (for example, where ostomy supplies can be purchased in the community) (1,6).
- Have participated in wound and ostomy care before discharge (6).
- Be aware of signs, symptoms, and complications that should be reported to a health care provider after discharge (4,5,6,8).
- Be able to independently manage the daily care of the colostomy, including stoma inspection, peristomal skin care, colostomy irrigations, pouch application, and pouch emptying (6).
- Be aware of specific dietary alterations required before discharge (3,7).
- Maintain weight within recommended ranges for height and bone structure (7).

Other possible nursing diagnoses

Anxiety, ineffective individual coping, fear, anticipatory grieving, bowel incontinence, altered role performance, self-esteem disturbance, altered sexuality patterns, social isolation

Potential complications

Fluid and electrolyte imbalance, sepsis, mechanical bowel obstruction, thrombophlebitis or deep vein thrombosis

Patient teaching

Colostomy skin care

- Protect the peristomal skin from contact with the effluent (fecal) drainage at all times.

(Text continues on page 203.)

PLAN OF CARE	PREADMIT PHASE	INPATIENT CARE Day 1	Day 2
DIAGNOSTIC TESTS	• Digital rectal examination • Stool guaiac test • Urinalysis (UA) • Chest X-ray (CXR) • Electrocardiogram (ECG) • Carcinoembryonic antigen • Colon X-rays • Ultrasound • Computed tomography of the abdomen • Flexible sigmoidoscopy • Colonoscopy, barium enema • Complete blood count (CBC) with differential, electrolytes (lytes), blood chemistries, coagulation profile, blood urea nitrogen (BUN) and creatinine (Cr), liver function tests, amylase • Enterostomal therapy (ET) nurse consulted for markings related to placement of ostomy	• CBC, serum chemistries and lytes, arterial blood gases (ABGs), BUN, Cr, blood type and screen • Pulse oximetry q 8 hr • UA • CXR	• CBC, serum chemistries and lytes, BUN, Cr, ABGs as needed • UA • Pulse oximetry q 12 hr
MEDICATIONS	• Oral cathartics for at least 24 hours before operation • Enemas to clean bowel • I.V. or oral antibiotics as prescribed • Analgesics as prescribed • Evaluate or administer home medications as ordered	• Serum I.V. fluids as ordered (dextrose 5% in half-normal saline [$D_5\frac{1}{2}NS$ with multivitamins [MVI] and potassium chloride [KCl]) • I.V. piggyback (IVPB) antibiotics • IVPB antiemetics as needed • Subcutaneous heparin injections • I.V. push (IVP)/IVPB analgesics • PCA if indicated • Home medications as ordered • IVPB antibiotics • IVPB antiemetic as needed	• PCA • I.V. fluids as ordered ($D_5\frac{1}{2}NS$ with MVI and KCl)
PROCEDURES	• Monitor vital signs (VS) q 4 hr. • Evaluate hydration status. • Initiate I.V. access if needed. • Monitor and document nasogastric (NG) drainage if present. • Apply antiembolism (TED) stockings. • If obstruction is present preoperatively, initiate I.V. fluids and NG suction.	• Check VS every 30 minutes for 4 hours, every hour for 4 hours, then q 4 hr. • Initiate respiratory therapy, TCDB, and incentive spirometry (IS) q 2 hr. • Have patient splint incision during respiratory exercises. • Evaluate surgical wounds and dressing (stoma), abdominal incision, and perineal incision (if present). • Elevate head of bed (HOB) to 30 degrees. • Apply TED stockings.	• Check VS q 4 hr. • Have patient TCDB and use IS q 2 hr. • Have patient splint incision during respiratory exercises. • Evaluate stoma for stomal ischemia (stoma should be very red and moist). • Evaluate peristomal skin. • Elevate HOB to 30°. • Secure ostomy pouch. • Apply TED stockings. • Monitor I.V. site care.
DIET	• Give diet high in calories, protein, and carbohydrates, and low in residue if tolerated. • Switch to full or clear liquid diet 24 hours before surgery. • Give nothing by mouth (NPO) if on NG suction. • Initiate total parenteral nutrition as ordered if indicated. • Keep NPO past midnight before surgery. • Obtain baseline weight.	• NPO; NG tube to intermittent suction; monitor drainage. • Weigh patient daily.	• Clamp NG tube to discontinue (D/C) and begin clear liquid diet. • D/C NG tube if no nausea and vomiting or excess residual obtained and positive bowel sounds auscultated. • After NG tube has been discontinued, begin clear liquid diet. • Weigh patient.

CLINICAL PATHWAY ■ Colostomy

198   Colostomy

Days 3 to 4	Days 5 to 7	Days 8 to 10	Day 11
• Serum chemistries and lytes, BUN, Cr • If increased temperature, culture of sputum, urine, stool, wound, and central lines • CXR • Pulse oximetry as needed	• CBC, chemistries, lytes if previous tests were abnormal	• Same as previous day	• Same as previous day
• Oral antibiotics and analgesics as ordered • Home medications • Antiemetics and antipyretics • Saline or heparin lock I.V.	• Oral antibiotics and analgesics • Home medications	• Continue home medications. • Continue oral analgesics as needed.	• Same as previous day
• Check VS q 4 hr. • Have patient TCDB and use IS q 2 hr. • Have patient splint incision during respiratory exercises. • Evaluate surgical wounds; change dressings as needed. • Evaluate stoma and pouch system. • Evaluate peristomal skin. • Elevate HOB to 30 degrees. • Apply TED stockings. • Monitor I.V. site care.	• Check VS q 4 hr. • Have patient TCDB and use IS q 2 hr. • Evaluate surgical wounds; change dressings as needed. • Evaluate stoma and pouch system. • Evaluate peristomal skin. • Elevate HOB to 30 degrees. • Continue with TED stockings. • Give I.V. site care.	• D/C saline or heparin lock. • Consider removal of staples from surgical incisions. • D/C TED stockings.	• Consider removal of staples from surgical incisions.
• Give diet as tolerated (DAT) • Encourage oral fluid intake. • Weigh patient.	• Same as previous day	• Give DAT. • Encourage fluid intake.	• Same as previous day

(continued)

PLAN OF CARE	PREADMIT PHASE	INPATIENT CARE Day 1	Day 2
ACTIVITY	• Evaluate activity tolerance before the operation. • Allow for adequate rest periods to minimize fatigue.	• Have patient turn in bed from side to side q 2 hr. • Have patient perform ankle exercises.	• Have patient turn in bed from side to side q 2 hr. • Have patient perform ankle exercises. • Help patient get up in bedside chair morning and afternoon.
ELIMINATION	• Measure intake and output (I & O). • Evaluate color, amount, consistency, and odor of stool. • Observe for blood, pus, or mucus in stool. • Observe for concentrated urine or increased urine specific gravity. • Document results of enemas, cathartics, and laxatives.	• Measure I & O. • Observe and document amount, color, and consistency of drainage from indwelling urinary catheter postoperatively. • Observe stoma for color and drainage q 2 hr and as needed, and document. • Observe rectal area for color and amount of drainage. • Observe and measure NG tube drainage.	• Measure I & O. • D/C urinary catheter as ordered. • Measure time of first voiding after catheter is discontinued. • Observe stoma q 4 hr and as needed for color and drainage. • Document amount and type of drainage from rectal area. • Observe and measure NG tube drainage before discontinuing.
HYGIENE	• Provide meticulous skin care, especially over bony prominences. • Provide prompt cleaning of anorectal area after administration of cathartics, enemas, or laxatives.	• Provide meticulous oral and perineal hygiene at least q 4 hr and as needed. • Provide skin care at least q4hr and as needed.	• Same as Day 1
PATIENT TEACHING	• Explain respiratory therapy, and give preoperative demonstration; request return demonstration of turning, coughing, and deep breathing (TCDB) exercises. • Observe return demonstration of incentive spirometry (IS) exercises. • Teach patient how to splint incision. • Teach use of patient-controlled analgesia (PCA) if ordered. • Explain disease process and need for surgery. • With ET nurse, begin teaching about colostomy care and perineal wound care.	• Reinforce and implement teaching about TCDB and IS exercises, ankle exercises, need for TED stockings, and splinting of incision. • Begin teaching patient and family about postoperative wound and ostomy care, including correct terminology, types of supplies needed, and where to locate supplies.	• Consider visit from ostomy society volunteer. • Allow patient and family to begin performing care of the ostomy, including care of the peristomal skin, pouch application, emptying of pouch, odor control, and regulation of bowel function via colostomy irrigations.
DISCHARGE PLANNING	*ET consult:* *Social services consult:* *Pastoral care consult:* *Home health consult:* *Respiratory therapy consult:* • Discuss home care supplies and needs.	*Social services consult:* • Determine patient's and family's ability to procure ostomy supplies on discharge.	• Refer patient to community support services and programs such as American Cancer Society, Can Surmount, I Can Cope, and local ostomy society.

Days 3 to 4	Days 5 to 7	Days 8 to 10	Day 11
• Have patient turn in bed from side to side q 2 hr. • Have patient perform ankle exercises. • Have patient walk in room with assistance.	• Have patient get up in chair with assistance. • Have patient progress to walking in hall.	• Continue TCDB exercises.	• As tolerated.
• Measure I & O. • Evaluate output from stoma: consistency, color, odor. • Measure output from stoma.	• Measure I & O. • Have patient and family evaluate stoma output. • Have patient and family measure output from stoma.	• Monitor and measure urine output. • Have patient and family evaluate stoma output. • Have patient and family measure output from stoma.	• Have patient and family evaluate stoma output. • Have patient and family measure output from stoma.
• Same as Day 2	• Same as Day 2	• Provide meticulous oral and perineal hygiene at least q 4 hr and as needed. • Provide skin care at least q 4 hr and as needed.	• Provide skin care at least q 4 hr and as needed.
• Teach about dietary modifications that may be necessary with a colostomy (that is, fluid intake of 2 to 3 qt [2 to 3 L]/day unless contraindicated; decreased intake or elimination of foods that can cause diarrhea or constipation, such as nuts, popcorn, fresh fruits and vegetables with the skin on, coconut, and so forth). • Allow patient and family to begin performing care of the ostomy, including care of the peristomal skin, pouch application, emptying of pouch, odor control, and regulation of bowel function via colostomy irrigations.	• Teach about signs and symptoms to report to health care professional after discharge: diarrhea; bleeding from stoma or surgical incisions; stoma which is pale, blue, or dusky in color; abdominal rigidity or distension; signs of infection; excoriation of peristomal area. • Explore effects of stoma on sexuality.	• Reinforce previous teaching. • Have patient give return demonstration on pouch emptying.	• Teach about schedule of home health visits and reasons for visits.
Social services: • Consult durable medical equipment company and resources for home health supplies and equipment such as bedside commodes, shower bench, walker, and hospital beds.	• Consult psychologist as needed to discuss sexuality and sexual functioning concerns.	• Arrange for home health nurse to visit patient and family before discharge from hospital.	• Discharge to home with return appointment to surgeon and oncologist if needed.

(continued)

PLAN OF CARE	HOME CARE Visit 1	Visit 2	Visit 3
DIAGNOSTIC TESTS	▪ Complete blood count ▪ Blood chemistries ▪ Electrolytes (lytes) ▪ Blood urea nitrogen ▪ Chest X-ray		▪ Lytes
MEDICATIONS	▪ Evaluate use and compliance with pre-scribed antibiotics, analgesics, antiemetics. ▪ Determine over-the-counter (OTC) med-ication use. ▪ Observe for undissolved medications in ostomy pouch.	▪ Observe for adverse effects of prescription and OTC drugs, particularly diarrhea or constipa-tion. ▪ Inspect ostomy pouch for undis-solved medications.	▪ Same as previous visit
PROCEDURES	▪ Determine specific ostomy type and location (for example, single barrel vs. double barrel; transverse, ascending, or descending). ▪ Evaluate patient's ability to manage ostomy care. ▪ Inspect surgical wounds and dressings. ▪ Take baseline vital signs (VS).	▪ Inspect peristomal skin for signs of yeast infection, bacterial infection, and excoriation. ▪ Evaluate color and size of stoma. ▪ Evaluate healing of surgical wounds. ▪ Check VS.	▪ Same as previous visit
DIET	▪ Take baseline weight. ▪ Determine daily caloric intake. ▪ Evaluate 24-hour diet recall for appro-priate calorie, vitamin, mineral, protein, and low residue intake.	▪ Weigh patient. ▪ Determine if body weight has been maintained or if loss or gain has occurred. ▪ Evaluate daily dietary consump-tion.	▪ Same as previous visit
ACTIVITY	▪ Determine level of activity since dis-charge. ▪ Determine patient's tolerance for activity. ▪ Perform home safety evaluation.	▪ Determine level of activity since discharge. ▪ Determine patient's tolerance for activity.	▪ Same as previous visit
ELIMINATION	▪ Assess quality, amount, and odor of colostomy effluent. ▪ Inspect urine amount, concentration, and color.	▪ Recommend dietary and fluid adjustments based on colosto-my and urine outputs.	▪ Same as previous visit
HYGIENE	▪ Inspect oral, perineal, and general body hygiene. ▪ Consider home health aide.	▪ Inspect oral, perineal, and gen-eral body hygiene.	▪ Same as previous visit
PATIENT TEACHING	▪ Reinforce prior teaching. ▪ Reteach concepts as necessary. ▪ Request return demonstration on peris-tomal skin prep and care, pouch empty-ing, pouch application, and ostomy irri-gation.	▪ Reinforce prior teaching. ▪ Reteach concepts as necessary. ▪ Request return demonstration on peristomal skin prep and care, pouch emptying, pouch application, and ostomy irriga-tion. ▪ If radiation or chemotherapy is to follow, begin teaching specific to these therapies.	▪ Same as previous visit
DISCHARGE PLANNING	▪ Evaluate amount and quality of home care supplies, such as skin barrier and pouches.	▪ Determine compliance with fol-low-up visits to health care providers such as surgeon, medical oncologist, and radia-tion oncologist.	▪ Provide patient and family with written information on how to contact local support agencies such as American Cancer Society and Ostomy Society.

- Clean the peristomal skin as needed with a moist, soft cloth and mild soap. Remove any excess skin barrier that has been applied to peristomal skin. Pat skin dry—do not rub.
- When the colostomy pouch is off, the stoma can be lightly covered with gauze to prevent seepage of fecal material.
- Inspect peristomal skin for redness, abrasion, irritation, and growth of yeast.
- Notify enterostomal therapy nurse or doctor if any of these occur.
- Reapply skin barrier around stoma after peristomal skin has been cleaned and patted dry. Skin barrier can consist of a wafer, powder, paste, or a combination of barriers.

Drainage pouch
- The stoma must be measured before applying the pouch.
- After the stoma has been measured, the pouch opening is cut. The pouch opening should be precisely ⅛" (0.3 cm) larger than the stoma.
- After the opening has been cut, peel the adhesive backing from the pouch and apply to clean peristomal skin that has had skin barrier applied.
- Press down on the pouch for 30 seconds to ensure good adhesive contact to the skin.
- Remove and drain the drainage appliance when it is one-quarter to one-third full.
- Disposable and odor-resistant pouches are commercially available.

Signs and symptoms
- Reinforce inspection of the stoma. The stoma should be pink to brick red in color. Notify enterostomal therapy nurse or doctor immediately if stoma color is blue, brown, or black in color.

Activity
- Discuss importance of maintaining a regular exercise program.
- Discuss importance of progressive increase in activity level and eliminating or participating cautiously in contact sports.

Medication
- Instruct patient on dosage, time of administration, purpose, and adverse effects.
- Explain need to avoid OTC drugs unless ordered by doctor; avoid alcohol use.
- Explain need to notify doctor of chronic constipation or diarrhea.

Nutrition
- Explain importance of maintaining a well-balanced diet.
- Explain importance of drinking 2 to 3 qt (2 to 3 L)/day.
- Provide a list of low residue foods, such as cooked, refined, or strained cereal; tender, steamed vegetables and fruits; plain desserts.
- Eliminate foods that may cause discomfort, such as raw fruits and vegetables (especially fruits with skin), whole grain cereals and breads, nuts, coconut, raisins, popcorn.

Lifestyle modifications
- Teach correct procedure for colostomy irrigation as needed.
- Teach patient to plan ahead for supplies for vacations, extended business trips, and so forth.

Critical thinking activities
1. Discuss whether the sexuality and sexual functioning concerns of older adults with colostomies are addressed as frequently as those of younger adults with colostomies.
2. Discuss the role the economic status of the ostomy patient plays in the occurrence rate of complications such as peristomal skin infections.

3. Describe how ostomy teaching should be prioritized between the inpatient and home care settings.
4. Explain the purpose of the surgical creation of a temporary colostomy.
5. Describe indications that peristalsis has returned following ostomy creation.
6. Discuss characteristics of a healthy stoma and peristomal skin.
7. Develop a teaching plan to assist an individual with a colostomy to deal with flatus.
8. List dietary and pharmacologic options that could be utilized to manage diarrhea or constipation in an individual with a colostomy.

Suggested research topics
- Coping strategies for colostomy
- Compliance with therapy
- Compliance with care routine
- Effectiveness of colostomy care instruction

Ileostomy

DRG: 148 Mean LOS: 11.2 days

Surgical removal of the entire colon, rectum, and anus, and closure of the anus (total proctocolectomy) results in the need for a diversion for stool. As part of the total proctocolectomy procedure, the end of the terminal ileum is brought out through the abdominal wall, forming a permanent stoma or ostomy. This stoma is termed an ileostomy.

A variation of total proctocolectomy with creation of a permanent ileostomy is total proctocolectomy with creation of a continent ileostomy, or Kock's pouch. In this procedure, an internal pouch is created in the distal segment of the ileum. This internal pouch serves as a reservoir for stool. During surgery, a one-way nipple valve is constructed through the stomal opening so that eventually the patient can insert a catheter through the stomal opening and through the one-way valve to drain the fecal contents of the internal pouch.

The continent ileostomy may be an alternative for individuals who do not wish to wear an external pouch over the stoma. The stoma created as part of the continent ileostomy procedure is flush with the abdominal wall and can be covered with only a cap or gauze dressing to absorb mucous drainage. However, the complication rate associated with a continent ileostomy is higher than for the traditional ileostomy.

Because of the removal of the entire colon, the stool that drains from the ileostomy is liquid to semi-formed and contains digestive enzymes. Initially, output of stool may be as high as 1,500 to 2,000 ml/day. Therefore, the major physiologic complications associated with ileostomy include fluid and electrolyte disturbances and impaired skin integrity.

Subjective assessment findings

Health history
Bowel elimination patterns, including frequency of diarrhea or constipation; episodes of abdominal or rectal cramping; history of colonic impactions; personal or family history of colon polyps or cancer; history of recent trauma to the abdomen; history of inflammatory bowel disease; dietary intake of fiber

Medication history
Prescription and over-the-counter cathartics, enemas, laxatives, and antidiarrheals

Functional health patterns
Nutritional-metabolic: anorexia, abdominal fullness, unexplained loss of > 10% of body weight, nausea with vomiting after eating
Elimination: frequent diarrhea or constipation; thin, ribbonlike stool; sensation of rectal pressure or cramping; blood in stool
Cognitive-perceptual: pain experienced with defecation, fear, anxiety

(Text continues on page 211.)

CLINICAL PATHWAY

PLAN OF CARE	PREADMIT PHASE	INPATIENT CARE Day 1	Day 2
DIAGNOSTIC TESTS	• Complete blood count (CBC) • Electrolytes (lytes) • Serum chemistries • Blood urea nitrogen (BUN), creatinine (Cr) • Prothrombin time/International Normalized Ratio • Activated partial thromboplastin time • Blood type and screen • Carcinoembryonic antigen • Liver function tests, amylase levels • Stool guaiac test • Chest X-ray (CXR) • Colon X-rays • Computed tomography scan of abdomen • Colonoscopy • Electrocardiogram • Flexible sigmoidoscopy • Digital rectal examination	• CBC, serum chemistries and lytes, BUN, Cr • Arterial blood gases (ABGs) • Pulse oximetry q 8 hr • CXR • UA	• CBC, lytes, serum chemistries, ABGs • Pulse oximetry q 12 hr • UA, urine osmolarity • Lytes
MEDICATIONS	• Oral cathartics, antibiotics, enemas (may be done in the home setting); use caution if patient is weakened or dehydrated, and with the elderly when administering tap water enemas until return is clear. • Home medications and nothing by mouth (NPO) after midnight before surgery.	• I.V. piggyback (IVPB) antibiotics • IVPB antiemetics as needed • Subcutaneous (S.C.) heparin • I.V. push (IVP)/IVPB analgesics • I.V. fluids (dextrose 5% in half-normal saline with potassium chloride and multivitamins • Patient-controlled analgesia (PCA) for pain control if present; monitor use	• Electrolyte replacement, especially sodium (Na) and potassium (K), if needed • IVPB antibiotics and antiemetics • S.C. heparin • IVP/IVPB analgesics • PCA for pain control if present
PROCEDURES	• Enterostomal therapy (ET) nurse marks stoma site selection for surgeon. • Obtain baseline weight. • Evaluate preoperative hydration status. • Evaluate results of cathartic, enemas, and laxatives. • Apply antiembolism (TED) stockings.	• Check vital signs (VS) every 30 minutes for 4 hours, every hour for 4 hours, then q 4 hr. • Evaluate surgical stoma wounds, tubes, drains and dressings in abdominal and perianal areas. • Monitor I.V. access site. • Elevate head of bed (HOB) to 30 degrees. • Continue with TED stockings. • Provide indwelling urinary catheter care. • Maintain patency of NG tube to intermittent suction. • Initiate respiratory therapy (RT): TCDB and incentive spirometry (IS) q 2 hr while awake. • Have patient splint incision during respiratory exercises.	• Check VS q 4 hr. • Evaluate stoma for stomal ischemia (stoma should be brick red and moist). • Evaluate peristomal skin. • Evaluate surgical stoma wounds, tubes, drains and dressings in abdominal and perianal areas. • Provide indwelling urinary catheter care. • Monitor I.V. access site. • Maintain HOB 30 degrees. • Continue with TED stockings. • Maintain patency of NG tube; attach NG tube to intermittent suction. • Secure ostomy pouch (consult ET nurse). • Encourage TCDB and IS q 4 hr while awake.
DIET	• Give diet high in calories, protein, and carbohydrates and low in residue if tolerated. • Begin full or clear liquid diet 24 hours before surgery. • Give NPO if on nasogastric (NG) suction. • Initiate total parenteral nutrition if indicated; keep NPO after midnight before surgery.	• NPO • NG and suction • Weigh patient.	• NPO; NG suction • Weigh patient.

Days 3 to 4	Days 5 to 7	Days 8 to 10	Day 11
• Urine osmolarity • If temperature spike occurs, CBC and culture of wounds, incisions, urine, sputum, and blood • Pulse oximetry • CXR	• Lytes • Urine osmolarity	• Lytes	• As indicated
• Electrolyte replacement, especially Na and K, if needed • IVPB antibiotics and antiemetics • S.C. heparin • IVP/IVPB analgesics • Saline or heparin lock I.V. • PCA for pain control if present	• Electrolyte replacement, especially Na and K, if needed. • Antibiotics and analgesics to P.O. as ordered • Resume home medications. • D/C PCA or epidural catheter for pain management.	• Continue home medications and oral analgesics as needed.	• Same as previous day
• Evaluate stoma for stomal ischemia. • Evaluate peristomal skin. • Secure ostomy pouch. • Evaluate surgical stoma wounds, tubes, drains, and dressings in abdominal and perianal areas. • Monitor I.V. access site. • Continue with TED stockings. • Consider sitz bath for perianal area. • Maintain patency of NG tube; attach NG tube to intermittent suction • Encourage TCDB and IS q 4 hr while awake.	• Monitor skin turgor and sensation of thirst. • Evaluate surgical wounds, tubes, drains, and dressings in abdominal and perianal areas. • Maintain TED stockings. • Consider sitz bath for perianal area. • Clamp NG tube as ordered by doctor if no nausea and vomiting is present, no excess residual is obtained, positive bowel sounds are auscultated, and fecal output is noted per ileostomy. • Encourage TCDB and IS q 4 hr while awake.	• D/C saline or heparin lock as ordered. • Consult with surgeon for removal of surgical drains and staples. • Monitor skin turgor and sensation of thirst. • Evaluate surgical wounds, tubes, drains, and dressings in abdominal and perianal areas. • Maintain TED stockings. • Consider sitz bath for perianal area. • Continue TCDB exercises.	• Monitor skin turgor and sensation of thirst. • Evaluate surgical wounds, tubes, drains and dressings in abdominal and perianal areas. • Maintain TED stockings. • Continue TCDB exercises.
• NPO; NG suction *Dietary consult:* • Discuss nutritional implications of ileostomy. • Weigh patient.	• After D/C NG tube, begin clear liquid diet; progress diet as tolerated (DAT). • Continue dietary teaching. • Weigh patient.	• Give DAT. • Encourage P.O. fluid intake.	• Same as previous day

(continued)

PLAN OF CARE	PREADMIT PHASE	INPATIENT CARE *Day 1*	*Day 2*
ACTIVITY	• Evaluate activity tolerance preoperatively. • Allow for adequate rest periods to minimize fatigue. • Practice turning, coughing, and deep breathing (TCDB) exercises.	• Have patient turn in bed from side to side q 2 hr. • Have patient perform ankle exercises.	• Have patient turn in bed from side to side q 2 hr. • Have patient continue ankle exercises. • Tell patient to splint incision during respiratory exercises. • Help patient get up in bedside chair morning and afternoon.
ELIMINATION	• Evaluate color, consistency, and odor of stool. • Observe for concentrated urine or increased urine specific gravity.	• Observe and document amount, color, and concentration of urine from indwelling urinary catheter. • Observe ileostomy stoma q 2 hr for color and drainage. • Observe perirectal area for drainage; note color and amount. • Monitor amount, color, and consistency of NG tube drainage. • Measure intake and output (I & O).	• Observe and document amount, color, and concentration of urine from indwelling urinary catheter • Observe ileostomy stoma q 2 hr for color and drainage. • Observe perirectal area for drainage; note color and amount. • Monitor amount, color, and consistency of NG tube drainage. • Measure I & O.
HYGIENE	• Provide prompt cleaning of anorectal area after administration of cathartics, enemas, laxatives and evacuation of stool. • Describe need for postoperative hygiene of anorectal area and peristomal areas.	• Provide meticulous oral and perineal hygiene at least q 4 hr and as needed. • Provide skin care to nares around NG tube q 4 hr and as needed. • Provide urinary catheter care every shift and as needed.	• Same as Day 1
PATIENT TEACHING	• Anticipate and discuss with patient type of procedure to be performed and why, and postoperative use of drains, tubes, sumps, and catheters. • With ET nurse, begin teaching about ileostomy care and perineal wound care. • If appropriate, instruct patient and family on bowel preparation regimen to be done at home.	• Reinforce and implement TCDB and IS exercises, as well as ankle exercise. • Discuss need for TED stockings and splinting of incision. • Begin incremental teaching of patient and family about postoperative wound and ostomy care, including correct terminology, types of equipment and supplies needed, and where to locate supplies.	• Visit from United Ostomy Association volunteer. • Continue teaching related to care of ostomy and peristomal skin. • Demonstrate skin cleaning, skin preparation, pouch application, and pouch emptying. • Have patient provide return demonstration on mannikin or model.
DISCHARGE PLANNING	• Preoperative visit by a United Ostomy Association trained volunteer. *ET nurse consult:* *Social services consult* • Review home care supplies and needs. • *Pastoral care consult* • *Home health consult* • *Respiratory therapy consult* • *Dietary consult*	*Social services:* • Determine patient's and family's ability to procure ostomy and other supplies in their community on discharge.	*Social services:* • Consult durable medical equipment company for home health supplies such as hospital bed with overbed trapeze, bedside commode, shower bench, and walker, as needed.

Days 3 to 4	Days 5 to 7	Days 8 to 10	Day 11
• Have patient turn in bed from side to side q 2 hr. • Have patient continue ankle exercises. • Tell patient to splint incision during respiratory exercises. • Have patient walk in room with assistance. • Have patient get up in chair with assistance.	• Have patient turn in bed from side to side q 2 hr. • Have patient continue ankle exercises. • Tell patient to splint incision during respiratory exercises. • Have patient progress to walking in hall.	• Have patient progress walking.	• Same as previous day
• Evaluate ileostomy output frequently; initially fecal output may be as high as 1,500 to 2,000 ml/24 hr. • Notify doctor if effluent increases in volume and becomes watery, necessitating pouch emptying every 20 to 30 minutes. • Discontinue (D/C) urinary catheter • Monitor, amount, color, and consistency of NG tube drainage. • Measure I & O.	• Evaluate ileostomy output frequently. • Monitor amount, color, and concentration of urine output.	• Evaluate ileostomy output frequently. • Measure I & O.	• Assess ileostomy and urine output.
• Consider sitz bath for perianal area cleaning and hygiene every shift as ordered. • Provide care to skin and nares.	• Same as previous day	• Consider sitz bath for perianal area cleaning and hygiene every shift as ordered.	• Provide care to skin. • Consider sitz bath for perianal area cleaning and hygiene every shift as ordered.
• Have patient and family give return demonstration on actual ostomy of skin care, appliance application, and pouch emptying. • Discuss odor control, food blockages, fungal infections, and other possible complications of the ileostomy.	• Teach complications related to ileostomy: diarrhea, fecal blockage of stoma, peristomal skin irritation, stenosis of the stoma, urinary calculi development, cholelithiasis, changes in appearance and color of stoma.	• Reinforce previous teaching. • Demonstrate ostomy care. • Have patient provide return demonstration.	• Teach about schedule of home health visits and reasons for visit.
• Refer patient and family to community support services sponsored by the United Ostomy Association, the American Cancer Society, and other organizations.	• Discuss specific restrictions to be adhered to after discharge, such as restrictions on heavy lifting, driving, return to work. • Discuss when it's safe to resume sexual activity.	*Home health nurse:* • Visit patient and family before discharge from hospital.	• Discharge to home with return appointment to surgeon (and oncologist if needed).

(continued)

PLAN OF CARE	HOME CARE Visit 1	Visit 2	Visit 3
DIAGNOSTIC TESTS	• Complete blood count • Blood urea nitrogen, creatinine • Electrolytes (lytes) • Urinalysis, urine osmolarity	• Urine osmolarity	• Lytes • Urine osmolarity
MEDICATIONS	• Caution patient not to use over-the-counter (OTC) or prescription laxatives. • Evaluate use and compliance with prescribed antibiotics, analgesics, and antiemetics. • Observe for undissolved medications in ostomy pouch (especially enteric-coated medicines).	• Observe for adverse effects of prescription and OTC drugs, particularly diarrhea or constipation. • If still on antibiotics, observe peristomal skin for signs of fungal or yeast superinfection.	• Observe for adverse effects of prescription and OTC drugs, particularly diarrhea or constipation. • If still on antibiotics, observe peristomal skin for signs of fungal or yeast superinfection. • Inspect ostomy pouch for undissolved or partially dissolved medications.
PROCEDURES	• Evaluate patient's ability to perform care of ostomy. • Inspect and evaluate perianal and abdominal wounds, staples, dressing, tubes, and drains as appropriate. • Take baseline vital signs (VS).	• Inspect stoma for signs of pallor, discoloration, bleeding, strangulation, hernia, or retraction. • Inspect peristomal skin for signs of yeast infection, bacterial infection, or contact with fecal drainage. • Evaluate healing of all surgical wound sites. • Check VS.	• Same as previous visit
DIET	• Evaluate hydration status by assessing mucous membranes and skin turgor. • Obtain 24-hour diet recall from patient. • Evaluate for evidence of food blockage of stoma. • Evaluate for nausea and vomiting (N/V). • Weigh patient.	• Evaluate hydration status by assessing mucous membranes and skin turgor. • Obtain 24-hour diet recall from patient. • Evaluate for evidence of food blockage of stoma. • Evaluate for N/V. • Weigh patient; from patient weight record determine if body weight loss or gain has occurred. • Evaluate daily food and fluid consumption. • Determine "problem foods" for patient.	• Same as previous visit
ACTIVITY	• Perform a home safety assessment. • Determine patient's level and tolerance of activity since discharge.	• Increase activity level as appropriate. • Determine need for assistive equipment. • Same as previous visit.	
ELIMINATION	• Determine quality, consistency, and amount of ileostomy effluent in 24 hours (should be approximately 800 to 1,000 ml/24 hr). • Determine color, concentration, and amount of urine output in previous 24 hours.	• Recommend dietary or fluid adjustments based on ostomy and urine outputs.	• Same as previous visit
HYGIENE	• Evaluate peristomal and perirectal skin areas for signs of redness, excoriation, and denuding.	• Consider home health aide to assist with hygiene as needed.	• Same as previous visit
PATIENT TEACHING	• Use correct terminology for wounds, equipment, and supplies. • Ask for return demonstrations on care of the ostomy as appropriate.	• Use correct terminology for wounds, equipment, and supplies. • Ask for return demonstrations on care of the ostomy; reteach concepts as needed.	• Same as previous visit
DISCHARGE PLANNING	• Evaluate amount, quality, and appropriateness of home care supplies. • Replenish supplies as needed.	• Determine compliance with follow-up visits to health care provider.	• Provide patient and family with written information and telephone numbers of local support groups, agencies, and organizations.

Objective assessment findings

Physical findings

Elimination: color, odor, and consistency of stool; presence of blood, mucus, or pus in stool; location, duration, and frequency of rectal pain

Gastrointestinal: abdominal distension, abdominal masses, hyperactive or hypoactive bowel sounds

Integumentary: pallor, poor skin turgor, skin infections, skin disruption in rectal area

Diagnostic tests

Complete blood count, serum electrolytes, serum chemistries, blood urea nitrogen, creatinine, partial thromboplastin/International Normalized Ratio, activated partial thromboplastin time, carcinoembryonic antigen, liver function tests, amylase levels, stool guaiac test, chest X-ray, colon X-ray, computed tomography of abdomen, colonoscopy, electrocardiogram, flexible sigmoidoscopy, digital rectal examination

Related nursing diagnoses

1 Anxiety
2 Body image disturbance
3 Pain
4 Constipation
5 Ineffective individual coping
6 Fear
7 Anticipatory grieving
8 Impaired home maintenance management
9 Bowel incontinence
10 Ineffective management of therapeutic regimen (community, family, or individual)
11 Altered nutrition: less than body requirements
12 Risk for personal identity disturbance
13 Altered role performance
14 Self-esteem disturbance
15 Altered sexuality patterns
16 Risk for impaired skin integrity
17 Impaired tissue integrity

Expected outcomes

The following expected outcomes pertain to the patient or family. Numbers in parentheses refer to related nursing diagnoses above.

- Integrate ostomy into self-concept and body image (1,2,5,7,12,13,14).
- Incorporate self-management of the ostomy within activities of daily living (3,6,8,10,12,13,14).
- Have ostomy effluent that is within normal limits in terms of amount, consistency, and color of drainage (4,9).
- Have peristomal skin remain intact without evidence of redness, abrasions, or denuded or eroded areas (16,17).
- Be knowledgeable about community support services and resources related to ostomy care before discharge (that is, where ostomy supplies can be purchased in their community) (8,10).
- Have sexuality and reproductive concerns addressed before discharge (14,15).
- Achieve and maintain fluid and electrolyte balance before discharge (11).
- Be aware of signs, symptoms, and complications that should be reported to a health care provider after discharge (8,10).
- Know dietary instructions specific to ileostomy before discharge (8,9,10,11).
- Manage the daily care of the ileostomy, including inspection of the stoma, peristomal skin care, pouch application, and pouch emptying (8,9,10).

Other possible nursing diagnoses

Altered family processes, risk for caregiver role strain, risk for injury, social isolation

Potential complications

Fluid and electrolyte imbalance

Patient teaching

Nutrition

- Initially, a fluid intake of at least 3 qt (3 L)/day is recommended to prevent dehydration.
- Be cautious about fluid intake, especially during periods of hot weather, when engaging in exercise, when perspiring excessively, and during episodes of diarrhea (normal output for an ileostomy is 27 to 33 oz [800 to 1,000 ml]/day).
- Include in the diet foods to manage diarrhea (low-residue foods), including applesauce and strained fruit juices, dry cereals without bran, lean tender meats, creamy peanut butter; limit milk products to 2 cups (473 ml)/day or eliminate them altogether during diarrheal episodes.
- Include in the diet foods to manage constipation, including whole grain cereals, raw fruits and vegetables, and bread and crackers containing whole grain flour or bran.
- Avoid foods that may cause blockage of the stoma, including nuts, popcorn, coconut, and fibrous fruits and vegetables such as celery and watermelon.
- All foods consumed should be chewed thoroughly and eaten slowly.

Medications

- The patient with an ostomy should never take a laxative because of the possibility of severe fluid and electrolyte imbalance.
- Enteric-coated pills or tablets should be taken with caution by a patient with an ileostomy. Observe for undissolved medication in the ostomy pouch (especially enteric-coated).

Signs and symptoms

- Instructions on sodium, potassium, and fluid depletion.
- Instructions on signs that would indicate blockage of the stoma; that is decreased fecal drainage, vomiting, abdominal distension and pain.

Coping

- Patient and family should be taught that the recovery process is often long.
- Patient teaching should include frank discussions about impact on sexual function and sexuality. Sexual function may be altered but sexuality does not have to be adversely affected.

Critical thinking activities

1. Compare long-term home maintenance costs of traditional versus continent ileostomy.
2. List all the supplies that would be necessary to demonstrate an ileostomy appliance change for a patient with a newly constructed ileostomy.
3. Discuss why ostomy irrigations are contraindicated for individuals with an ileostomy.

Suggested research topics

- Coping strategies for ileostomy
- Compliance with therapy
- Effectiveness of teaching methods for ileostomy care

PART 10

Pressure ulcers

Pressure ulcers

DRG: 271   Mean LOS: 6.6 days

Pressure ulcers (PUs) are wounds caused by unrelieved pressure, usually over bony prominences, that result in damage to skin and underlying tissues. Prevention and treatment have confounded caregivers for years; however, several recent achievements have fostered considerable progress. First, moist wound healing has been accepted as *the* standard of wound care. Second, standards for the treatment and prevention of PUs have been disseminated — *Treatment of Pressure Ulcers, Clinical Practice Guideline, No. 15* (1994) and *Pressure Ulcers in Adults: Prediction and Prevention, Clinical Practice Guideline, No. 3* (AHCPR, 1992). Third, a standard classification system for PUs has been adopted worldwide (National Pressure Ulcer Advisory Panel, 1989).

In a landmark study, Winter (1962) discovered that moist wounds heal faster than dry wounds that form scabs. Scab formation delays re-epithelialization because epithelial cells located at wound edges must burrow beneath the scab to resurface the wound. In the past, wound care consisted of keeping the wound dry and protected with gauze dressings. Today, dressings facilitate the healing process by providing a moist healing environment. The most common dressings now used to promote moist healing are wet gauze or occlusive dressings. Benefits to healing PUs with moist dressings are prevention of eschar formation, decreased pain, less wound infection, and increased quality of life.

The recommendations of the Agency for Health Care Policy and Research (AHCPR) guide clinicians as they develop comprehensive PU treatment and prevention programs. The guidelines explain assessment parameters, tissue load management, ulcer care, management of bacterial colonization and infection, surgical alternatives, PU education, and quality improvement.

The most common sites for PUs are the sacrum, heels, greater trochanters, ischial tuberosities, ankles, and elbows. The National Pressure Ulcer Advisory Panel (NPUAP) proposed a four-stage PU classification system based on the depth of the ulcer. Accurate staging and description of PUs are necessary to treat and monitor PU healing. The following criteria are used to correctly classify PUs by stage:

Stage I: Nonblanchable erythema of intact skin; the heralding lesion of skin ulceration. In individuals with darker skin, discoloration of the skin, warmth, edema, induration, or hardness may also be indicators.

Stage II: Partial-thickness skin loss involving epidermis or dermis. The ulcer is superficial and presents as an abrasion, blister, or shallow crater.

Stage III: Full-thickness skin loss involving damage to or necrosis of subcutaneous tissue; damage may extend down to, but not through, underlying fascia. The ulcer presents clinically as a deep crater with or without undermining of adjacent tissue.

Stage IV: Full-thickness skin loss with extensive destruction, tissue necrosis, or damage to muscle, bone, or supporting structures (for example, tendon, joint capsule). Undermining and sinus tracts may also be associated with Stage IV PUs.

Several cautions are necessary when using the NPUAP staging system:
- When eschar or slough is present in the wound, a PU cannot be accurately staged until the devitalized tissue is removed.

- Do not use reverse staging to describe a PU as it heals. It is incorrect to describe a Stage IV PU that begins to heal as a Stage III ulcer.
- Stage I PUs may be difficult to detect in darkly pigmented individuals.
- Extra vigilance is required to detect and prevent PUs under casts, orthopedic devices, and support hose.
- Management of advanced PUs is an involved, long-term process. A progressive approach to preventing and treating PUs encompasses a comprehensive, systematic, interdisciplinary, and ongoing educational program for patients, caregivers, families, and health care providers.

Through concerted implementation of recommendations outlined in *Clinical Practice Guideline, No. 3* and *No. 15*, the personal and economic costs of PUs can be significantly reduced.

Subjective assessment findings

Health history
Anemia, malnutrition, dehydration, incontinence, fever, alteration in sensory perception or level of consciousness, diabetes, stroke, spinal cord injury, advanced age, bed rest or immobility, infection, low diastolic blood pressure, premature ventricular contraction, recent surgery, musculoskeletal injury (with casting, bracing, splinting), immune deficiencies, collagen or vascular disease

Medication history
Use of narcotics, hypnotics, corticosteroids, muscle paralyzers, vitamin or mineral supplements

Functional health patterns
Health perception–health management: self-care problems
Nutritional-metabolic: anorexia, weight loss, edema, impaired healing ability, past or current PU
Elimination: incontinence
Activity-exercise: chair-bound, bed-bound, immobility, paralysis, paresis
Cognitive-perceptual: decreased mental status; altered pain sensation; insensate; altered memory, judgment, cognition, or communication; pain in PU area
Role-relationship pattern: death or change in health status of caregiver
Coping-stress tolerance: depression, psychosis, alcohol or drug use

Objective assessment findings

Physical findings
Cardiovascular: peripheral edema, dehydration, capillary refill
General: PU risk assessment tool, fever, polypharmacy or overmedication, social support, depression, home care resources (availability of skilled caregiver, finances, equipment)
Integumentary: PU site — stage, size, edges, sinus tract, tunneling, undermining, necrotic tissue, exudate, periwound skin color, edema, maceration, induration, granulation tissue, epithelialization; skin — intactness, color or discoloration, temperature, diaphoresis, infection (*Candida*, bacterial), hydration, edema, induration; bony prominences — skin intactness, color, temperature, changes in skin tone (for example, red, blue, purple), blisters, denudation
Neurologic: mental status changes, pain sensation
Nutritional: current weight, previous weight, percent weight change, ideal body weight, height, current body mass index (BMI), previous BMI, percent BMI change, creatine height index; serum albumin, total protein, prealbumin, serum transferrin, total lipid count, oral or cutaneous signs of vitamin or mineral deficiencies

Diagnostic tests
Complete blood count, serum chemistry

(Text continues on page 222.)

CLINICAL PATHWAY

PLAN OF CARE	PREADMIT PHASE	INPATIENT CARE Day 1
DIAGNOSTIC TESTS	• Complete blood count (CBC) with differential, electrolytes, hemoglobin (Hgb), fasting blood sugar (FBS), albumin, total lymphocyte count (TLC), transferrin	• CBC with differential, electrolytes, Hgb, FBS, albumin, TLC, transferrin • Electrocardiogram • Urine culture and sensitivity, osmolarity • Chest X-ray
MEDICATIONS	• Assess current prescription and over-the-counter (OTC) medications	• Multivitamin every day • Antispasmodic in spinal cord–injured patients
PROCEDURES	• Take baseline vital signs (VS). • Assess skin.	• Perform PU risk assessment, using a valid risk assessment scale. • Check VS q 4 hr. *PU care:* • Clean PU and surrounding skin with mild soap and lukewarm water, rinse well, and pat dry. • Gently apply silicone-based lotion or lubricant (do not massage red areas) or protect reddened area with one or combination of: – thin coat of skin sealant applied in two to three layers and allowed to dry thoroughly between layers – transparent film dressing changed q 5 to 7 days or if dislodged – thin hydrocolloid dressing changed q 5 to 7 days or if dislodged (if sacral PU, windowpane with micropore tape). • Avoid massage over bony prominences. • Manage pain by covering the wound, repositioning, and analgesics. *Managing tissue loads:* • Avoid positioning on PU and using donut ring devices. • Use positioning device to raise PU off surface (head, heel). • Post written repositioning schedule. • Avoid positioning immobile patients on trochanters or ischial tuberosities. • Prevent direct contact between bony prominences (knees, ankles). • Do not raise head of bed (HOB) > 30 degrees unless contraindicated by medical condition, or tube feeding. • Limit lateral position to < 30 degrees • Reposition bed-bound patients at least q 2 hr, chair-bound patients hourly. • Teach chair-bound patients to shift weight q 15 min. • Have patient perform range-of-motion (ROM) exercises q 4 hr while awake. • Support feet with foot board. • Lift patient; avoid pulling or sliding. *Support surfaces:* • Implement pressure-reducing support surface based on patient's risk for developing PU: – comfort only and no risk: sheepskin, high-density or 3" to 4" (7.5- to 10-cm) convoluted foam – medium risk: air-filled static or alternating-pressure overlay or pads – high risk: low air-loss bed, dynamic flotation mattress – ultra-high risk: air-fluidized bead bed. • Provide pressure-reducing cushion for chair-bound patients.
DIET	• Assess current diet. • Take baseline weight.	• Give diet high in protein and calories unless contraindicated. • Ensure adequate hydration (about 2.5 qt [2.5L]/day unless contraindicated). • Assess skin turgor and mucous membranes. • Weigh patient.

Day 2	Days 3 to 6
• As indicated	• As indicated
• Same as Day 1	• Same as Day 1
• Complete focused physical assessment daily, including VS, level of consciousness, and mental status. • Perform comprehensive PU status assessment daily. • Check VS q 8 hr. *PU care:* • Same as Day 1 • Evaluate dressing; change as needed. *Managing tissue loads:* • Provide same care as Day 1; increase turning schedule if areas of skin color change do not disappear in 1 hour. *Support surfaces:* • Assess patient response to pressure reduction measures. • Check that support surface is not "bottoming out."	• Same as Day 2
• Same as Day 1	• Same as Day 1 • Assess nutritional status at least every 3 months.

(continued)

PLAN OF CARE	PREADMIT PHASE	INPATIENT CARE *Day 1*
ACTIVITY	• Assess activity level, ability to assist in moving self, contractures, and joint pain.	• Ambulatory: Encourage patient to walk t.i.d. • Ambulatory with assistance: Reposition and encourage repositioning in bed or chair. – Assist patient to walk t.i.d. • Up in chair with assistance: Assist patient to get up in chair b.i.d. to t.i.d. – Assist patient to perform ROM exercises. – Encourage patient to shift weight q 15 min when up in chair. – Change patient position hourly when in chair. – Cover chair with sheet or blanket. • Immobile or bed-bound: Assist patient to perform ROM exercises q 4 hr while awake. – Assist patient to turn, cough, and deep breathe (TCDB) q 2 hr. – Position patient in alignment, with body weight evenly distributed. – Encourage patient to perform active or passive ROM, stretching, isometric, or light weight-training exercises.
ELIMINATION	• Assess elimination pattern, laxative intake, and previous bowel, bladder, or kidney surgery.	• Keep skin clean and dry. • Apply moisture barrier after each voiding and bowel movement. • Assess for and treat incontinence. • Assess need for male external catheter, fecal pouch, antidiarrheal medication, and disimpaction. • Use reusable underpads. • Establish voiding schedule. • Measure intake and output.
HYGIENE	• Assess self-care ability, cleanliness, grooming needs, and body odor.	• Provide complete care or assist as needed. • Inspect skin and bony prominences daily. • Keep skin clean with mild soap and lukewarm water, rinse well, and pat dry. • Avoid hot water and excessive friction. • Apply humectants, emollients, or moisturizers for dry skin.
PATIENT TEACHING	• Assess cognition, memory, and understanding. • Teach prevention of pressure ulcers (PUs). • Teach treatment of PUs.	• Orient to hospital routines and unit. • Initiate PU teaching to patient and family. • Involve patient and family in care planning.
DISCHARGE PLANNING	• Assess support systems.	*Social services consult:* • Assess need for home health nursing, home health aide, physical therapy, or nursing home care.

• Same as Day 1	• Same as Day 1

• Same as Day 1	• Same as Day 1

• Same as Day 1	• Same as Day 1

• Evaluate learning. • Evaluate caregiver's understanding of care.	• Instruct patient and family on preventive measures, and assess ongoing need for change in plan of care and need for new teaching.

Social services: • Arrange for home health care, durable medication equipment, and supplies, or arrange for nursing home referral.	*Social services:* • Notify home health agency or nursing home of PU treatment and prevention plan; arrange for patient transfer.

(continued)

PLAN OF CARE	HOME CARE *Visit 1*	*Visit 2*	*Visit 3*
DIAGNOSTIC TESTS	• Review recent hospital laboratory data; draw blood for complete blood count, electrolytes.	• Draw blood for fasting blood sugar.	• Review results of lab work with patient and family.
MEDICATIONS	• Multivitamin supplement daily	• Same as first visit	• Same as first visit
PROCEDURES	• Perform complete admission history and physical assessment to establish baseline data. • Complete initial wound assessment, and document location, size, color, edges, exudate, peri-wound skin color, temperature, edema, maceration, induration, blisters, pain. • Manage pressure ulcer (PU) pain with wound covering, repositioning, and analgesics. • Instruct caregiver and patient to keep pain log using pain scale and to record pain intensity and effect of dressing, turning, and medication. • Mutually establish treatment goals with caregiver and patient.	• Perform comprehensive PU assessment, including ongoing assessment for complications and monitoring for worsening of PU. • Complete wound assessment. • Evaluate PU pain management. • Check vital signs and mental status. • Review treatment goals and document progress in meeting goal.	• Same as previous visit • Assess skin over bony prominences for signs and symptoms of tissue breakdown. • Revise goals as needed; document progress in meeting goals. • Reevaluate effectiveness of pain management; adjust plan as necessary.
DIET	• Assess current diet, fluid intake, appetite, and feeding ability. • Encourage diet high in protein and calories unless contraindicated. • Ensure adequate fluids to about 2.5 qt (2.5L)/day unless contraindicated. • Assess skin turgor and mucous membranes • Take baseline weight.	• Same as first visit • Initiate food and fluid intake record. • Weigh patient.	• Same as previous visit • Assess adequacy of intake. • Initiate dietary consult as needed. • Report significant unexpected weight gain or loss over time (change up or down of 3 lb/wk) to doctor.
ACTIVITY	• Assess activity level and safety: ability to ambulate and assist moving self in bed, and chair. • Assess for contractures, joint mobility, and pain. • Evaluate home environment for safety; teach measures to prevent falls. • Evaluate need for assistive devices. • Encourage patient to perform exercise regimen: active or passive range of motion (ROM), stretching, isometric, or light weight training. • Confirm assessments and initiate physical therapy (PT) consult as needed.	• Assess caregiver and patient compliance.	• Assess patient's and caregiver's understanding of PU prevention regimen. • Initiate PT consult as needed. • Assess caregiver and patient compliance.
ELIMINATION	• Assess elimination pattern, laxative use, and incontinence. • Initiate instruction on skin care following voiding and bowel movement (BM) • Keep skin clean and dry. • Apply moisture barrier after each voiding or BM. • Assess and treat incontinence. • Assess need for male external catheter, fecal pouch, antidiarrheal medication, or disimpaction. • Use reusable (not disposable) underpads. • Establish voiding schedule.	• Continue to instruct patient and caregiver on skin care following BM or voiding.	• Evaluate effectiveness of caregiver, patient, and home health aide (HHA) implementation of skin protection following BM and voiding.
HYGIENE	• Assess self-care ability, cleanliness, grooming needs, and body odor.	• Assess skin for dryness, cleanliness, intactness, rashes, color changes, and itching.	• Same as previous visit • Evaluate effectiveness of skin care regimen in maintaining skin cleanliness and integrity.
PATIENT TEACHING	• Orient to home health care agency and services. • Involve caregiver, patient, and family in ongoing care planning and meeting treatment goals. • Initiate PU teaching: risk factors, prevention, staging, prevention of infection, care, healing.	• Teach importance of regular follow-up visits with health care providers; continue PU teaching. • Review wound care teaching with caregiver and patient.	• Document patient's and caregiver's understanding and performance.

Pressure ulcer (stage I) *(continued)*

CLINICAL PATHWAY

PLAN OF CARE	HOME CARE

HOME CARE

Visit 1 | *Visit 2* | *Visit 3*

PATIENT TEACHING
(continued)

Visit 1

PU care:
- Teach caregiver to clean PU and surrounding skin with mild soap and lukewarm water, rinse well, and pat dry.
- Teach caregiver to gently apply silicone-based lotion or lubricant or to protect PU with one or combination of:
  – thin coat of skin sealant applied in two to three layers and allowed to dry thoroughly between layers
  – transparent film dressing changed q 5 to 7 days or if dislodged
  – thin hydrocolloid dressing changed q 5 to 7days or if dislodged (if sacral PU, windowpane with micropore tape).
- Tell caregiver and patient to avoid massage over bony prominences.
- Warn caregiver not to use occlusive dressing if PU is infected.
Managing tissue loads:
- Provide written instructions to:
  – avoid positioning on PU and donut ring devices
  – use positioning device to raise PU off surface (head, heel)
  – post written repositioning schedule
  – avoid positioning immobile patients on trochanters or ischial tuberosities
  – prevent direct contact of bony prominences (knees, ankles) by padding with a pillow or blanket.
- Do not raise head of bed > 30 degrees unless contraindicated by medication, condition, or tube feeding.
- Limit lateral position to < 30 degrees
- Reposition bed-bound patients at least q 2 hr, chair-bound patients hourly.
- Teach chair-bound patients to shift weight q 15 min.
- Have patient do ROM exercises q 4 hr while awake.
- Have patient support feet with foot board.
- Lift patient; avoid pulling or sliding
- Manage moisture, perspiration, and humidity.
Support surfaces:
- Work with caregiver, patient, and payer for reimbursement of medically necessary equipment.
- Teach need for pressure-reducing support surface based on patient condition and risk for developing PU:
  – comfort only or no risk: sheepskin, high-density convoluted foam
  – medium risk: air-filled static or alternating-pressure overlay or pads
  – high risk: low air-loss bed, dynamic flotation mattress
  – ultra-high risk: air-fluidized bead bed.
- Provide pressure-reducing cushion for chair-bound patients.
- Initiate teaching to prevent additional PUs or worsening of current PU.
- Instruct patient who can walk on importance of ambulating in home at least t.i.d.
- Teach caregiver or home health aide (HHA) to help patient who can walk with assistance with walking t.i.d.
- Teach caregiver or HHA to reposition patient and encourage repositioning in bed and chair.

Visit 2

- Provide caregiver and patient with written PU care instructions.
- Review teaching related to PU stages, risk factors, conditions necessary for healing (nutrients, fluid, pressure relief, uninfected wound, correct dressing changed as often as necessary).
- Evaluate patient and caregiver learning with return demonstration.
Managing tissue loads:
- Assess caregiver and patient understanding of moisture, pressure, friction, and shear in PU etiology.
- Assess caregiver and patient ability to reduce and distribute tissue loading.
Support surfaces:
- Same as first visit
- Assess patient's and caregiver's comprehension, follow-through, and compliance with teaching.

Visit 3

Managing tissue loads:
- Assess patient care and caregiver competence and understanding.
Support surfaces:
- Same as previous visit
- Initiate support surface intervention.
- Evaluate ongoing effectiveness of pressure reduction in PU prevention.

(continued)

PLAN OF CARE	HOME CARE Visit 1	Visit 2	Visit 3
PATIENT TEACHING (continued)	▪ Teach caregiver or HHA of patient who gets up in chair with assistance about complete ROM exercises b.i.d. to q.i.d. ▪ Teach patient to shift weight q 15 min when up in chair. ▪ Teach caregiver or HHA to change patient's position hourly when in chair. ▪ Cover chair with sheet or blanket. ▪ Teach caregiver or HHA of patient who is immobile or on bed rest to have patient complete ROM exercises q 4 hr while awake. ▪ Teach patient to turn, cough, and deep breathe q 2 hr. ▪ Teach caregiver or HHA to position patient in alignment, with body weight evenly distributed. ▪ Teach caregiver or patient individualized bathing schedule and routine: – keep skin clean with mild soap and lukewarm water; rinse well, and pat dry – avoid hot water and excessive friction – apply humectants, emollients, or moisturizers for dry skin – apply cornstarch or powder between skin folds; wash skin folds twice daily.	▪ Evaluate teaching effectiveness. ▪ Answer patient's, caregiver's, and family's questions. ▪ Continue teaching caregiver and patient PU care and prevention.	▪ Instruct patient and family in preventive measures, and assess ongoing need for change in plan of care and need for new or additional teaching. ▪ Evaluate caregiver, patient, and HHA implementation of skin care regimen. ▪ Assess resources: availability and skill of caregiver, patient understanding, equipment needs.
DISCHARGE PLANNING	▪ Assess need for HHA; wound, ostomy, continence (WOC) nurse; nutritionist; social service; and physical therapist. ▪ Arrange HHA visit. ▪ Assess resources, including availability and skill of caregiver, patient understanding, and equipment needs.	▪ Assess caregiver's need for rest and sleep and ability to provide care. ▪ Discuss HHA service.	▪ Determine progress toward meeting goals of care. ▪ Establish plan for remainder of "healing time." ▪ Evaluate HHA care.

Related nursing diagnoses

1 Impaired skin integrity
2 Risk for impaired skin integrity
3 Impaired tissue integrity
4 Risk for infection
5 Altered nutrition: less than body requirements
6 Altered nutrition: more than body requirements
7 Impaired physical mobility
8 Pain
9 Self-care deficit (bathing/hygiene, feeding, dressing/grooming, or toileting)
10 Knowledge deficit
11 Ineffective management of therapeutic regimen (community, family, or individual)

Expected outcomes

The following expected outcomes pertain to the patient or family. Numbers in parentheses refer to related nursing diagnoses above.

▪ Demonstrate healing of PU within reasonable time frame depending on PU size, patient condition, and presence or absence of PU complications (1,3).

- Demonstrate uncomplicated healing of PU without development of wound infection (4).
- Have skin remain intact without development of PUs, discoloration, induration, pallor, or mottling (2).
- Demonstrate adequate nutrition to compensate for wound fluid losses and to support wound healing (5,6).
- Demonstrate use of adaptive devices to increase mobility and manage tissue loads (7).
- Report an increase in muscle strength and endurance (7).
- Describe measures that decrease pain (8).
- Report decreased pain intensity (8).
- Perform activities of daily living at expected optimal level or report satisfaction with outcomes when assistance required (9).
- Identify PU causative factors, preventive measures, and rationale for treatment regimen (10,11).
- Participate in and demonstrate understanding of interdisciplinary treatment plan: PU care and prevention, nutrition and fluid requirements, skin care, prevention of wound infection, support surfaces and managing tissue loads, turning and repositioning schedule, and pain management (10,11).
- Express understanding of and satisfaction with postdischarge care plan (10,11).

Other possible nursing diagnoses

Altered peripheral tissue perfusion, sensory-perceptual alteration (tactile), impaired memory, incontinence

Potential complications

Sepsis, opportunistic infection, osteomyelitis, cellulitis

Patient teaching

Risk factors
- Extrinsic predisposing factors: unrelieved pressure on vulnerable areas, moisture or excessive perspiration, friction, shear, inappropriate positioning, poor lifting and moving techniques
- Intrinsic predisposing factors: malnutrition (overweight or underweight), immunosuppression, altered mental status, weakness or debility, incontinence, immobility or paralysis, decreased sensation, chronic diseases (cancer, stroke, anemia, diabetes, peripheral vascular disease, cardiac disease, atherosclerosis), fever, and age over 65 years

Signs and symptoms
- Define PU as an area of skin or lower tissues where blood flow has been blocked by unrelieved pressure that has caused tissue to die.
- Explain that PUs occur over bony areas: tailbone, hips, buttocks, heels, ankles, elbows, knees.
- Teach patient and family early signs of skin breakdown: blanchable redness, warmth, discomfort, or pain. Tell darkly pigmented patients to assess for darker areas of skin tone using a halogen or natural light.
- Notify health care provider if signs and symptoms of infection occur: chills, fever, increase in drainage, foul odor, pus, increase in pain, redness, swelling.

Stages
- Stage I: changes in skin color (red, blue, purple) and warmth that does not go away when pressure is relieved; the first sign that a deeper PU is possible; painful; usually occurs over a bony prominence
- Stage II: a superficial break in the skin that appears as an abrasion, blister, or shallow crater; results when unrelieved pressure causes the skin to die; painful; can become infected

(Text continues on page 230.)

PLAN OF CARE	PREADMIT PHASE	INPATIENT CARE *Day 1*
DIAGNOSTIC TESTS	Complete blood count (CBC) with differential, electrolytes, hemoglobin (Hgb), fasting blood sugar (FBS), albumin, total lymphocyte count (TLC), transferrin	• CBC with differential, electrolytes, Hgb, FBS, albumin, TLC, transferrin • Electrocardiogram • Urine culture and sensitivity, osmolarity • Chest X-ray
MEDICATIONS	• Assess current prescription and over-the-counter (OTC) medications.	• Multivitamin every day • Antispasmodic in spinal cord–injured patients
PROCEDURES	• Take baseline vital signs (VS). • Assess skin.	• Perform pressure ulcer (PU) risk assessment, using valid PU risk assessment sca • Check VS q 4 hr. *PU care:* • Clean PU and surrounding skin gently with normal saline solution (NSS); pat pe wound skin dry. • Select dressing that will keep wound moist, exudate controlled, and periwound skin dry. • Cover PU with transparent film, polyurethane foam, or hydrocolloid dressing; change q 3 to 7 days if leaking or dislodged or according to wound care produ manufacturer directive. • Avoid massage over bony prominences. • Avoid occlusive dressing if PU is infected. • Measure wound weekly; take picture with grid if available. • Manage pain by covering wound, repositioning, and analgesics. *Managing tissue loads:* • Avoid positioning on PU and using donut ring devices. • Use positioning device to raise PU off surface (head, heel). • Post written repositioning schedule. • Avoid positioning immobile patients on trochanters or ischial tuberosities. • Prevent direct contact between bony prominences (knees, ankles). • Do not raise head of bed > 30 degrees unless contraindicated by medical cond or tube feeding. • Limit lateral position to < 30 degrees. • Reposition bed-bound patients at least q 2 hr, chair-bound patients hourly. • Teach chair-bound patients to shift weight q 15 min. • Have patient perform range-of-motion (ROM) exercises q 4 hr while awake. • Support feet with foot board. • Lift patient; avoid pulling or sliding. *Support surfaces:* • Implement pressure-reducing support surface based on risk for developing PL – comfort only and no risk: sheepskin, high-density or 3″ to 4″ (7.5- to 10-cm) voluted foam – medium risk: air-filled static or alternating-pressure overlay or pads – high risk: low air-loss bed, dynamic flotation mattress – ultra-high risk: air-fluidized bead bed. • Provide pressure-reducing cushion for chair-bound patients. *Wound, ostomy, continence (WOC) nurse consult:* • Consider electrical stimulation in nonhealing, clean PU receiving correct care unless contraindicated.
DIET	• Assess current diet and oral intake.	• Give diet high in protein and calories unless contraindicated. • Ensure adequate hydration (about 2.5 qt (2.5 L)/day unless contraindicated. • Consult dietitian. • Assess skin turgor and mucous membranes. • Weigh patient.

Day 2	Days 3 to 6
- As indicated	- As indicated
- Same as Day 1	- Same as Day 1
- Perform focused physical assessment every day, including VS, level of consciousness, and mental status. - Check VS q 8 hr. - Perform comprehensive PU status assessment every day. *PU care:* - Same as Day 1 - Evaluate dressing for intactness; change as needed. *Managing tissue loads:* - Provide same care as Day 1; increase turning schedule if areas of skin color change do not disappear in 1 hour. *Support surfaces:* - Assess patient response to pressure reduction measures.	- Check VS q 8 hr. *PU care:* - Same as Day 2 *Managing tissue loads:* - Same as Day 2 *Support surfaces:* - Same as Day 2
- Same as Day 1	- Same as Day 1

(continued)

PLAN OF CARE	PREADMIT PHASE	INPATIENT CARE *Day 1*
ACTIVITY	• Assess activity level, ability to assist in moving self, contractures, and joint pain.	*Physical therapy (PT) consult:* • Ambulatory: Encourage patients to walk t.i.d. • Ambulatory with assistance: Assist patient to walk t.i.d. – Reposition or encourage repositioning in bed or chair. • Up in chair with assistance: Assist patient to perform ROM exercises and shift weight q 15 min when up in chair. – Change patient's position hourly when in chair. – Cover chair with sheet or blanket. • Immobile/Bed rest: Encourage patients to perform ROM exercises q 4 hr while awake. – Assist patient to turn, cough, and deep breathe (TCDB) q 2 hr. – Position patient in alignment with body weight evenly distributed. – Encourage patient to perform exercise regimen: active or passive ROM, stretching, isometric, or light weight-training exercises.
ELIMINATION	• Assess elimination pattern, laxative intake, and previous bowel, bladder, and kidney surgery.	• Keep skin clean and dry. • Apply moisture barrier after each voiding or bowel movement. • Assess and treat incontinence. • Assess need for male external catheter, fecal pouch, antidiarrheal medication, or disimpaction. • Use reusable underpads. • Establish voiding schedule. • Measure intake and output.
HYGIENE	• Assess self-care ability, cleanliness, grooming needs, and body odor.	• Provide complete care or assist as needed. • Inspect skin and bony prominences daily. • Keep skin clean with mild soap and lukewarm water; rinse well, and pat dry. • Avoid hot water and excessive friction. • Apply humectants, emollients, or moisturizers for dry skin.
PATIENT TEACHING	• Assess cognition, memory, and understanding. • Teach need for inpatient care.	• Orient to hospital routines and unit. • Initiate PU teaching to patient or family. • Involve patient or family in care planning.
DISCHARGE PLANNING	• Evaluate social support.	*Social services consult:* • Assess need for home health nursing, home health aide, PT, or nursing home care.

Day 2	Days 3 to 6
• Same as Day 1	• Same as Day 1
• Same as Day 1	• Same as Day 1
• Same as Day 1	• Same as Day 1
• Continue PU teaching. • Evaluate teaching effectiveness. • Answer patient's or family's questions.	• Same as Day 2
Social services: • Arrange for home health care, durable medication equipment, and supplies, or arrange for nursing home referral.	*Social services*: • Notify home health agency or nursing home of PU treatment and prevention plan; arrange for patient transfer.

(continued)

CLINICAL PATHWAY ■ Pressure ulcer (stage II) *(continued)*

PLAN OF CARE	HOME CARE Visit 1	Visit 2	Visit 3
DIAGNOSTIC TESTS	▪ Review recent hospital laboratory data; draw blood for complete blood count and electrolytes.	▪ Draw blood for fasting blood sugar.	▪ Review results of lab work with patient or family
MEDICATIONS	▪ Multivitamin supplement daily	▪ Same as first visit	▪ Same as first visit
PROCEDURES	▪ Perform complete admission history and physical assessment to establish baseline data. ▪ Complete initial wound assessment, and document location, size, color, edges, exudate, peri-wound skin color, temperature, edema, maceration, induration, blisters, and pain. ▪ Mutually establish treatment goals with caregiver or patient. ▪ Manage PU pain by covering wound, repositioning, and analgesics. ▪ Instruct caregiver or patient to keep pain log using a pain scale to record pain intensity and effect of dressing, turning, and medication.	▪ Perform focused physical assessment, including vital signs and mental status. ▪ Perform comprehensive PU assessment, including ongoing assessment for complications and monitoring for worsening of PU: increase in wound drainage, change in character or color of wound drainage (purulent yellow or green, sanguineous), increase in wound size. ▪ Review treatment goals and document progress in meeting goals.	▪ Evaluate PU pain management; adjust plan as necessary ▪ Same as Visit 2
DIET	▪ Assess current diet, fluid intake, appetite, and ability to feed self. ▪ Give diet high in protein and calories unless contraindicated. ▪ Ensure adequate fluids to approximately 2.5 qt (2.5 L)/day unless contraindicated. ▪ Assess skin turgor and mucous membranes. ▪ Take baseline weight.	▪ Same as first visit ▪ Initiate food or fluid intake record. ▪ Weigh patient.	▪ Assess adequacy of intake. ▪ Initiate dietary consult as needed. ▪ Report significant unexpected weight loss or gain over time and vitamin or mineral deficiencies.
ACTIVITY	▪ Assess activity level and safety: ability to ambulate and assist moving self into bed and chair. ▪ Assess for contractures, joint mobility, and pain. ▪ Evaluate home environment for safety; teach measures to prevent falls. ▪ Evaluate need for assistive devices. ▪ Encourage patient to perform exercise regimen: stretching, isometric exercises, or light weight-training.	▪ Confirm assessments and initiate physical therapy (PT) consult as needed. ▪ Assess caregiver or patient compliance.	▪ Assess patient's or caregiver's understanding of PU prevention regimen. ▪ Initiate PT consult as needed. ▪ Assess caregiver or patient compliance.
ELIMINATION	▪ Assess elimination pattern, laxative use, and incontinence. ▪ Initiate instruction on skin care following voiding or bowel movement (BM): ▪ Keep skin clean and dry. ▪ Apply moisture barrier after each voiding or BM. ▪ Assess and treat incontinence. ▪ Assess need for male external catheter, fecal pouch, antidiarrheal medication, or disimpaction. ▪ Use reusable (not disposable) underpads. ▪ Establish voiding schedule. ▪ Measure intake and output (I & O).	▪ Continue instructing patient or caregiver on skin care after voiding or BM. ▪ Evaluate skin care regimen after voiding or BM. ▪ Measure I & O.	▪ Evaluate effectiveness of caregiver, patient, and home health aide (HHA) implementation of skin protection following BM and voiding. ▪ Evaluate effectiveness of voiding schedule. ▪ Measure I & O.
HYGIENE	▪ Assess self-care ability, cleanliness, grooming needs, and body odor.	▪ Assess skin for dryness, cleanliness, intactness, rash, color changes, and itching.	▪ Same as previous visit ▪ Evaluate effectiveness of skin care regimen.

PLAN OF CARE	HOME CARE Visit 1	Visit 2	Visit 3
PATIENT TEACHING	• Orient to home health care agency and services. • Involve caregiver, patient, or family in ongoing care planning and meeting treatment goals. • Initiate PU teaching: risk factors, prevention, staging, prevention of infection, care, and healing. *PU care:* • Begin teaching by having caregiver observe care and hear explanations. • Teach caregiver to clean PU and surrounding skin with saline solution and pat periwound skin dry. • Teach caregiver to gently apply silicone-based lotion or lubricant without massage and to protect discolored skin areas with one or combination of: – thin coat of skin sealant, applied in two to three layers and allowed to dry thoroughly between layers – transparent film dressing, changed q 5 to 7 days or if dislodged – thin hydrocolloid dressing, changed q 5 to 7 days or if dislodged (if sacral PU, windowpane with micropore tape). • Tell caregiver and patient to avoid massage over bony prominences. • Warn caregiver not to use occlusive dressing if PU is infected. *Managing tissue loads:* • Provide written instructions to: – avoid positioning on PU and donut ring devices. – use positioning device to raise PU off surface (head, heel). – post written repositioning schedule. – avoid positioning immobile patients on trochanters, ischial tuberosities. – prevent direct contact of bony prominences (knees, ankles) by padding with pillow or blanket. • Do not raise head of bed > 30 degrees unless contraindicated by medication, condition, or tube feeding. • Limit lateral position to < 30 degrees. • Reposition bed-bound patients at least q 2 hr, chair-bound patients hourly. • Teach chair-bound patients to shift weight q 15 min. • Have patient do ROM exercises q 4 hr while awake. • Have patient support feet with foot board. • Lift patient; avoid pulling or sliding • Manage moisture, perspiration, and humidity. *Support surfaces:* • Work with caregiver, patient, and payer for reimbursement of medically necessary equipment. • Teach need for pressure-reducing support surface based on patient condition and risk for developing PU: – comfort only or no risk: sheepskin, high-density convoluted foam – medium risk: air-filled static or alternating-pressure overlay or pads – high risk: low air-loss bed, dynamic flotation mattress – ultra-high risk: air-fluidized bead bed. • Provide pressure-reducing cushion for chair-bound patients. • Initiate teaching to prevent additional PUs or worsening of current PU.	• Teach importance of regular follow-up visits with health care providers; reinforce PU teaching. • Implement further wound care teaching to caregiver and patient. • Provide caregiver or patient with written PU care instructions. • Begin teaching related to PU stages, risk factors, conditions necessary for healing (nutrients, fluid, pressure relief, uninfected wound, correct dressing changed as often as necessary). *Managing tissue loads:* • Assess caregiver's or patient's understanding of moisture, pressure, friction, and shear in PU etiology. • Assess caregiver's or patient's ability to reduce and distribute tissue loading. *Support surfaces:* • Assess comprehension, follow-through, and compliance. • Review bathing schedule and routine with caregiver and patient.	• Evaluate teaching. • Answer patient's, caregiver's, or family's questions. • Continue teaching caregiver and patient PU care and prevention. • Document patient's or caregiver's understanding and performance. *Managing tissue loads:* • Assess patient care and caregiver competence and understanding. *Support surfaces:* • Initiate support surface intervention. • Continue ongoing evaluation of effectiveness of pressure reduction in PU prevention. • Instruct in preventive measures, and assess ongoing need for change in plan of care and need for additional or new teaching. • Evaluate caregiver or patient comprehension, follow-through, and compliance with teaching.

(continued)

PLAN OF CARE	HOME CARE Visit 1	Visit 2	Visit 3
PATIENT TEACHING *(continued)*	• Instruct patient who can walk on importance of ambulating in home at least t.i.d. • Teach caregiver or home health aide (HHA) to help patient who can walk with assistance to walk t.i.d. • Teach caregiver or HHA to reposition patient and encourage repositioning in bed and chair. • Teach caregiver or HHA of patient who gets up in chair with assistance about complete ROM exercises t.i.d. to q.i.d. • Teach patient to shift weight q 15 min when up in chair. • Teach caregiver or HHA to change patient position hourly when in chair. • Cover chair with sheet or blanket. • Teach caregiver or HHA of patients who are immobile or need bed rest to encourage patient to complete ROM exercises q 4 hr while awake. • Teach patient to turn, cough, and deep breathe q 2 hr. • Teach caregiver or HHA to position patient in alignment, with body weight evenly distributed • Teach caregiver or patient about individual bathing schedule and routine: – keep skin clean with mild soap and lukewarm water; rinse well, and pat dry – avoid hot water and excessive friction – apply humectants, emollients, or moisturizers for dry skin – apply cornstarch or powder between skin folds; wash skin folds b.i.d.		
DISCHARGE PLANNING	• Assess resources: availability and skill of caregiver, patient understanding, equipment needs and finances. • Assess need for HHA; wound, ostomy, continence (WOC) nurse; nutritionist; social service; and physical therapist (PT). • Arrange HHA visit.	• Assess caregiver's need for rest and sleep and ability to provide care. • Discuss HHA service.	• Evaluate HHA care. • Determine progress toward meeting goals of care.

• Stage III : a deep ulcer due to the death of skin and fatty tissue from pressure that extends down to the muscle; may be covered with a hard black, dead crust; easily infected
• Stage IV: a very deep ulcer with extensive destruction and death of tissue that extends down through muscle into bone; drains much fluid and may cause a generalized infection

Healing and treatment
• Explain the need for adequate nutrition and fluids; a clean, moist, uninfected wound; the correct dressing changed as frequently as needed; pressure relief obtained through a combination of a turning schedule, positioning, and pressure-reducing support surface.
• Explain the goals of the PU treatment plan: to promote healing within expected time frame, to prevent deterioration of the ulcer, to prevent occurrence of new ulcer.
• Correct patient factors that interfere with wound healing.
• Involve patient and family in PU care and preventive program.

Medications
- Debriding agents
- Systemic and topical antibiotics
- Vitamin and mineral supplements
- Products that stimulate tissue growth and wound healing

Assessment and care
- Describe general PU assessment parameters: stage, size, drainage, pain, healing, wound tissue color description (red, yellow, or black).
- Describe procedures to prevent and control infection: hand washing; clean, dry bed linens and clothes; cleaning, irrigating, and packing solutions; disposal of soiled dressing; call about or change dressing if soiled, leaking, or displaced.
- Explain purpose and type of dressing(s), packing, and frequency of dressing change.
- Describe debridement purpose and method(s), and tell patient that stable heel ulcers with dry eschar need not be debrided.
- Tell how to protect reddened areas with 2 or 3 coats of thin skin sealant, dry thoroughly between coats; use transparent film dressing or thin hydrocolloid dressing.
- Explain to patient and caregivers rationale for not massaging over bony prominences.
- Teach how to maintain skin care, and prevent friction and shear.
- Tell patient to eat a diet high in protein and calories that promotes healing.

Roles of interdisciplinary team
- Wound, ostomy, and continence nurse
- Physical therapist
- Dietitian
- Surgeon
- Clinical nurse specialist
- Home health nurse, home health aide
- Occupational therapist
- Social worker

Preventing recurrence
- Establish individualized skin care protocol.
- Inspect skin daily, especially over bony prominences.
- Maintain clean, dry, supple skin.
- Apply moisture barrier after each voiding or bowel movement.
- Wash moist areas of perineum, axilla, and under breasts twice a day.
- Use mild soap and tepid water; rinse well; pat skin dry.
- Apply lotion or cream after bathing.
- Use reusable (not disposable) underpads.
- Apply male external catheter as needed.
- Apply fecal containment device as needed.
- Prevent urinary and fecal incontinence.
- Keep sheets and clothes wrinkle-free.

Pressure reduction
- Establish and post written turning schedule.
- Do not massage over bony prominences.
- Avoid donut ring devices.
- Use device to raise heels off surface at all times.
- Place pillow between legs and ankles.

(Text continues on page 247.)

Pressure ulcer (stage III)

PLAN OF CARE	PREADMIT PHASE	INPATIENT CARE Day 1
DIAGNOSTIC TESTS	• Complete blood count (CBC) with differential, electrolytes, hemoglobin (Hgb), fasting blood sugar (FBS), albumin, total lymphocyte count (TLC), transferrin	• CBC with differential, electrolytes, Hgb, FBS, albumin, TLC, transferrin • Electrocardiogram • Urine culture and sensitivity, osmolarity • Chest X-ray • Vitamin C, A, B assay; zinc, magnesium, iron assay • Blood and wound fluid cultures and Gram stains • PU tissue biopsy • Evaluate patient for osteomyelitis in nonhealing PUs: white blood cell count, erythrocyte sedimentation rate, X-ray
MEDICATIONS	• Assess current prescription and over-the-counter (OTC) medications	• High-potency vitamin and mineral supplement daily if deficient • Antispasmodic in spinal cord–injured patient • Systemic antibiotics and noncytotoxic topical antiseptics • No topical antibiotics or antiseptics in clean wounds • Systemic antibiotic therapy in patients with bacteremia, sepsis, advancing cellulitis, or osteomyelitis
PROCEDURES	• Take baseline vital signs (VS). • Assess skin and pressure ulcer (PU). • Signs and symptoms (S/S) of wound infection	• Perform comprehensive history and physical assessment. • Check VS q 4 hr. • Perform PU risk assessment using valid PU risk assessment scale. • Perform comprehensive PU status assessment daily. • Select dressing that will keep wound moist, exudate controlled, and periwound skin dry. • Avoid massage over bony prominences. *PU care:* • Debride necrotic tissue using surgical, sharp, autolytic, enzymatic, or mechanical means. • Clean PU and surrounding skin gently with normal saline solution (NSS); pat periwound skin dry. • Irrigate wound, undermining, and tunnels with NSS using 35-ml syringe with 19G angiocath. • Loosely fill dead space, undermining, and tunnels with saline- or gel-moistened gauze. • Manage exudate with absorbent dressing (moist gauze, calcium alginate, foam, hydrocolloid, paste or granules, copolymer starch). • Apply secondary cover dressing. • Depending on type of dressing, change daily to t.i.d. as needed to prevent strikethrough, leakage, and skin maceration. • Monitor dressing near anus for rolled edges. *Infected PU care:* • Avoid occlusive dressing if PU is infected. • Clean wound and surrounding skin with NSS; pat skin dry. • Irrigate wound, undermining, and tunnels with NSS using 35-ml syringe with 19G angiocath. • Loosely pack wound, undermining, and tunnels with gauze moistened with noncytotoxic concentration of topical antiseptic. • Cover with secondary dressing. • Depending on type of dressing, change daily to t.i.d. as needed to prevent strikethrough, leakage, and skin maceration. • Consider whirlpool b.i.d. for PUs with thick exudate, slough, or necrotic tissue. *Managing tissue loads:* • Avoid positioning on PU and using donut ring devices. • Use positioning device to raise PU off surface (head, heel). • Post written repositioning schedule. • Avoid positioning immobile patients on trochanters or ischial tuberosities. • Prevent direct contact between bony prominences (knees, ankles). • Do not raise head of bed > 30 degrees unless contraindicated by medical condition or tube feeding. • Limit lateral position to < 30 degrees. • Reposition bed-bound patients at least q 2 hr, chair-bound patients hourly. • Teach chair-bound patients to shift weight q 15 min. • Have patient perform range-of-motion (ROM) exercises q 4 hr while awake. • Support patient's feet with foot board.

Day 2	Days 3 to 6
• Sinography (sinus tract) • Urine urea nitrogen • Creatinine height index • 24-hour creatinine	• Repeat CBC with differential, electrolytes, and FBS as necessary
• Same as Day 1	• Same as Day 1 • Monitor for S/S of secondary infection: diarrhea, nausea, and rash; medicate as appropriate
• Perform physical assessment every day, including VS, level of consciousness, and mental status. • Check vital signs q 4 hr. • Provide comprehensive PU status assessment daily. *PU care:* • Same as Day 1 • Evaluate dressing for intactness; change daily to t.i.d. as needed. • Debride necrotic tissue using surgical, sharp, autolytic, enzymatic, or mechanical means. *Infected PU care:* • Same as Day 1 *Managing tissue loads:* • Provide same care as Day 1; increase turning schedule if discolored areas of skin do not disappear in 1 hour. *Support surfaces:* • Assess patient's response to pressure-reduction measures.	*PU care:* • Same as Day 2 *Infected PU care:* • Same as Day 2 *Managing tissue loads:* • Same as Day 2 *Support surfaces:* • Same as Day 2

(continued)

PLAN OF CARE	PREADMIT PHASE	INPATIENT CARE Day 1
PROCEDURES *(continued)*		▪ Lift patient; avoid pulling or sliding. *Support surfaces:* ▪ Implement pressure-reducing or pressure-relieving support surface based on risk for developing PU and available turning surfaces: – medium risk: air-filled static or alternating pressure overlay or pads – high risk: low air-loss bed, dynamic floatation mattress – ultra-high risk: air-fluidized bead bed ▪ Provide pressure-reducing cushion for chair-bound patients. *Wound, ostomy, continence (WOC) nurse consult; surgical consult:* ▪ Consider electrical stimulation in nonhealing, clean PU receiving correct care unless contraindicated. ▪ Consider surgical repair (flaps or grafts) for clean PUs that do not respond to optimal care.
DIET	▪ Assess current diet and oral intake.	▪ Give diet high in protein and calories unless contraindicated. ▪ Ensure adequate hydration (about 2.5 qt (2.5 L)/day unless contraindicated). ▪ Give oral nutritional supplements. ▪ Assess skin turgor and mucous membranes. *Dietary consult:* ▪ Assess need for enteral or parenteral nutrition ▪ Weigh patient.
ACTIVITY	▪ Assess activity level, ability to assist in moving self, contractures, and joint pain.	*Physical therapy (PT) consult:* ▪ Ambulatory: Encourage patient to walk t.i.d. ▪ Ambulatory with assistance: Assist patients with walking t.i.d. – Reposition or encourage repositioning in bed or chair. ▪ Up in chair with assistance: Assist patients perform ROM exercises. – Encourage patient to shift weight q 15 min when up in chair. – Change patient position hourly when in chair. – Cover chair with sheet or blanket. ▪ Immobile/Bed rest: Assist to perform ROM exercises q 4 hr while awake. – Have patient turn, cough, and deep breathe q 2 hr. – Position patient in alignment with body weight evenly distributed. – Encourage patient to perform exercises: active or passive ROM, stretching, isometric, or light weight-training.
ELIMINATION	▪ Assess elimination pattern, laxative intake, and previous bowel, bladder, or kidney surgery.	▪ Measure intake and output. ▪ Keep skin clean and dry. ▪ Apply moisture barrier after each voiding or bowel movement. ▪ Assess for and treat incontinence. ▪ Assess need for male external catheter, fecal pouch, antidiarrheal medication, or disimpaction. ▪ Use reusable underpads. ▪ Establish voiding schedule.
HYGIENE	▪ Assess self-care ability, cleanliness, grooming needs, and body odor.	▪ Provide complete care or assist as needed. ▪ Inspect skin and bony prominences daily. ▪ Keep skin clean with mild soap and lukewarm water, rinse well, and pat dry. ▪ Avoid hot water and excessive friction. ▪ Apply humectants, emollients, or moisturizers for dry skin.
PATIENT TEACHING	▪ Assess cognition, memory, and understanding. ▪ Teach need for inpatient care.	▪ Orient to hospital routines and unit. ▪ Initiate PU teaching to patient or family. ▪ Involve patient or family in care planning.
DISCHARGE PLANNING	*Social services consult:* ▪ Assess insurance, level of care required, social support, caregiver status, post-hospitalization plans, and financial status.	*Social services consult:* ▪ Assess need for home health nursing, home health aide, PT, WOC nurse, or nursing home care.

Day 2	Days 3 to 6
• Same as Day 1 • Determine calorie or protein requirements. • Weigh patient.	• Same as Day 2 • Assess nutritional status at least q 3 months. • Determine nitrogen balance. • Correct malnutrition. • Weigh patient.
• Same as Day 1	• Same as Day 1
• Same as Day 1	• Same as Day 1
• Same as Day 1	• Same as Day 1
• Continue teaching about PU etiology, skin assessment, movement, turning schedule, activity or support surface, skin care, nutrition, and PU care and prevention.	• Continue teaching and evaluate learning.
Social services: • Arrange for home health or nursing home care, durable medical equipment, and supplies.	• Notify home health agency or nursing home of PU treatment plan, prevention regimen, and patient needs. • Complete discharge paperwork.

(continued)

PLAN OF CARE	HOME CARE Visit 1	Visit 2	Visit 3
DIAGNOSTIC TESTS	• Review recent hospital laboratory data. • Draw blood for complete blood count, electrolytes, fasting blood sugar, and serum albumin • Assess wound and patient for signs and symptoms (S/S) of wound infection.	• Review results of lab work with patient or caregiver. • Continue ongoing assessment for wound infection.	• Review results of lab work with patient or caregiver. • If wound appears infected, obtain wound fluid for Gram stain or obtain wound culture.
MEDICATIONS	• High-potency multivitamin and mineral supplement daily • Systemic antibiotic with wound infection • No topical antibiotics or antiseptics in clean wounds • Systemic antibiotic therapy in patients with bacteremia, sepsis, advancing cellulitis, or osteomyelitis	• Same as first visit	• Same as first visit
PROCEDURES	• Perform complete admission history and physical assessment to establish baseline data. • Complete initial wound assessment and document location, size, color, edges, exudate, sinus tract, tunneling, undermining, necrotic tissue, periwound skin color, temperature, edema, maceration, induration, and pain • Mutually establish treatment goals with patient or caregiver. *•Pressure ulcer (PU) care:* • Clean PU and surrounding skin with normal saline solution (NSS); pat skin dry. • Irrigate wound, undermining, and tunnels with NSS using 35-ml syringe with 19G angiocath. • Loosely fill dead space, undermining, and tunnels with saline- or gel-moistened gauze. • Manage exudate with absorbent dressing (moist gauze, calcium alginate, foam, hydrocolloid, paste or granules, copolymer starch). • Apply secondary cover dressing. • Depending on type of dressing, change dressing daily to t.i.d. as needed to prevent strike-through, leakage, and skin maceration. (Teach family to change second dressing.) • Monitor dressing near anus for rolled edges. • Avoid massage over bony prominences. • Determine need to debride necrotic tissue. *Infected PU care:* • Teach patient or caregiver purposes for infected wound care. • Obtain order for systemic antibiotics and noncytotoxic topical antiseptic.	• Perform comprehensive PU assessment, including ongoing assessment for complications and monitoring for worsening of PU. • Perform focused physical assessment, including vital signs, mental status, and intake and output (I &O). • Review treatment goals, and document progress in meeting goals. *PU care:* • Same as first visit • Debride necrotic tissue using autolytic, enzymatic, or sharp debridement. *Infected PU care:* • Continue with wound care regimen. • Evaluate wound for decrease S/S of infection. • Assess effectiveness of pain management regimen.	• Complete wound assessment • When patient is on systemic antibiotics, monitor for S/S of secondary infection: diarrhea, nausea, and rash. • Revise treatment plan and goals as needed; document progress in meeting goals. *PU care:* • Same as previous visit • Using valid PU assessment tool (for example, Bates-Jenson Pressure Sore Assessment Tool), assess wound for healing: size (length, width, depth); periwound skin color, intactness, edema, maceration, induration; wound edges (open or closed); character and amount of exudate; formation of granulation tissue; re-epithelialization; necrotic tissue, slough; evidence of sinus tract, tunneling, or undermining. *Infected PU care:* • Assess PU odor, exudate, and wound bed for response to systemic and local therapy. • Revise antibiotic therapy based on wound culture if necessary. • Reevaluate effectiveness of pain management; adjust plan as necessary.

PLAN OF CARE	HOME CARE Visit 1	Visit 2	Visit 3
PROCEDURES *(continued)*	• Avoid occlusive dressing if PU is infected. • With aseptic technique, clean wound and surrounding skin with NSS; pat skin dry • Irrigate wound, undermining, and tunnels with NSS using 35-ml syringe with 19G angiocath. • Loosely fill wound dead space, undermining, and tunnels with gauze moistened with noncytotoxic concentration of topical antiseptic. • Cover with nonocclusive secondary dressing to manage exudate (calcium alginate, foam, gauze). • Depending on type of dressing, change dressing daily to t.i.d. as needed to prevent strike-through, leakage, and skin maceration. (Teach family to change second dressing.) • Consider using a dressing that can be left in place for several days; as recommended by the Agency for Health Care Policy and Research. • Manage PU pain by covering wound, repositioning, analgesic medication, or nonpharmacologic intervention (imagery, relaxation techniques, music therapy). • Instruct caregiver or patient to keep a pain log using a pain scale to record pain intensity and effect of dressing, turning, and medication.		
DIET	• Assess current diet, fluid intake, appetite, and ability to feed self. • Give diet high in protein and calories unless contraindicated. • Ensure adequate fluids to approximately 2.5 qt (2.5 L)/day unless contraindicated. • Assess skin turgor and mucous membranes. • Take baseline weight.	• Same as first visit • Initiate food and fluid intake record. • Weigh patient.	• Same as first visit • Assess adequacy of intake. • Initiate nutritional consult if necessary. • Assess nutritional status q 3 months. • Report unexpected significant weight gain or loss (change up or down of 3 lb [1.4 kg]/wk) to doctor.
ACTIVITY	• Assess activity level: ability to ambulate and assist moving self in bed and chair. • Assess for contractures, joint mobility, and pain. • Evaluate home environment for safety. • Teach measures to prevent falls. • Evaluate need for assistive devices. • Encourage patient to perform exercise regimen: active or passive range-of-motion (ROM) exercises, isometrics, stretching, or light weight training.	• Confirm assessments and initiate PT consult as needed. • Assess patient or caregiver compliance.	• Reinforce PU prevention instructions. • Initiate PT consult if needed. • Assess patient or caregiver compliance.

CLINICAL PATHWAY

(continued)

PLAN OF CARE	HOME CARE Visit 1	Visit 2	Visit 3
ELIMINATION	• Assess elimination pattern, laxative use, and incontinence. • Initiate instruction on skin care after voiding or bowel movement (BM). • Keep skin clean and dry. • Apply moisture barrier after each voiding or BM. • Assess and treat incontinence. • Assess need for male external catheter, fecal pouch, antidiarrheal medication, or disimpaction. • Use reusable (not disposable) under-pads. • Establish voiding schedule. • Measure input and output (I & O).	• Continue patient or caregiver instruction on skin care after voiding or BM. • Measure I & O.	• Evaluate caregiver, patient, or HHA implementation of skin protection after voiding or BM. • Evaluate effectiveness of voiding schedule. • Measure I & O.
HYGIENE	• Assess self-care ability, cleanliness, grooming needs, and body odor. • Teach caregiver or patient bathing schedule and routine. • Keep skin clean with mild soap and lukewarm water, rinse well, and pat dry. • Avoid hot water and excessive friction. • Apply humectants, emollients, or moisturizers for dry skin. • Apply cornstarch or power between skin folds; wash skin folds b.i.d.	• Assess skin for dryness, cleanliness, intactness, rashes, and itching.	• Same as previous visit • Evaluate effectiveness of skin care regimen.
PATIENT TEACHING	• Orient to home health care agency and services. • Involve caregiver or patient in ongoing care planning and meeting treatment goals. • Initiate PU teaching: stages, risk factors, prevention, prevention of infection, PU care to promote healing, conditions necessary for healing (nutrients, fluid, pressure relief, uninfected wound, correct dressing changed as often as necessary). • Provide written PU information. *Managing tissue loads:* • Provide written instructions to: – avoid positioning on PU and donut ring devices – use positioning device to raise PU off surface (head, heel) – post written repositioning schedule – avoid positioning immobile patients on trochanters and ischial tuberosities – prevent direct contact between bony prominences (knees, ankles) by padding with a pillow or blanket. • Do not raise head of bed to > 30 degrees unless contraindicated by medical condition or tube feeding. • Limit lateral position to < 30 degrees. • Reposition bed-bound patients at least q 2 hr, chair-bound patients hourly.	• Teach importance of regular follow-up visits with health care providers. • Continue teaching, assessing comprehension, follow-through, and compliance.	• Answer patient's, caregiver's, or family questions. • Continue teaching caregiver and patient PU care and prevention.

PLAN OF CARE	HOME CARE Visit 1	Visit 2	Visit 3
PATIENT TEACHING *(continued)*	• Teach chair-bound patients to shift weight q 15 min. • Encourage performing ROM exercises q 4 hr while awake. • Support patient's feet with foot board. • Lift patient; avoid pulling or sliding. • Manage moisture or perspiration and humidity. *Support surfaces:* • Work with caregiver, patient, or payer for reimbursement of medically necessary equipment. • Teach need for pressure reducing support surface based on patient's condition and risk for developing PU: – comfort only or no risk: sheepskin, convoluted high-density foam – medium risk: air-filled static or alternating-pressure overlay or pads – high risk: low air-loss bed, dynamic floatation mattress – ultra-high risk: air-fluidized bead bed. • Provide pressure-reducing cushion for chair-bound patients. • Initiate teaching to prevent further PUs or worsening of current PU. • Instruct patient who can walk on importance of ambulating in home at least t.i.d. • Teach caregiver or home health aide (HHA) to help patient who can walk with assistance to walk t.i.d. • Teach caregiver or HHA to reposition or encourage repositioning in bed or chair. • Teach caregiver or HHA to patient who can get to chair with assistance to have patient complete ROM exercises t.i.d. to q.i.d. • Teach patient to shift weight q 15 min when up in chair. • Teach caregiver or HHA to change patient position hourly when in chair. • Cover chair with sheet or blanket. • Teach caregiver or HHA of patient who is immobile or requires bed rest to encourage patient to complete ROM exercises q 4 hr while awake. • Teach patient to turn, cough, deep breathe q 2 hr. • Teach caregiver or HHA to position patient in alignment, with body weight evenly distributed.	*Managing tissue loads:* • Assess caregiver's or patient's understanding of moisture, pressure, friction, and shear in PU etiology. • Assess caregiver's or patient's ability to reduce and distribute tissue loading. *Support surfaces:* • Assess comprehension, follow-through, and compliance.	*Managing tissue loads:* • Assess patient care and caregiver competence and understanding. • Assess skin over bony prominences for S/S of tissue breakdown. *Support surfaces:* • Initiate support surface intervention. • Evaluate PU preventive measures, and assess need for change in plan of care and need for additional or new teaching.
DISCHARGE PLANNING	• Assess resources: availability and skill of caregiver, patient understanding, and equipment needs. • Assess need for HHA; wound, ostomy, continence (WOC) nurse; nutritionist; social service; and physical therapist (PT). • Arrange HHA visit.	• Assess caregiver need for rest and sleep and ability to provide care. • Discuss HHA service.	• Evaluate HHA care. • Determine progress toward meeting goals of care.

Pressure ulcer (stage IV)

PLAN OF CARE	PREADMIT PHASE	INPATIENT CARE Day 1
DIAGNOSTIC TESTS	• Complete blood count (CBC) with differential, electrolytes, hemoglobin (Hgb), fasting blood sugar (FBS), albumin, total lymphocyte count (TLC), transferrin	• CBC with differential, electrolytes, Hgb, FBS, albumin, TLC, transferrin • Electrocardiogram • Urine culture and sensitivity, osmolarity • Chest X-ray • Vitamin C, A, B assay; zinc, magnesium, iron assay • Blood and wound fluid cultures and Gram stains • PU tissue biopsy • Evaluate patient for osteomyelitis in nonhealing PUs: white blood cell count, erythrocyte sedimentation rate, X-ray
MEDICATIONS	• Assess current prescription and over-the-counter medications	• High-potency vitamin and mineral supplement daily if deficient • Antispasmodic in spinal cord–injured patient • Systemic antibiotics and noncytotoxic topical antiseptics • No topical antibiotics or antiseptics in clean wounds • Systemic antibiotic therapy in patients with bacteremia, sepsis, advancing cellulitis, or osteomyelitis
PROCEDURES	• Take baseline vital signs (VS). • Assess skin and pressure ulcer (PU). • Signs and symptoms (S/S) of wound infection	• Perform comprehensive history and physical assessment. • Check vital signs q 4 hr. • Perform PU risk assessment using valid PU risk assessment scale. • Perform comprehensive PU status assessment daily. • Select dressing that will keep wound moist, exudate controlled, and periwound skin dry. • Avoid massage over bony prominences. *PU care:* • Debride necrotic tissue using autolytic, enzymatic, or sharp debridement. • Clean PU and surrounding skin gently with normal saline solution (NSS); pat periwound skin dry. • Irrigate wound, undermining, and tunnels with NSS using 35-ml syringe with 19G angiocath. • Loosely fill dead space, undermining, and tunnels with saline- or gel-moistened gauze. • Manage exudate with absorbent dressing (moist gauze, calcium alginate, foam, hydrocolloid, paste or granules, copolymer starch). • Apply secondary cover dressing. • Depending on type of dressing, change dressing daily to t.i.d. as needed to prevent strike-through, leakage, and skin maceration. • Monitor dressing near anus for rolled edges. *Infected PU care:* • Avoid occlusive dressing if PU is infected. • Clean wound and surrounding skin with NSS; pat skin dry. • Irrigate wound, undermining, and tunnels with NSS using 35-ml syringe with 19G angiocath. • Loosely fill dead space, undermining, and tunnels with saline- or gel-moistened gauze. • Manage exudate with absorbent dressing (moist gauze, calcium alginate, foam, hydrocolloid, paste or granules, copolymer starch). • Cover with secondary cover dressing. • Depending on type of dressing, change dressing daily to t.i.d. as needed to prevent strike-through, leakage, and skin maceration. • Consider whirlpool b.i.d. for PUs with thick exudate, slough, and necrotic tissue. *Managing tissue loads:* • Avoid positioning on PU and donut ring devises. • Use positioning device to raise PU off surface (head, heel). • Post written repositioning schedule. • Avoid positioning immobile patients on trochanters or ischial tuberosities. • Prevent direct contact between bony prominences (knees, ankles). • Do not raise head of bed to > 30 degrees unless contraindicated by medical condition or tube feeding. • Limit lateral position to < 30 degrees. • Reposition bed-bound patients at least q 2 hr, chair-bound patients hourly. • Teach chair-bound patients to shift weight q 15 min. • Have patient perform range-of-motion (ROM) exercises q 4 hr while awake. • Support patient's feet with foot board. • Lift patient; avoid pulling or sliding.

Day 2	Days 3 to 6
• Urine urea nitrogen • Creatinine height index • 24-hour creatinine	• Repeat CBC with differential, electrolytes, and FBS as necessary • Computed tomography scan (abscess) • Sinography (sinus tract) around abscess.
• Same as Day 1	• Same as Day 1 • Monitor for S/S of secondary infection (diarrhea, nausea, rash) and medicate accordingly.
• Perform physical assessment every day, including VS, level of consciousness, and mental status. • Check VS q 4 hr. • Perform comprehensive PU status assessment daily. *PU care:* • Same as Day 1 • Evaluate dressing for intactness; change daily to t.i.d. as needed. *Infected PU care:* • Same as Day 1 *Managing tissue loads:* • Provide same care as Day 1; increase turning schedule if discolored areas do not disappear in 1 hour. *Support surfaces:* • Assess patient's response to pressure reduction measures.	• Same as Day 2 • Check VS q 4 hr. *PU care:* • Same as Day 2 *Infected PU care:* • Same as Day 2 *Managing tissue loads:* • Same as Day 2 *Support surfaces:* • Same as Day 2

(continued)

PLAN OF CARE	PREADMIT PHASE	INPATIENT CARE *Day 1*
PROCEDURES *(continued)*		*Support surfaces:* ▪ Implement pressure-reducing or pressure-relieving support surface based on risk for developing PU and available turning surfaces: – medium risk: air-filled static or alternating-pressure overlay or pads – high risk: low air-loss bed, dynamic floatation mattress – ultra-high risk: air-fluidized bead bed ▪ Provide pressure-reducing cushion for chair-bound patient. *Wound, ostomy, continence (WOC) nurse consult; surgical consult:* ▪ Consider electrical stimulation in nonhealing, clean PU receiving correct care unless contraindicated. ▪ Consider surgical repair (graft or flap) for clean PUs that do not respond to optimal care.
DIET	▪ Assess current diet and oral intake.	▪ Give diet high in protein and calories unless contraindicated. ▪ Ensure adequate hydration (approximately 2.5 qt (2.5 L)/day unless contraindicated). ▪ Give oral nutritional supplements. ▪ Assess skin turgor and mucous membranes. *Dietary consult:* ▪ Assess need for enteral or parenteral nutrition. ▪ Weigh patient.
ACTIVITY	▪ Assess activity level, ability to assist in moving self, contractures, and joint pain.	*Physical therapy (PT) consult:* ▪ Ambulatory: Encourage patient to walk three times a day. ▪ Ambulatory with assistance: Assist patient with walking three times a day. – Reposition or encourage repositioning in bed or chair. ▪ Up in chair with assistance: Assist patient perform range-of-motion (ROM) exercises. – Encourage patient to shift weight q15min when up in chair. – Change patient position q hr when in chair. – Cover chair with sheet or blanket. ▪ Immobile/Bed rest: Have patient who is immobile or requires bed rest perform ROM exercises q 4 hr while awake. – Have patient turn, cough, and deep breathe q 2 hr. – Position in alignment with body weight evenly distributed. – Encourage patient to perform exercise regimen, such as active or passive ROM, stretching, isometric, or light weight-training exercises.
ELIMINATION	▪ Assess elimination pattern, laxative intake, and previous bowel, bladder, or kidney surgery. ▪ Measure intake and output (I & O).	▪ Keep skin clean and dry. ▪ Apply moisture barrier after each voiding or bowel movement. ▪ Assess for and treat incontinence. ▪ Assess need for male external catheter, fecal pouch, antidiarrheal medication, or disimpaction. ▪ Use reusable underpads. ▪ Establish voiding schedule. ▪ Measure I & O.
HYGIENE	▪ Assess self-care ability, cleanliness, grooming needs, body odor.	▪ Provide complete care or assist as needed. ▪ Inspect skin and bony prominences daily. ▪ Keep skin clean with mild soap and lukewarm water, rinse well, and pat dry. ▪ Avoid hot water and excessive friction. ▪ Apply humectants, emollients, or moisturizers for dry skin.
PATIENT TEACHING	▪ Assess cognition, memory, and understanding. ▪ Teach need for inpatient care.	▪ Orient to hospital routines and unit. ▪ Initiate PU teaching to patient or family. ▪ Involve patient or family in care planning.
DISCHARGE PLANNING	*Social services consult:* ▪ Assess insurance, level of care required, social support, caregiver status, post-hospitalization plans, and financial status.	*Social services consult:* ▪ Assess need for home health care, home health aide, PT, WOC nurse, or nursing home care.

- Same as Day 1
- Determine calorie or protein requirements.
- Weigh patient.

- Same as Day 2
- Determine nitrogen balance.
- Correct malnutrition.

- Same as Day 1

- Same as Day 1

- Same as Day 1

- Same as Day 1

- Same as Day 1

- Same as Day 1

- Continue teaching about PU etiology, skin assessment, movement or turning schedule activity or support surface, skin care, nutrition, and PU care and prevention.

- Continue teaching and evaluate learning.

Social services:
- Arrange for home health or nursing home care, durable medical equipment, and supplies.

- Notify nursing home or home health agency of PU treatment plan, prevention regimen, and patient's needs.
- Complete discharge paperwork.

(continued)

PLAN OF CARE	HOME CARE Visit 1	Visit 2	Visit 3
DIAGNOSTIC TESTS	• Review recent hospital laboratory data. • Draw blood for complete blood count, electrolytes, and fasting blood sugar. • Assess wound and patient for signs and symptoms (S/S) of wound infection.	• Review results of lab work with patient or caregiver. • Continue ongoing assessment for wound infection.	• Review results of lab work with patient or caregiver. • If wound appears infected, obtain wound fluid for Gram stain or obtain wound culture.
MEDICATIONS	• High-potency multivitamin and mineral supplement daily • Systemic antibiotic with wound infection • Topical antibiotic ointment (triple antibiotic, silver sulfadiazine) in clean, nonhealing, exudative pressure ulcers (PUs) after 2 to 3 weeks of correct care • No topical antibiotics or antiseptics in clean wounds • Systemic antibiotic therapy in patients with bacteremia, sepsis, advancing cellulitis, or osteomyelitis • Analgesics if nonpharmacologic treatments are not sufficient	• Same as first visit • Assess wound for decreased S/S of infection and medicate as appropriate.	• Same as previous visit • Assess wound for decreased S/S of infection.
PROCEDURES	• Perform complete admission history and physical assessment to establish baseline data. • Complete initial wound assessment, and document location, size; color, edges, exudate, sinus tract, tunneling, undermining, necrotic tissue, periwound skin color, temperature, edema, maceration, induration, and pain. • Mutually establish treatment goals with patient or caregiver. • Determine need to debride necrotic tissue using autolytic, enzymatic, or sharp debridement. *PU care:* • Clean PU and surrounding skin with normal saline solution (NSS); pat skin dry. • Irrigate wound, undermining, and tunnels with NSS using 35-ml syringe with 19G angiocath. • Loosely fill dead space, undermining, and tunnels with saline- or gel-moistened gauze. • Manage exudate with absorbent dressing (moist gauze, calcium alginate, foam, hydrocolloid, paste or granules, copolymer starch). • Apply secondary cover dressing. • Depending on type of dressing, change dressing daily to t.i.d. as needed to prevent strike-through, leakage, and skin maceration. • Monitor dressing near anus for rolled edges. • Avoid massage over bony prominences. *Infected PU care:* • Teach patient or caregiver purposes for infected wound care. • Obtain order for systemic antibiotics and noncytotoxic topical antiseptics. • Avoid occlusive dressing if PU is infected. • Using aseptic technique, clean wound and surrounding skin with NSS; pat skin dry. • Irrigate wound, undermining, and tunnels with NSS using 35-ml syringe with 19G angiocath. • Loosely pack wound, undermining, and tunnels with gauze moistened with noncytotoxic concentration of topical antiseptic. • Cover with nonocclusive secondary dressing to manage exudate (calcium alginate, foam, gauze).	• Perform comprehensive PU assessment, including ongoing assessment for complications and monitoring for worsening of PU. • Perform focused physical assessment, including vital signs and mental status. • Measure PU size weekly. • Review treatment goals, and document progress in meeting goals. *PU care:* • Same as first visit • Debride necrotic tissue as needed using autolytic, enzymatic, or sharp debridement. *Infected PU care:* • Reinforce teaching. • Continue with wound care regimen. • Evaluate wound for decreasing S/S of infection. • Assess effectiveness of pain management regimen.	• Same as previous visit • When patient is on systemic antibiotics, monitor for S/S of secondary infection: diarrhea, nausea, and rash. • Revise treatment plan and goals as needed; document progress in meeting goals. • Debride necrotic tissue as needed using autolytic, enzymatic, or sharp debridement. *PU care:* • Same as previous visit • Using valid PU assessment tool (for example, Bates-Jenson Pressure Sore Assessment Tool), assess wound for healing: size (length, width, depth); periwound skin color, intactness, edema, maceration, induration; wound edges (open or closed); character and amount of exudate; formation of granulation tissue; re-epithelialization; necrotic tissue, slough; evidence of sinus tract, tunneling, or undermining. *Infected PU care:* • Assess PU odor, exudate, and wound bed for response to systemic and local therapy. • Revise antibiotic therapy based on wound culture if necessary. • Reevaluate effectiveness of pain management; adjust plan as necessary.

PLAN OF CARE	HOME CARE Visit 1	Visit 2	Visit 3
PROCEDURES *(continued)*	• Change dressing daily to t.i.d. as needed to prevent strike-through, leakage, and skin maceration. (Teach family to change second dressing.) • Consider using a dressing that can be left in place for several days as recommended by Agency for Health Care Policy and Research. • Manage PU pain by covering wound, repositioning, analgesics, or nonpharmacologic intervention (imagery, relaxation techniques, music therapy) • Instruct caregiver or patient to keep pain log using pain scale and to record pain intensity and effect of dressing, turning, and medication.		
DIET	• Assess current diet, fluid intake, appetite, and ability to feed self. • Encourage diet high in protein and calories unless contraindicated. • Ensure adequate fluids to approximately 2.5 qt (2.5 L)/day unless contraindicated. • Assess skin turgor and mucous membranes. • Take baseline weight.	• Same as first visit • Initiate food and fluid intake record. • Weigh patient.	• Same as previous visit • Assess adequacy of intake. • Initiate dietary consult if necessary. • Assess nutritional status q 3 months. • Report significant unexpected weight gain or loss (change up or down of 3 lb/wk) to doctor.
ACTIVITY	• Assess activity level: ability to ambulate and assist moving self in bed or chair. • Assess for contractures, joint mobility, and pain. • Evaluate home environment for safety; teach measures to prevent falls. • Evaluate need for assistive devices. • Encourage patient to perform exercise regimen: stretching, isometric, or light weight-training exercises.	• Confirm assessments and initiate physical therapy (PT) consult as needed. • Assess patient or caregiver compliance.	• Reinforce PU prevention instructions. • Initiate PT consult if needed. • Assess patient or caregiver compliance.
ELIMINATION	• Assess elimination pattern, laxative use, and incontinence. • Initiate instruction on skin care following voiding or bowel movement (BM). • Keep skin clean and dry. • Apply moisture barrier after each voiding or BM. • Assess and treat incontinence. • Assess need for male external catheter, fecal pouch, antidiarrheal medication, or disimpaction. • Use reusable (not disposable) underpads. • Establish voiding schedule. • Measure intake and output (I & O).	• Continue instruction to patient or caregiver on skin care after voiding or BM. • Measure I & O.	• Evaluate caregiver, patient or HHA implementation of skin protection after voiding or BM. • Measure I & O.
HYGIENE	• Assess self-care ability, cleanliness, grooming needs, and body odor. • Teach caregiver or patient bathing schedule and routine. • Keep skin clean with mild soap and lukewarm water, rinse well, and pat dry • Avoid hot water and excessive friction • Apply humectants, emollients, or moisturizers for dry skin • Apply cornstarch or power between skin folds; wash skin folds b.i.d.	• Assess skin for dryness, cleanliness, intactness, rash, and itching.	• Same as previous visit

(continued)

PLAN OF CARE	HOME CARE *Visit 1*	*Visit 2*	*Visit 3*
PATIENT TEACHING	• Orient to home health care agency and services. • Involve caregiver or patient in ongoing care planning and meeting treatment goals. • Initiate PU teaching: stages, risk factors, prevention, prevention of infection, PU care to promote healing, conditions necessary for healing (nutrients, fluid, pressure relief, uninfected wound, correct dressing changed as often as necessary). • Provide written PU information. *Managing tissue loads:* • Provide written instructions to: – avoid positioning on PU and donut ring devices – use positioning device to raise PU off surface (head, heel) – post written repositioning schedule – avoid positioning immobile patients on trochanters, ischial tuberosities – prevent direct contact between bony prominences (knees, ankles) with a pillow or blanket. • Do not raise head of bed to > 30 degrees unless contraindicated by medical condition or tube feeding. • Limit lateral position to < 30 degrees. • Reposition bed-bound patients at least q 2 hr, chair-bound patients hourly. • Teach chair-bound patients to shift weight q 15 min. • Have patient perform range-of-motion (ROM) exercises q 4 hr while awake. • Support patient's feet with foot board. • Lift patient; avoid pulling or sliding. • Manage moisture or perspiration and humidity. *Support surfaces:* • Work with caregiver, patient, or payer for reimbursement of medically necessary equipment. • Teach need for pressure-reducing support surface based on patient condition and risk for developing PU: – comfort only or no risk: sheepskin, convoluted high-density foam – medium risk: air-filled static or alternating-pressure overlay or pads – high risk: low air-loss bed, dynamic floatation mattress – ultra-high risk: air-fluidized bead bed • Provide pressure-reducing cushion for chair-bound patient. • Initiate teaching to prevent further PUs or worsening of current PU. • Instruct patient who can walk on importance of ambulating in home at least t.i.d. • Teach caregiver or home health aide (HHA) to assist patient who can walk with assistance to walk t.i.d. • Teach caregiver or HHA to reposition or encourage repositioning in bed or chair. • Teach caregiver or HHA of patient who gets up in chair with assistance to have patient perform complete ROM exercises t.i.d. to q.i.d. • Teach patient to shift weight q 15 min when up in chair. • Teach caregiver or HHA to change patient position hourly when in chair. • Cover chair with sheet or blanket.	• Teach importance of regular follow-up visits with health care providers. • Continue teaching, assessing comprehension, follow-through, and compliance. *Managing tissue loads:* • Assess caregiver's or patient's understanding of moisture, pressure, friction, and shear in PU etiology. • Assess caregiver's or patient's ability to reduce and distribute tissue loading. *Support surfaces:* • Assess comprehension, follow-through, and compliance.	• Answer patient's, caregiver's, or family's questions. • Continue teaching caregiver and patient PU care and prevention. • Document patient's or caregiver's understanding and performance. *Managing tissue loads:* • Assess patient care and caregiver competence and understanding. • Assess skin over bony prominences for S/S of tissue breakdown. *Support surfaces:* • Initiate support surface intervention. • Evaluate PU preventive measures.

PLAN OF CARE	HOME CARE *Visit 1*	*Visit 2*	*Visit 3*
PATIENT TEACHING *(continued)*	▪ Teach caregiver or HHA of a patient who is immobile or requires bed rest to perform ROM exercises q 4 hr while awake. ▪ Teach patient to turn, cough, and deep breathe q 2 hr. ▪ Teach caregiver or HHA to position patient in alignment, with body weight evenly distributed.		
DISCHARGE PLANNING	▪ Assess resources: availability and skill of caregiver, patient understanding, and equipment needs. ▪ Arrange for home health aide (HHA) visits. ▪ Discuss HHA service with patient or caregiver.	▪ Assess caregiver's need for rest, sleep, and ability to provide care. ▪ Evaluate HHA care.	▪ Determine progress toward meeting goals of care.

- Reposition bed-bound patient at least every 2 hours with body weight evenly distributed.
- Reposition chair-bound patient every hour.
- Encourage weight-shifting every 15 minutes when in chair.
- Teach chair push-ups every hour for chair-bound patients.
- Encourage patient to perform range-of-motion exercises every 2 hours while awake to prevent contractures and improve circulation; program could include stretching, isometrics, and light weight training to improve strength and circulation.

Preventing friction and shear
- Use genuine sheepskin pads, elbow and heel protectors, and high-density 3- to 4-inch foam.
- Limit elevation head of bed to < 30 degrees unless contraindicated.
- Limit side-lying position to < 30 degrees.
- Support feet with footboard.
- Lift patient; avoid pulling and sliding.
- Use trapeze and turning sheets for repositioning patient.

Nutrition
- Maintain optimal nutrition with high-protein, high-calorie diet unless contraindicated: 30 to 50 calories/kg/day; 1.25 to1.5 grams protein/kg/day.

- Ensure adequate hydration of 2.5 qt (2.5 L)/day unless contraindicated.
- Provide multivitamin supplement with vitamin C, A, K, and B-complex.
- Provide magnesium, iron, copper, and zinc supplement if deficient. Assess need for parenteral or enteral nutrition.

Critical thinking activities

1. Describe the risk factors for predicting PUs that will not heal and for predicting patients who are at risk for nonhealing ulcers.
2. Detail the criteria that can be used by clinicians, surveyors, and payers that describe PU healing over time.
3. Explain the predictive validity of the National Pressure Ulcer Advisory Panel proposal to revise the definition for Stage I PUs.
4. Describe in detail the risk assessments for Stage I PUs that vary according to skin pigmentation.
5. Describe the risk assessment scores that are valid for the elderly and persons with darkly pigmented skin.
6. Discuss the relationship between vasoconstrictive medication and the development of PUs.
7. Describe the effect of topical oxygen therapy on PU healing.
8. Discuss how attitudes of staff affect the prevention, prevalence (total number of cases), and incidence (rate of occurrence) of PUs.
9. Describe how dressing type affects the rate of healing of PUs.
10. Discuss the direct and indirect costs of hospital and home care of PUs.
11. Describe the effect of electrical stimulation on PU healing.

Suggested research topics

- Coping strategies for PUs
- Compliance with therapy
- Effectiveness of programs to prevent PUs
- Effectiveness of describing PUs according to stages
- Effectiveness of various dressings in healing PUs

PART 11

Psychiatric disorders

Alzheimer's type dementia

Depression

Panic disorder without agoraphobia (anxiety)

Alzheimer's type dementia

DRG: 429 Mean LOS: 5.9 days

Dementia is a maladaptive cognitive response that produces a loss of intellectual function. Impairment in memory, judgment, and abstract thought are the major features of dementia and represent the loss of intellectual function. Dementia is usually a progressive degenerative disorder that affects the person's whole life and the lives of those closest to him or her. Patients experience the insidious loss of the essence of who they are and their "being" at all levels of the self: physical, emotional, social, cognitive, and spiritual. Dementia ultimately results in death.

Dementia may occur at any age, but most often affects the elderly, those persons age 65 or older. It is estimated that 4 million people suffer from dementia and that by the year 2030, the incidence will increase to 5.5 million. Furthermore, the cost of caring for patients with dementia will increase from $58 billion to $759 billion by 2030. This puts a serious financial strain on families of dementia patients, who presently pay 70% of the cost, and on the health care delivery system. The most common and best-known form of dementia is "dementia of the Alzheimer's type." At present, only palliative treatment is available for the disorder, which is the fourth leading cause of death among people age 65 or older and is more common in women than in men. Other forms of dementia include multi-infarct dementia, Pick's disease, Creutzfeldt-Jakob disease, and encephalopathy in acquired immunodeficiency syndrome.

Dementia results from structural and neurochemical changes in the brain. Although the cause of Alzheimer's disease is unknown, research finding demonstrate the following brain changes: increased number of neurofibrillary tangles and plaques in the cerebral cortex; deterioration of temporal, parietal, and occipital regions of the cerebral cortex; decreased levels of acetylcholine, norepinephrine, serotonin, and somatostatin; decreased corticotropin-releasing hormone; inhibition of the hypothalamic-pituitary axis with subsequent disruption of hormone release; high levels of aluminum in the brain; and the accumulation of amyloid in the center of plaques and in the walls of blood vessels in the brain.

Pseudodementia is an extreme condition in which clinical features resemble dementia, but there is no organic brain dysfunction or defect of intelligence. This type is most often due to depression.

Subjective assessment findings

Health history
Brain trauma, brain lesions, neurologic disorder, nutritional deficiencies, metabolic or endocrine disorders, hypoxia ischemia, exposure to volatile agents or insecticides, ingestion of drugs or heavy metals, infections such as syphilis, encephalitis

Medication history
Tacrine (Cognex), vitamin B_{12} deficiency, anemia

Functional health patterns
Health perception–health maintenance: use of aluminum in cooking, family history of Alzheimer's
Activity-exercise: unsteady gait
Sleep-rest: insomnia

Cognitive-perceptual: confusion, memory impairment (loss), forgetfulness, indecisiveness
Self-perception: altered perception of self, other, environment
Coping: denies any problems with memory; fear, anxiety, emotional distress

Objective assessment findings

Psychosocial assessment

Physical appearance: disheveled, body odor, dirty, unsteady gait, erect posture
Affect: labile, blunted affect, inappropriate affect, tearful, withdrawn, irritable, hostile, euphoric, sad, anxious, fearful
Behaviors: pacing, wandering or roaming at night, undressing in public places, ritualistic behaviors, unsteady gait, hoarding
Cognitive: disorientation, aphasia, paraphasia, anomia, apraxia, palilalia, confabulation, delusional thinking, paranoia, suspicious, hallucination, short attention span, decreased concentration, impaired memory, short- and long-term memory loss, deterioration of general intellect, nocturnal confusion (sundown syndrome), inability to acquire or use new information, impaired judgment, indecisiveness, inability to problem solve
Physical: oral health, ability to chew and swallow, weight changes, bowel and bladder dysfunction, insomnia, ability to carry out activities of daily living (ADLs) independently
Family assessment: support system for patient and family, relationship of caregiver to patient, physical and mental health of caregiver, impact of responsibilities on caregiver, level of change on caregiver, financial resources that support caregiver, knowledge in regard to legal help
Mental Status Exam: Short Portable Mental Status Questionnaire (SPMSQ), Alzheimer's Disease Assessment Scale

Diagnostic tests

Neurologic assessment, pharmacologic assessment, mental status exam, chest X-ray, electrocardiogram, computed tomography scan, magnetic resonance imaging, complete blood count with differential, thyroid function studies, electrolytes, liver function studies, vitamin B levels, blood cultures, lumbar puncture

Related nursing diagnoses

1 Altered thought processes
2 Impaired memory
3 Risk for injury
4 Self-care deficit (bathing/hygiene, feeding, dressing/grooming, or toileting)
5 Sleep pattern disturbance
6 Altered health maintenance
7 Impaired verbal communication
8 Impaired physical mobility
9 Anxiety
10 Fear
11 Ineffective family coping: Compromised
12 Impaired home maintenance management

Expected outcomes

The following expected outcomes pertain to the patient or family. Numbers in parentheses refer to related nursing diagnoses above.
- Have diminished confusion (1).
- Maintain memory at optimal level (2).
- Not become injured (3).

(Text continues on page 257.)

PLAN OF CARE	PREADMIT PHASE	INPATIENT CARE *Day 1*	*Day 2*
DIAGNOSTIC TESTS	• Chest X-ray • Electrocardiogram • Complete blood count with differential • Electrolytes • Thyroid function tests • Liver function tests • Blood cultures • Vitamin B levels • Erythrocyte sedimentation rate • Magnetic resonance imaging • Computed tomography scan of head (if not done within 6 months)	• Lumbar puncture	• As indicated
MEDICATIONS	• Tacrine (Cognex) • Pharmacologic assessment	• Tacrine (Cognex) • Antipsychotic (low dose)	• Same as Day 1
PROCEDURES	• Perform neurologic assessment and mental status examination.	• Give milieu therapy: provide structure; involve patient in care; provide low-glare lighting; decrease noise level; give reality orientation, validation therapy, remotivation therapy, and reminiscence therapy. • Check vital signs q.i.d.	• Same as Day 1
DIET	• Give diet as tolerated (DAT).	• Give DAT • Weigh patient before breakfast. • Give nutritional supplements as needed. • Give finger foods as snacks. • Provide adequate time for meals. • Verbally direct patient through each step of the eating process. • Give one food at a time.	• Same as Day 1
ACTIVITY	• Evaluate for sundown syndrome (wandering or roaming at night). • Evaluate pacing to be sure patient is not at risk for injury.	• Establish nonstimulating bedtime ritual. • Provide quiet. • Provide minimal light. • Provide consistency at bedtime. • Give warm milk. • Give back rub. • Play soft classical music. • Provide an area to pace. • Set boundaries on pacing area (for example, use stop signs, red tape, closed or locked doors). • Schedule rest times.	• Same as Day 1
ELIMINATION	• Evaluate for bowel and bladder Incontinence (eventually all patients lose cognitive ability to use toilet).	• Use protective undergarment such as adult diapers. • Change undergarment q 4 hr or as necessary. • Assess for skin breakdown.	• Same as Day 1
HYGIENE		• Provide consistent bathing routine. • Provide privacy. • Orient patient to what to do. • Verbally direct patient through steps. • Assist patient when necessary.	• Same as Day 1

Day 3	Day 4	Day 5
• As indicated	• As indicated	• As indicated
• Same as Day 1	• Same as Day 1	• Same as Day 1
• Same as Day 1	• Same as Day 1	• Same as Day 1
• Same as Day 1	• Same as Day 1	• Same as Day 1
• Same as Day 1	• Same as Day 1	Same as Day 1
• Same as Day 1	• Same as Day 1	• Same as Day 1
• Same as Day 1	• Same as Day 1	• Same as Day 1

PLAN OF CARE	PREADMIT PHASE	INPATIENT CARE *Day 1*	*Day 2*
PATIENT TEACHING	• Give family essential information about program and how patient will progress through it.	*Family caregiver:* • Discuss disease process, stage, and medication.	*Family caregiver:* • Assess learning from Day 1. • Continue learning from Day 1. • Discuss how to modify the environment for safety. • Teach communication skills with demented patients.
DISCHARGE PLANNING	*Social services consult:* • Consider home health care, partial program, or adult day care.	*Psychological consult:* • Discuss counseling (self-esteem and coping) for both patient and caregiver.	*Social services:* • Arrange for home health care, partial program, or adult day care.

Day 3	Day 4	Day 5
Family caregiver: • Assess learning from Day 2. • Continue learning from Day 2. • Teach how to maintain patient's nutrition. • Teach how to deal with eating problems. • Teach how to promote sleep and rest.	*Family caregiver:* • Assess learning from Day 3. • Continue learning from Day 3. • Teach how to access support system for caregiver: instrumental support, expressive support, support groups, respite care, and community resources.	*Family caregiver:* • Assess learning from Day 4. • Continue learning from Day 4. • Teach how to access support groups for patient.
• Assist caregiver in setting up a structured program for patient.	• Assist caregiver in developing a program of care and support for self.	• With caregiver, evaluate the structured program for the patient and self.

(continued)

PLAN OF CARE	HOME CARE Visit 1	Visit 2	Visit 3
DIAGNOSTIC TESTS	• If indicated	• If indicated	• If indicated
MEDICATIONS	• Give Tacrine (Cognex). • Give antipsychotic (low dose). • Assess for effectiveness of medications and adverse effects. • Assess for proper administration (when it is given, with or without food, and so forth).	• Assess for compliance with medication regimen. • Assess for effectiveness of medications and adverse effects.	• Same as previous visit
PROCEDURES	• Check vital signs. • Assess home for safety factors. • Assess mental status. • Assess structured environment. • Assess reality orientation. • Assess reminiscence therapy.	• Same as previous visit	• Same as previous visit
DIET	• Assess nutritional status, especially intake. • Assess for chewing or swallowing problems.	• Reassess same as previous visit. • Refer to nutritional consult if needed.	• Same as previous visit
ACTIVITY	• Assess for sleep activity. • Monitor pacing area for safety. • Establish exercise program (consult with doctor or physical therapy).	• Reassess same as previous visit.	• Same as previous visit
ELIMINATION	• Assess skin integrity. • Assess for bowel movement pattern.	• Same as previous visit	• Same as previous visit
HYGIENE	• Assess for urinary problems. • Assess hygiene.	• Same as previous visit	• Same as previous visit
PATIENT TEACHING	• Teach caregiver to recognize signs and symptoms of the progressive stages of dementia and to prioritize care. • Teach caregiver how to manage emotions (recognize feelings and deal with them through support groups or counselor). • Teach caregiver to build a collaborative partnership with health care provider to help deal with the personal, social, and financial problems the caregiver will encounter.	• Assess learning from last visit. • Teach caregiver how to control and prevent crisis. • Teach caregiver how to overcome denial through expressing emotions and support groups. • Teach caregiver how to balance needs (caregiver's as well as patient's) with resources. • Teach problem-solving techniques to the caregiver.	• Assess learning from last visit. • Assess for further teaching needs of the caregiver. • Reinforce all teaching with caregiver.
DISCHARGE PLANNING	• Reinforce the use of support groups for patient and caregiver. • Help with making contacts with community support services. • Plan a family meeting to obtain help from patient's other family members if feasible. • Facilitate identification of needs, and plan schedule for intervention from family members.	• Reinforce previous visit.	• Help caregiver evaluate possible options for the patient's final days. • If possible, include the patient in the decision-making process.

- Not experience any skin breakdown (3).
- Remain as independent in ADLs as physical resources will permit (4).
- Sleep 6.5 to 7 hours at night (5).
- Maintain adequate nutrition and fluid intake (6).
- Maintain fluid and electrolyte balance (6).
- Verbalize the disease process of Alzheimer's (7).
- Verbalize ways to maintain optimal health (7,11).
- Maintain optimal independence per physical status (4,8).
- Have a decrease in anxiety (9).
- Feel safe and secure in the environment (9,10).
- Have a decrease in fear (10).
- Be able to balance obligations and responsibilities with minimal disruptions in family members' lives (11).
- Agree to adhere to treatment plan (12).

Other possible nursing diagnoses

Altered role performance, bowel incontinence, diversional activity deficit, ineffective individual coping, impaired social interaction, risk for fluid volume deficit, sensory/perceptual alterations (visual, auditory, kinesthetic, gustatory, tactile, or olfactory), social isolation

Potential complications

Cardiovascular disease, adverse effects of medication therapy

Patient teaching

Patients with dementia have irreversible cognitive deficits and are often unable to participate in the teaching and learning process. Thus, teaching is primarily done with the family caregiver.

Disease process of dementia of the Alzheimer's type

- Early stage: characterized by forgetfulness; trouble concentrating; trouble coping with everyday problems; changes in personality, most commonly apathy, irritability, or sudden outburst of anger; language disturbance; limited problem-solving abilities; limited ability to learn new things
- Middle stage: trouble eating, childlike behavior, failure to perform self-care activities unassisted, trouble communicating and following directions, emotional disinhibition, bowel and bladder incontinence, wandering, pacing and agitation, visual hallucinations, difficulty recognizing family and friends, meaningless words and actions, catastrophic reactions, sundown syndrome
- Late stage: characterized by loss of all cognitive ability, loss of voluntary body functions, extreme difficulty swallowing, significant weight loss, verbal communication limited to guttural sound or mutism, bedridden state, stupor, coma, death

Safety

- Provide adequate low-glare lighting.
- Remove potential dangers (for example, throw rugs).
- Be consistent in environment and routine.
- Use cues (for example, calendars, pictures, clocks) and labels on doors and pictures to promote orientation.
- Provide area for pacing and provide boundaries such as stop signs, locks, and red or yellow tape on the floor to prevent patient from getting lost.
- Schedule rest times.
- Use large block letters to label clothes and objects to promote name recognition.
- Label or use symbols or colors to help patients locate rooms.
- Decrease noise levels.

Communication

- Treat the person with respect and dignity (do not talk down to the patient with terms such as "Pops" or "Honey").
- Approach patient from the front.
- Identify yourself and address the patient by name.
- Speak slowly, clearly, and concisely in a normal unhurried tone of voice.
- Use simple short familiar words.
- Emphasize verbal content with nonverbal gestures to reinforce verbal content.
- Speak in a positive manner (for example, say "Do this." Rather than "Do not do this.").
- Cover one point at a time.
- Use nonverbal communication such as gestures. Make sure verbal and nonverbal communication are congruent.
- Encourage reminiscence and capitalize on long-term memory when communicating.

Nutrition

- Schedule consistent meal times.
- Provide a quiet constant environment with minimal distractions.
- Verbally direct patient through each step of the eating process.
- Serve soft food or food appropriate to patient's state of health, preferences, and so forth.
- Provide finger foods.
- Make food and fluid available and visible.
- Give one food at a time.

Rest

- Establish a nonstimulating bedtime ritual.
- Provide quiet.
- Provide minimal light.
- Provide consistency at bedtime.
- Take to toilet before bedtime.

Support

- Teach the caregiver about the various instrumental support that is available (financial, legal, home repair assistance, hands-on care for the patient).
- Be an advocate and recommend that patients and families obtain legal advice for such things as power of attorney, living will, living trust, conservatorship, will, guardianship, and other legal matters.
- Provide a list of support groups for caregivers and encourage the caregiver to attend meetings.
- Teach the caregiver about respite care.
- Teach the caregiver about resource programs in the community for Alzheimer's patients and caregivers such as psychiatric home care, adult care, outpatient geriopsychiatric clinics, home health care, legal services, and psychiatric hospitals.

Medications

- Teach the family the name, dosage, time of administration, purpose, side effects, and adverse reactions of tacrine.
- Teach the family the titrating process of tacrine (6-week intervals when increasing the dosage).
- Teach the family the importance in obtaining transaminase levels during the titrating process and for maintenance dosages.
- Teach the family that tacrine interacts with other drugs and a doctor should monitor all drugs given to the patient.
- Teach the family to monitor pulse and to notify the doctor if the patient becomes bradycardic.

- Teach the family to monitor for GI bleeding and to notify the doctor if overt or covert bleeding occurs.
- Teach the family that tacrine's beneficial effects diminish over time as Alzheimer's disease progresses.

Critical thinking activities

1. Describe the most effective way to differentiate between dementia and pseudodementia.
2. List the best methods for maintaining memory in demented patients.
3. List and describe the best methods for decreasing symptoms of sundown syndrome.
4. List and describe the best supports for the sandwich generation (middle-aged persons who care for children and demented parents).
5. Discuss the etiologic theories that are hypothesized to cause dementia of the Alzheimer's type.
6. Explain the difference between alexia, acalculia, agraphia, agnosia, astereognosis, auditory agnosia, aphasia, and apraxia, and discuss the techniques used in the assessment process to identify the data for these symptoms.
7. Discuss the differences between dementia and delirium.
8. Discuss nursing interventions that would be used with demented patients who use confabulation, and give the principles and rationale for using these interventions.
9. Identify the issues that would be essential in the assessment of the family of an Alzheimer's patient and discuss the relevance of these factors in relation to care of the patient.
10. Compare and contrast the counseling techniques used with demented patients to those used with patients who have depression, schizophrenia, and anxiety disorders.

Suggested research topics

- Coping strategies for Alzheimer's
- Effectiveness of support groups for Alzheimer's
- Coping strategies for caregivers

Depression

DRG: 426 Mean LOS: 3.9 days

Depression is an emotion characterized by extreme sadness and grief. The term *depression* can denote a variety of phenomena: a sign, symptom, syndrome, emotional state, reaction, disease, or clinical condition. Furthermore, depression is viewed in a continuum and ranges from normal depressive reactions such as grief to mild and moderate depressive states to severe depression with or without psychotic features. In this chapter, depression is viewed as a clinical condition that is severe, maladaptive, and incapacitating.

Depression is the most common and most treatable of all mental illness, affecting one in four people. The lifetime risk of major depressive illness for men is nearly 13%; for women, it is 21%. Furthermore, depression is more common among first-degree relatives of persons with depression. Although depression can occur at any age, the most common age of onset is between ages 25 and 44. There has been an increase in depression in children and adolescents and in those over age 60. Depression appears unrelated to ethnicity, education, income, or marital status.

Substance abuse and anxiety disorders are often concomitant with depression, and the comorbidity of depression and substance abuse is approximately 30%. Depression often accompanies major medical illnesses, such as cardiac problems, cancer, diabetes, epilepsy, multiple sclerosis, and cerebral vascular accidents. Depression is also associated with suicide. In fact, the rate of suicide for depressed people is 18%. Risk factors for suicide include a history of mood disorders, depression, general medical illness, substance abuse, anxiety, and stress. Thus, depression is a mental health problem encountered not only in mental health care delivery settings, but also in primary and specialty health care delivery settings.

Although the exact cause of depression is unknown, it is believed that biological, psychosocial, and sociocultural factors, whether singularly or in combination, play a role in its development. It most likely has a biological basis (and may even be inherited), and the degree and the duration of the disorder are influenced by psychosocial and sociocultural factors. In people with depression, levels of the neurotransmitters serotonin and norepinephrine are decreased while cortisol levels are increased. It is unknown if these imbalances cause depression or if depression itself influences the imbalances. For these reasons, a combination of biological and psychological treatments render the best therapy. For mild forms of depression, psychotherapy alone may be sufficient.

Subjective assessment findings

Health history
Previous depressive episode (number, severity, symptoms, hospitalization, treatment), previous psychiatric problems (type, symptoms, treatment), family history of psychiatric problems, history of suicide attempt

Medication history
Terminal medical problems (for example, cancer, acquired immunodeficiency syndrome), chronic medical problems (for example, diabetes, cardiac disorders), physical trauma (for example, car accident, amputation)

Functional health patterns

Nutrition: decreased appetite, weight loss without dieting, increased appetite, weight gain
Elimination: constipation
Activity-exercise: decreased energy, loss of interest in pleasurable activities
Sleep-rest: insomnia, difficulty falling asleep, midnight awakenings, early morning awakenings, hypersomnia
Cognitive: confusion, inability to concentrate, indecisiveness, obsessive thoughts, suicidal or self-destructive thoughts, slowed thoughts, negative and pessimistic thoughts, difficulty answering, self-doubt, self-blame, somatizing
Self-perception: depressed, apathetic, helpless, hopeless, angry, anxious, low self-esteem, powerless, overwhelmed
Role: withdrawal from family and friends, problems with interpersonal relationships, occupational problems, legal problems
Sexuality: decreased sexual desire, decreased responsiveness, impotence
Coping: ineffective coping, loss of control, use of drugs or alcohol

Objective assessment findings

Psychosocial assessment

Physical appearance: poor personal hygiene, dirty, disheveled, body odor, uncombed dirty hair, unshaved, dirty clothes, bandages on wrists, older or younger than age, deformities, prosthesis, slouched posture
Affect: gloomy, joyless, overwhelmed, powerless, bitter, dejected, despondent, sad, tired, labile, flat, blunted, apathetic, angry, hopeless, tearful, remorseful, anxious, helpless, guilty
Behaviors: crying, tearful, sighing, hypoactive, poor eye contact, passive dependent, robot-like movements, slow movements, slow shuffling gait, withdrawal, lack of spontaneity, irritable, agitated, pacing, wringing of hands, fidgeting
Cognitive: see "Functional Health Patterns"
Speech: mute, mumbles, whispers, soft, slow, slurred, monotone, poverty of speech
Physical: nutrition assessment, sleep patterns
General: physiologic, cognitive, affective, and behavioral symptom of depression

Mental status

Appearance: see "Psychosocial Assessement"
Mood and affect: see "Psychosocial Assessement"
Judgment: intact—depressed people have difficulty making decisions and concentration is decreased, which makes it appear as though judgment is impaired; can become impaired, especially if suicidal or psychotic
Insight: fair
Memory: intact

Suicide assessment

History of suicidal ideation or attempt, present suicidal ideations, plan, lethality of plan, contract for safety

Diagnostic tests

Urinalysis, complete blood count, thyroid profile, chemistry profile, electrocardiogram, other tests as ordered

(Text continues on page 265.)

PLAN OF CARE	PREADMIT PHASE	INPATIENT CARE *Day 1*
DIAGNOSTIC TESTS	▪ There is no preadmit phase because the person will only be admitted to the hospital if they are a threat to themselves or others; this would be an emergency commitment.	▪ Urinalysis ▪ Complete blood count ▪ Thyroid profile and chemistry profile ▪ Other laboratory or diagnostic tests as ordered related to comorbid conditions
MEDICATIONS	▪ Antidepressants	▪ Target symptoms ▪ Antidepressants as ordered ▪ Routine medications as ordered
PROCEDURES	▪ Assess for possible outpatient therapy.	▪ Check vital signs b.i.d. ▪ Give psychosocial assessment every shift and as needed. ▪ Perform suicide assessment per shift and as needed. ▪ Observe for safety via protocol. ▪ Give individual therapy, 15 minutes per shift. ▪ Provide group therapy. ▪ Initiate suicide precautions as indicated.
DIET	▪ Give diet as tolerated (DAT). ▪ Assess for overeating or undereating.	▪ Give DAT. ▪ Encourage small, frequent feedings from all food groups. ▪ Assess eating pattern. ▪ Give nutritional supplement as needed. ▪ Weigh patient before breakfast. ▪ Take calorie count. ▪ Provide preferred snacks and food. ▪ Provide adequate time for meals and snacks. ▪ Give low-tyramine diet if patient is taking monoamine oxidase inhibitor (MAOI).
ACTIVITY	▪ Have patient get out of bed. ▪ Assess for low energy levels. ▪ Assess for decreased interest in activities.	▪ Encourage recreation and therapeutic activity per recreational therapist and therapeutic activity department. ▪ Encourage patient to participate in the activities. ▪ Encourage patient to participate in simple exercise.
ELIMINATION	▪ Assess for constipation.	▪ Measure intake and output. ▪ Administer stool softener or laxative as per order. ▪ Increase fluid intake to 2 to 3 qt (2 to 3 L)/day.
HYGIENE	▪ Assess for poor hygiene.	▪ Assess hygiene of patient. ▪ Encourage daily bath and oral hygiene after each meal and at bedtime. ▪ Encourage female patients to use make-up and male patients to shave. ▪ Assist with any activities as needed.
PATIENT TEACHING	▪ Emergency admission	*Patient and family:* ▪ Explain symptoms of depression. ▪ Explain the basics of neurotransmitters as they relate to depression and antidepressant medication. ▪ Describe antidepressants (name, dosage, schedule, adverse effects, contraindications). ▪ Discuss length of time before therapeutic level is obtained. ▪ If patient is taking an MAOI, teach foods to avoid on a low-tyramine diet. ▪ Discuss psychoeducation sessions. ▪ Evaluate understanding of teaching.
DISCHARGE PLANNING	▪ Emergency admission	▪ Have social worker take psychosocial history. ▪ Assess social support. ▪ Assess family support. ▪ Establish discharge objectives with patient and family.

Day 2	Day 3
• Electrocardiogram • Abnormal values to be reported to doctor	• As indicated
• Same as Day 1	• Same as Day 1
• Same as Day 1	• Same as Day 1
• Same as Day 1	• Same as Day 1
• Same as Day 1	• Same as Day 1
• Same as Day 1	• Same as Day 1
• Same as Day 1	• Same as Day 1
Patient and family: • Teach stress management, including assertiveness training and identification of emotions and appropriate ways of dealing with those emotions. • Teach importance of a daily structured activity plan. • Teach social skills. • Provide psychoeducation sessions. • Evaluate understanding of teaching.	*Patient and family:* • Teach symptoms of relapse. • Teach how to recognize early signs of relapse. • Explain value of relapse action plan. • Provide psychoeducation sessions. • Evaluate understanding of teaching.
Social services consult: • Arrange for home health care as needed, • Assess for support and resource needs (that is, economic status to purchase medications). • Review discharge objectives with patient and family.	• Refer to home health care agency as needed. • Make appointment for follow-up with counselor, psychiatrist, or out-patient care. • Meet with caseworker and family to provide for continuity of care. • Review progress toward discharge objectives with patient and family.

(continued)

CLINICAL PATHWAY ■ **Major depression** *(continued)*

PLAN OF CARE	HOME CARE *Visit 1*	*Visit 2*	*Visit 3*
DIAGNOSTIC TESTS	• If indicated	• If indicated	• If indicated
MEDICATIONS	• Give antidepressants as prescribed. • Assess patient's knowledge of antidepressant (name, dosage, schedule, adverse effects, contraindications). • Assess effectiveness of antidepressants. • Assess compliance with antidepressants. • Stool softeners or laxatives as indicated.	• Give antidepressants as perscribed. • Assess effectiveness of antidepressants. • Assess for compliance with antidepressants. • Stool softeners or axatives as indicated.	• Same as previous visit
PROCEDURES	• Perform psychosocial assessment. • Perform suicide assessment. • Provide 1:1 intervention. • Have patient identify strengths and accomplishments. • Have patient identify goals to work on for next visit. • Teach patient about support groups for depression. • Teach patient about cognitive distortion log and have patient do a log as an assignment.	• Perform psychosocial assessment. • Perform suicide assessment. • Provide 1:1 intervention. • Patient evaluates goals from previous visit. • Discuss content of patient cognitive distortion log. Also role play situations from log and use assertiveness techniques. • Have patient identify goals to work on for next visit. • Have patient continue thought distortion log as homework assignment. • Monitor and increase social interactions. • Evaluate teaching from previous visits.	• Same as previous visit
DIET	• Give diet as tolerated (DAT). • Assess nutritional intake. • Give low tyramine diet if taking a monoamine oxidase inhibitor. • Refer to dietitian if indicated.	• Same as first visit	• Same as first visit
ACTIVITY	• Assess sleep activity. • Assess activity level.	• Same as first visit • Assess for spontaneity.	• Same as previous visit
ELIMINATION	• Encourage fluids 2 to 3 qt (2 to 3 L)/day	• Reinforce previous visit.	• Reinforce previous visit.
HYGIENE	• Encourage hygiene activities.	• Reinforce previous visit.	• Reinforce previous visit.
PATIENT TEACHING	• Teach prevention of relapse (recognize symptoms of depression when they first occur: change in mood, becoming more depressed, decrease in energy, isolating self, not participating in activities, tired, sleep disturbances, appetite changes, suicidal thoughts). • Teach not to stop taking antidepressants unless instructed to by doctor. • Teach how to set up structured daily schedule. • If symptoms do occur, teach the patient to see his doctor or therapist as soon as possible. • Review medication instruction and evaluate understanding.	• Evaluate understanding of previous teaching.	• Evaluate understanding of previous teaching.
DISCHARGE PLANNING	• Emphasize importance of ongoing outpatient care. • Emphasize importance of support group. • Emphasize importance of following antidepressant regimen.	• Reinforce previous visit.	• Reinforce previous visit.

Related nursing diagnoses

1 Risk for self-harm
2 Hopelessness
3 Ineffective individual coping
4 Impaired social interaction
5 Self-esteem disturbance
6 Altered thought processes
7 Fatigue
8 Self-care deficit (bathing/hygiene, feeding, dressing/grooming, or toileting)
9 Sleep pattern disturbance
10 Altered nutrition: More than body requirements
11 Altered nutrition: Less than body requirements

Expected outcomes

The following expected outcomes pertain to the patient or family. Numbers in parentheses refer to related nursing diagnoses above.

- Not harm self (1).
- Verbalize relief of target symptoms (2).
- Verbalize hope for the future (2).
- Use problem-solving skills (3).
- Use assertive techniques, for example, "I" statements (3).
- Demonstrate an ability to adequately cope with stressors (3).
- Utilize strengths and skills in managing current and ongoing stressors (3).
- Verbalize an understanding of a relapse action plan (3).
- Verbalize cues of relapse (3).
- Seek appropriate support groups and referrals to maintain well-being (3,4,5).
- Develop sustaining relationships with friends and family members (4).
- Actively participate in activities on the unit (4).
- Verbalize an understanding of depression (4,6).
- Make positive self-statements (5).
- Express a positive self-perception and self-esteem (5).
- Communicate feelings openly and honestly (5).
- Replace faulty cognitions with realistic interpretations of stressful situations and positive self-perceptions (6).
- Be able to reframe distorted thoughts (6).
- Verbalize an understanding of the antidepressants (6).
- Comply with medication regimen (6).
- Verbalize an understanding of the treatment program (6).
- Maintain adequate rest and activity behaviors (7).
- Attain maximum independent self-care (8).
- Initiate activities of daily living (8).
- Sleep undisturbed for 8 hours per night (9).
- Maintain optimal weight (10,11).
- Not experience constipation (10,11).

Other possible nursing diagnoses

Anxiety, impaired verbal communication, anticipatory grieving, sexual dysfunction

Potential complications

Adverse effects of antidepressant therapy, cardiovascular disease, urine retention, agranulocytosis

Patient teaching

Disease process
- **Causes:** biological, psychosocial, sociocultural
- **Symptoms:** physiologic, cognitive, affective, behavioral
- **Treatments:** psychotropic medications, especially antidepressants; psychotherapy; other treatments such as assertiveness training, exercise, problem solving

Medications
- Instruct patient on name, dosage, time of administration, purpose, and adverse effects of antidepressants.
- Teach the patient and patient's family about the lag time (3 to 4 weeks) before therapeutic effects of the antidepressant can be anticipated. Instruct the patient to keep taking the drug even if there are no noticeable effects. After 4 weeks, if there is no observable improvement, notify the doctor.
- Tell patient to avoid alcohol while taking antidepressants.
- Teach ways to counteract the adverse effects of antidepressants: sucking on hard candy for a dry mouth; eating a high-fiber diet (bran), increasing fruit and vegetable intake, and increasing fluids in the diet for constipation; rising slowly when getting up from a chair or bed because of orthostatic hypotension; using sunscreen and wearing protective clothing because of increased sensitivity to the sun; refraining from driving or operating machinery because of the drowsiness.
- Teach importance of not discontinuing the drug without discussing it with the prescriber.

Techniques to reduce depression
- Assertiveness training
- Social skills
- Cognitive restructuring
- Problem solving
- Relaxation
- Anger management
- Stress reduction
- Attendance at support groups

Preventing recurrence
- Educate the public about the disease concept of depression.
- Teach that depression is treatable and that recovery is the rule and not the exception.
- Encourage patients to adhere to medication regimen
- Reinforce knowledge about depression via reading material, videos, and question and answer sessions with appropriate health care providers.
- Explain the importance of follow-up care with the therapist or psychiatrist.
- Explain the importance of attendance at community support groups.
- Encourage the patient to express feelings in an open and honest manner.
- Remind the patient to use assertiveness techniques when appropriate.
- Suggest that the patient join a club, church, or organization within the community.
- Teach the patient to practice positive self-talk.
- Suggest that the patient exercise daily.
- Tell the patient to avoid fatigue and stressful situations.
- Tell the patient to avoid alcohol and other mood-altering drugs.
- Tell the patient to seek care at the first signs and symptoms of depression: feeling sad, anxious, despondent, pessimistic, negative, tired, irritable, fearful and hopeless, decrease in energy, isolating self, appetite changes and suicidal thoughts.

Education the family
- Take time out, away from the patient.

- Avoid martyrdom.
- Accept their own negative feelings.
- Teach about the disease concept of depression
- Teach about anitdepressants

Critical thinking activities
1. Discuss the relationship, if any, between the multiple roles of women (wife, mother, employee) in today's society and the diagnosis of depression.
2. Detail the difference between men and women in relation to depression, stress, social support, treatment, and relapse.
3. Discuss whether psychotherapy, psychopharmacology, or a combination provides the most effective treatment for depression.
4. Discuss which is the most effective treatment for depression: individual psychotherapy or group psychotherapy.
5. What is the difference between primary and secondary depression?
6. Describe how cultural, social, psychological, and biological influences relate to depression.
7. Describe health promotion and preventive interventions for populations at risk for depression.
8. Compare and contrast grief and depression in terms of etiologies, psychodynamics, assessment, treatments, and outcomes.
9. List the steps involved in conducting a suicide assessment and discuss responses that the nurse will take if the patient reports: (a) no suicidal ideations; (b) suicidal ideations without a plan;(c) suicidal ideations with an ill-defined plan; (d) suicidal ideations with a nonlethal plan; (e) suicidal ideations with a well-defined lethal plan.
10. Discuss the issues of "free choice" and "confidentiality" in relation to a depressed patient who is suicidal.

Suggested research topics
- Coping strategies for depression
- Compliance with therapy
- Effectiveness of psychotherapy
- Effectiveness of psychopharmacology

Panic disorder without agoraphobia (anxiety)

DRG: 425 Mean LOS: 3.5 days

Anxiety is a universal phenomena and can be defined as a subjective feeling of apprehension and helplessness that results from a threat to a person's being, self-esteem, or identity. Although some levels of anxiety may help a person establish a stronger self-esteem or identity, high levels can be detrimental. Excessive anxiety can interfere with interpersonal relationships and social or vocational functioning and therefore have a destructive effect on a person's activities of daily living (ADLs).

There are 11 different types of anxiety disorders, according to the *Diagnostic and Statistical Manual of Mental Disorders*, fourth edition. One of those anxiety disorders is panic disorder without agoraphobia. It is estimated that 3.8% of the population suffers from this disorder. In panic disorder without agoraphobia, the individual experiences the highest level of anxiety: panic. Panic is associated with awe, dread, and terror. A person experiencing a panic attack has disintegration of the personality, causing a loss of control and an inability to communicate or function. Physiologically, a person suffering from a panic attack experiences heart palpitations, chest pain, difficulty breathing, and a feeling of smothering or choking. The major underlying pathology of panic attack is anxiety. Although no physiologic pathology is associated with panic disorders, an individual experiencing a panic attack should have a thorough physical examination to rule out a coexisting cardiac or respiratory problem.

Individuals suffering from anxiety disorders such as panic without agoraphobia are rarely hospitalized for the disorder unless they become depressed, suicidal, or cannot carry out activities of daily living. Most cases are treated in the outpatient or home setting.

Subjective assessment findings

Health history
Panic attacks, family history of psychiatric problems (anxiety and substance abuse)

Medication history
No medical problems. Determine use of benzodiazepines.

Functional health patterns
Health perception–health maintenance: ego dystonia, "Something is wrong," "I get so scared, I can't function"
Activity-exercise: pacing, fidgeting, "can't sit still," trembling, shaking
Cognitive: confusion, preoccupation, rumination, distortion of perception, decreased attention span; fear of choking, smothering, dying, and "going crazy"
Perceptual pattern: depersonalization, chest pain, heart palpitations, heart pounding, shortness of breath, powerlessness, losing control, anxiety, overwhelmed
Role-relationships: withdrawal from social engagements, occupational responsibilities, family and friends, intrapersonal relations
Coping–stress tolerance: ineffective coping, loss of control, use of alcohol and drugs

Objective assessment findings

Psychosocial assessment

Physical appearance: clean, neatly groomed, anxious, sweating, shortness of breath, facial flushing, trembling and shaking

Affect: worried, focused on physical symptoms, scared, jittery, distressed, anxious, anguished, unsteady feelings

Behaviors: pacing, fidgeting, restless

Judgment: impaired during panic attack

Insight: good

Memory: intact

Physical: pulse and respirations elevated, blood pressure elevated

General: nervous, anxious person

Suicide assessment

History of suicidal ideation or attempt, present suicidal ideations, plan, lethality of plan, contract for safety

Diagnostic tests

Complete physical examination, urinalysis, complete blood count, thyroid profile, chemistry profile, electrocardiogram, other tests as indicated by physical examination

Related nursing diagnoses

1 Anxiety
2 Fear
3 Powerlessness
4 Hopelessness
5 Ineffective individual coping
6 Self-esteem disturbance

Expected outcomes

The following expected outcomes pertain to the patient or family. Numbers in parentheses refer to related nursing diagnoses above.

- Comply with medication regimen (1).
- Be able to control anxiety (1,3).
- Verbalize a reduction of anxiety (1,3,4,5).
- Have a reduction in panic attacks (1,2,5).
- Have a reduction in fear during a panic attack (2).
- Learn ways to decrease panic attacks (3,5).
- Be able to function without panic attacks (5).
- Express feelings of well-being (6).

Other possible nursing diagnoses

Impaired verbal communication, impaired social interaction, impaired adjustment, acute confusion, altered thought processes, altered role performance, risk for violence: self-directed or directed at others

Potential complications

Depression, neutropenia, blood dyscrasia, seizures, cardiovascular, urine retention, adverse effects of anti-anxiety therapy

(Text continues on page 273.)

PLAN OF CARE	PREADMIT PHASE	INPATIENT CARE *Day 1*
DIAGNOSTIC TESTS	• Complete physical examination • Chest X-ray • Electrocardiogram • Complete blood count, thyroid profile, chemistry profile • Other tests as indicated	• If indicated
MEDICATIONS	• Drug history	• Target symptoms • Antianxiety drugs as ordered • Antidepressants as ordered
PROCEDURES	• Perform suicide assessment. • Initiate exercise program (breathing, walking). • Begin outpatient therapy.	• Check vital signs b.i.d. • Perform psychosocial assessment every shift and as needed. • Perform suicide assessment every shift and as needed. • Observe for safety via protocol. • Perform individual therapy. • Give group therapy. • Take suicide precautions as indicated. • Have patient begin practicing relaxation techniques.
DIET	• Give diet as tolerated (DAT).	• Give DAT.
ACTIVITY	• Assess ability to perform activities of daily living.	• As tolerated
ELIMINATION		• Assess for deviation from normal.
HYGIENE		• Encourage self-care.
PATIENT TEACHING		*Patient and family:* • Discuss symptoms of panic disorder. • Teach about antianxiety and antidepressant medications: (name, dosage, schedule, adverse effects, contraindications, usual length of time before therapeutic level of antidepressant is obtained). • Describe psychoeducational sessions. • Explain breathing exercises. • Explain progressive muscle relaxation. • Explain visual imagery.
DISCHARGE PLANNING		*Social services consult:* • Assess home care needs.

Note: Patients with panic disorders with agoraphobia are rarely hospitalized because they are not a danger to themselves or others.

CLINICAL PATHWAY ■ **Panic disorder without agoraphobia**

Day 2	Day 3
• If indicated	• If indicated
• Antianxiety drugs as ordered • Antidepressants as ordered	• Same as previous day
• Same as Day 1	• Same as Day 1
• Same as Day 1	• Same as Day 1
• Same as Day 1	• Same as Day 1
• Same as Day 1	• Same as Day 1
• Same as Day 1	• Same as Day 1
• Reinforce previous teaching. • Evaluate previous teaching. • Introduce stress restructuring log.	• Reinforce previous teaching. • Evaluate previous teaching. • Introduce thought stopping. • Introduce concepts of assertiveness.
• Assess resources and support needs.	• Same as previous day

(continued)

PLAN OF CARE	HOME CARE Visit 1	Visit 2	Visit 3
DIAGNOSTIC TESTS	• If indicated	• If indicated	• If indicated
MEDICATIONS	• Assess effectiveness of antianxiety drugs. • Assess effectiveness of antidepressants. • Identify target symptoms.	• Assess effectiveness of antianxiety drugs. • Assess effectiveness of antidepressants. • Assess compliance with medication regimen. • Evaluate knowledge of medications from previous session.	• Same as previous visit
PROCEDURES	• Perform psychosocial assessment. • Perform suicide assessment. • Have patient perform progressive muscle relaxation. • Evaluate patient's goals for anxiety reduction. • Evaluate anxiety or stress reduction log. • Have patient practice breathing exercises. • Monitor outpatient therapy.	• Perform psychosocial assessment. • Perform suicide assessment. • Have patient perform self-evaluation of relaxation goals. • Discuss and evaluate anxiety and stress reduction log (cognitive restructuring). • Have patient perform role playing. • Review patient's goals for anxiety reduction. • Monitor outpatient therapy.	• Perform psychosocial assessment. • Perform suicide assessment. • Have patient perform self-evaluation: relaxation, goals, assertive behaviors, thought stopping. • Discuss and evaluate anxiety or stress reduction log (cognitive restructuring). • Have patient perform role playing. • Review patient's goals for anxiety reduction. • Monitor outpatient therapy.
DIET	• Give diet as tolerated (DAT). • Assess nutritional status.	• Give DAT.	• Same as previous visit
ACTIVITY	• Have patient perform activities as tolerated. • Assess sleep pattern. • Discuss exercise and start daily plan with patient (for example, walking or aerobics).	• Assess benefits of exercise program. • Continue with exercise.	• Same as previous visit
ELIMINATION	• Assess for any problems.	• Same as first visit	• Same as first visit
HYGIENE	• Assess for any problems.	• Same as first visit	• Same as first visit
PATIENT TEACHING	• Discuss disease process of panic disorder. • Review medications: antianxiety agents and antidepressants. • Discuss progressive muscle relaxation. • Review anxiety or stress log. • Teach about support groups.	• Evaluate learning from previous session. • Review thought stopping. • Discuss assertiveness.	• Evaluate learning from previous session. • Review problem-solving techniques and time management.
DISCHARGE PLANNING	• Emphasize importance of ongoing care. • Emphasize importance of support group. • Emphasized importance of compliance with medication regimen.	• Reinforce previous visit. • Emphasize assertiveness.	• Reinforce previous visit. • Emphasize time management and problem solving.

Patient teaching

Disease process
- **Causes:** biologic, psychosocial, sociocultural
- **Symptoms:** physiologic, cognitive, affective, behavioral
- **Treatments:** psychotropic medications (antianxiety drugs and antidepressants); psychotherapy; other treatments such as relaxation exercises, time management, problem solving, and support groups

Antianxiety medications
- Instruct patient on name, dosage, time of administration, purpose, and adverse effects of antianxiety drugs.
- Stress the importance of taking the drug as directed.
- Caution the patient about possible tolerance or psychological and physical dependence.
- Caution not to abruptly stop taking antianxiety drugs because it may lead to withdrawal symptoms.
- Teach about interactions between antianxiety drugs and other drugs, especially alcohol.
- Teach ways to counteract the adverse effects of antianxiety drugs.
- Tell the patient to avoid beverages containing caffeine because it decreases the effect of antianxiety drugs.

Antidepressant medications
- Instruct the patient on name, dosage, time of administration, purpose, and adverse effects of antidepressants.
- Teach the patient and family about the lag time (3 to 4 weeks) before therapeutic effects of antidepressants can be anticipated. Instruct the patient to keep taking the drug even if there are no noticeable effects. After 4 weeks, if there is no observable improvement, notify the doctor.
- Tell the patient to avoid alcohol while taking antidepressants.
- Stress the importance of not discontinuing the drug without discussing it with the prescriber.
- Teach ways to counteract the adverse effects of antidepressants, such as sucking on hard candy for a dry mouth; eating a high-fiber diet (bran), increasing fruit and vegetable intake, and increasing fluids in the diet for constipation; rising slowly when getting up from a chair or bed because of orthostatic hypotension; using sunscreen and wearing protective clothing because of increased sensitivity to the sun; avoiding driving or operating machinery because of the drowsiness.

Coping
- Breathing exercises
- Relaxation techniques
- Meditation
- Cognitive restructuring
- Thought stopping
- Visual imagery
- Assertiveness training
- Exercise
- Problem solving
- Time management
- Attendance at support groups

Preventing recurrence
- Explain that panic disorders are treatable and that recovery is the rule and not the exception.
- Stress the importance of adherence to the medication regimen.
- Remind the patient to use anxiety-reducing techniques at first sign of anxiety or stressful situations.
- Reinforce knowledge about panic disorders via reading material, videos, and question and answer sessions with appropriate health care providers.
- Explain the importance of attendance at community support groups.

- Encourage the patient to express feelings in an open and honest manner.
- Remind the patient to use assertiveness techniques when appropriate.
- Suggest that the patient exercise daily.
- Tell the patient to avoid fatigue and stressful situations.
- Tell the patient to avoid alcohol and other mood-altering drugs.
- Instruct the patient to seek professional care if experiencing feelings of being overwhelmed or other symptoms of losing control.

Educating the family
- Disease concept of panic disorder
- Medications and what to do if the patient has a drug reaction
- Techniques used in behavior therapy and to encourage the patient to perform the techniques

Critical thinking activities

1. Describe the relationship between cognitive and affective cues in anxiety disorders.
2. Discuss the effect on treatment outcomes when the family participates in a systematized program of behavioral therapy reinforcement with patients who have a panic disorder.
3. Detail the difference between panic disorder without agoraphobia and panic disorder with agoraphobia in relation to trait and state anxiety.
4. Discuss the ways in which culture influences the behaviors manifested in anxiety disorders.
5. Discuss the biologic manifestations of panic disorder in relation to the sympathetic and parasympathetic nervous system.
6. Explain the importance of self-evaluation of the nurse's own anxiety in relation to intervening with patients who are experiencing panic attacks.
7. Identify the assessment data for each of the four levels of anxiety (mild, moderate, severe, and panic) in relation to the affective, physiologic, behavioral, and cognitive signs and symptoms of anxiety.
8. Discuss the rationale and importance of doing a comprehensive health assessment with patients who have anxiety disorders, and list the possible coexisting disorders and possible disorders that would be ruled out from the data obtained from this assessment.
9. Compare and contrast psychobiological treatment, psychological treatment, and a combination for patients with panic disorder.
10. Explain the reasons biological theories need to be included in conjunction with psychosocial theories in developing psychoeducation programs for patients with anxiety disorder, their families, and significant others.

Suggested research topics
- Coping strategies for anxiety
- Compliance with therapy
- Effectiveness of behavior therapy

Appendices
Selected references
Index

NANDA-approved nursing diagnoses

The currently accepted classification system for nursing diagnoses is that of the North American Nursing Diagnosis Association (NANDA). It is organized around nine human response patterns: exchanging, communicating, relating, valuing, choosing, moving, perceiving, knowing, and feeling.

The complete taxonomic structure is listed here. The series of numbers before each diagnosis is its classification number, used to determine the placement of the diagnosis within the taxonomy. The number of digits delineates the level of abstraction of the nursing diagnosis (more specific diagnoses are assigned longer numbers).

Pattern 1. Exchanging (Mutual giving and receiving)

1.1.2.1	Altered nutrition: More than body requirements
1.1.2.2	Altered nutrition: Less than body requirements
1.1.2.3	Altered nutrition: Risk for more than body requirements
1.2.1.1	Risk for infection
1.2.2.1	Risk for altered body temperature
1.2.2.2	Hypothermia
1.2.2.3	Hyperthermia
1.2.2.4	Ineffective thermoregulation
1.2.3.1	Dysreflexia
1.2.3.2	Risk for autonomic dysreflexia
1.3.1.1	Constipation
1.3.1.1.1	Perceived constipation
1.3.1.1.2	Colonic constipation
1.3.1.2	Diarrhea
1.3.1.3	Bowel incontinence
1.3.1.4	Risk for constipation
1.3.2	Altered urinary elimination
1.3.2.1.1	Stress incontinence
1.3.2.1.2	Reflex urinary incontinence
1.3.2.1.3	Urge incontinence
1.3.2.1.4	Functional urinary incontinence
1.3.2.1.5	Total incontinence
1.3.2.1.6	Risk for urinary urge incontinence
1.3.2.2	Urinary retention
1.4.1.1	Altered (specify type) tissue perfusion (renal, cerebral, cardiopulmonary, gastrointestinal, peripheral)
1.4.1.2	Risk for fluid volume imbalance
1.4.1.2.1	Fluid volume excess
1.4.1.2.2.1	Fluid volume deficit
1.4.1.2.2.2	Risk for fluid volume deficit
1.4.2.1	Decreased cardiac output
1.5.1.1	Impaired gas exchange

1.5.1.2	Ineffective airway clearance
1.5.1.3	Ineffective breathing pattern
1.5.1.3.1	Inability to sustain spontaneous ventilation
1.5.1.3.2	Dysfunctional ventilatory weaning response (DVWR)
1.6.1	Risk for injury
1.6.1.1	Risk for suffocation
1.6.1.2	Risk for poisoning
1.6.1.3	Risk for trauma
1.6.1.4	Risk for aspiration
1.6.1.5	Risk for disuse syndrome
1.6.1.6	Latex allergy
1.6.1.7	Risk for latex allergy
1.6.2	Altered protection
1.6.2.1	Impaired tissue integrity
1.6.2.1.1	Altered oral mucous membrane
1.6.2.1.2.1	Impaired skin integrity
1.6.2.1.2.2	Risk for impaired skin integrity
1.6.2.1.3	Altered dentition
1.7.1	Decreased adaptive capacity: Intracranial
1.8	Energy field disturbance

Pattern 2. Communicating (Sending messages)

2.1.1.1	Impaired verbal communication

Pattern 3. Relating (Establishing bonds)

3.1.1	Impaired social interaction
3.1.2	Social isolation
3.1.3	Risk for loneliness
3.2.1	Altered role performance
3.2.1.1.1	Altered parenting
3.2.1.1.2	Risk for altered parenting
3.2.1.1.2.1	Risk for altered parent/infant/child attachment
3.2.1.2.1	Sexual dysfunction
3.2.2	Altered family processes
3.2.2.1	Caregiver role strain
3.2.2.2	Risk for caregiver role strain
3.2.2.3.1	Altered family process: Alcoholism
3.2.3.1	Parental role conflict
3.3	Altered sexuality patterns

Pattern 4. Valuing (Assigning relative worth)

4.1.1	Spiritual distress (distress of the human spirit)
4.1.2	Risk for spiritual distress
4.2	Potential for enhanced spiritual well-being

Pattern 5. Choosing (Selecting alternatives)

5.1.1.1	Ineffective individual coping
5.1.1.1.1	Impaired adjustment
5.1.1.1.2	Defensive coping

5.1.1.1.3	Ineffective denial
5.1.2.1.1	Ineffective family coping: Disabling
5.1.2.1.2	Ineffective family coping: Compromised
5.1.2.2	Family coping: Potential for growth
5.1.3.1	Potential for enhanced community coping
5.1.3.2	Ineffective community coping
5.2.1	Ineffective management of therapeutic regimen (individuals)
5.2.1.1	Noncompliance (specify)
5.2.2	Ineffective management of therapeutic regimen: Families
5.2.3	Ineffective management of therapeutic regimen: Community
5.2.4	Effective management of therapeutic regimen: Individual
5.3.1.1	Decisional conflict (specify)
5.4	Health-seeking behaviors (specify)

Pattern 6. Moving (Involving activity)

6.1.1.1	Impaired physical mobility
6.1.1.1.1	Risk for peripheral neurovascular dysfunction
6.1.1.1.2	Risk for perioperative positioning injury
6.1.1.1.3	Impaired walking
6.1.1.1.4	Impaired wheelchair mobility
6.1.1.1.5	Impaired wheelchair transfer ability
6.1.1.1.6	Impaired bed mobility
6.1.1.2	Activity intolerance
6.1.1.2.1	Fatigue
6.1.1.3	Risk for activity intolerance
6.2.1	Sleep pattern disturbance
6.2.1.1	Sleep deprivation
6.3.1.1	Diversional activity deficit
6.4.1.1	Impaired home maintenance management
6.4.2	Altered health maintenance
6.4.2.1	Delayed surgical recovery
6.4.2.2	Adult failure to thrive
6.5.1	Feeding self-care deficit
6.5.1.1	Impaired swallowing
6.5.1.2	Ineffective breast-feeding
6.5.1.2.1	Interrupted breast-feeding
6.5.1.3	Effective breast-feeding
6.5.1.4	Ineffective infant feeding pattern
6.5.2	Bathing or hygiene self-care deficit
6.5.3	Dressing or grooming self-care deficit
6.5.4	Toileting self-care deficit
6.6	Altered growth and development
6.6.1	Risk for altered development
6.6.2	Risk for altered growth
6.7	Relocation stress syndrome
6.8.1	Risk for disorganized infant behavior
6.8.2	Disorganized infant behavior
6.8.3	Potential for enhanced organized infant behavior

Pattern 7. Perceiving (Receiving information)

7.1.1	Body image disturbance
7.1.2	Self-esteem disturbance
7.1.2.1	Chronic low self-esteem
7.1.2.2	Situational low self-esteem
7.1.3	Personal identity disturbance
7.2	Sensory or perceptual alterations (specify visual, auditory, kinesthetic, gustatory, tactile, olfactory)
7.2.1.1	Unilateral neglect
7.3.1	Hopelessness
7.3.2	Powerlessness

Pattern 8. Knowing (Associating meaning with information)

8.1.1	Knowledge deficit (specify)
8.2.1	Impaired environmental interpretation syndrome
8.2.2	Acute confusion
8.2.3	Chronic confusion
8.3	Altered thought processes
8.3.1	Impaired memory

Pattern 9. Feeling (Being subjectively aware of information)

9.1.1	Pain
9.1.1.1	Chronic pain
9.1.2	Nausea
9.2.1.1	Dysfunctional grieving
9.2.1.2	Anticipatory grieving
9.2.1.3	Chronic sorrow
9.2.2	Risk for violence: Self directed or directed at others
9.2.2.1	Risk for self-mutilation
9.2.3	Post-trauma syndrome
9.2.3.1	Rape-trauma syndrome
9.2.3.1.1	Rape-trauma syndrome: Compound reaction
9.2.3.1.2	Rape-trauma syndrome: Silent reaction
9.2.4	Risk for post-trauma syndrome
9.3.1	Anxiety
9.3.1.1	Death anxiety
9.3.2	Fear

National resources

Part 2: Respiratory problems

Allergy and Asthma Network/Mothers of Asthmatics
1554 Chain Bridge Rd., Suite 200
Fairfax, VA 22030
Phone: 1-800-878-4403 or (703) 385-4403
Fax: (703) 352-4354
http://www.podi.com/health/aanma

American Academy of Allergy, Asthma, and
    Immunology
611 East Wells St.
Milwaukee, WI 53202
Phone: 1-800-822-ASTHMA or (414) 272-6071
http://www.aaaai.org

American Association for Respiratory Care
11030 Ables Lane
Dallas, TX 75229
Phone: (972) 243-2272
Fax: (972) 484-2720
webmaster@aarc.org

American College of Allergy, Asthma, and Immunology
85 W. Algonquin Rd., Suite 550
Arlington Heights, IL 60005
Phone: 1-800-842-7777 or (847) 427-1200
Fax: (847) 427-1294
http://allergy.mcg.edu

American Lung Association of Washington
2625 Third Ave.
Seattle, WA 98121-1213
Phone: (206) 441-5100
Fax: (206) 441-3277

American Thoracic Society
1740 Broadway
New York, NY 10019
Phone: (212) 315-8700

Asthma and Allergy Foundation of America
1125 15th St., NW, Suite 502
Washington, DC 20005
Phone: 1-800-7-ASTHMA or (202) 466-7643

Bureau of Tuberculosis Control
New York City Department of Health
125 Worth St.
New York, NY 10012
Phone: (212) 788-4155

Chronic Disease Prevention and Health Promotion
Centers for Disease Control and Prevention
1600 Clifton Rd., N.E.
Atlanta, GA 30333
Phone: (404) 639-3311

National Asthma Education Program Information
    Center
4733 Bethesda Ave., Suite 530
Bethesda, MD 20814
Phone: (301) 951-3260

National Center for Environmental Health
Centers for Disease Control and Prevention
1600 Clifton Rd., N.E.
Atlanta, GA 30333
Phone: (404) 639-3311

National Center for Infectious Diseases
Centers for Disease Control and Prevention
1600 Clifton Rd., N.E.
Atlanta, GA 30333
Phone: (404) 639-3311

National Center for Prevention Services
Centers for Disease Control and Prevention
1600 Clifton Rd., N.E.
Atlanta, GA 30333
Phone: (404) 639-3311

National Home Oxygen Patients Association
http://members.aol.com/nhopa/index.htm

National Institute for Occupational Safety and Health
Centers for Disease Control and Prevention
1600 Clifton Rd., N.E.
Atlanta, GA 30333
Phone: (404) 639-3311

National Tuberculosis Center
University of Medicine and Dentistry of New Jersey
Executive Office, Suite GB1
65 Bergen St.
Newark, NJ 07107-3001
Phone: (973) 972-3270
Fax: (973) 3268
Info Line: 1-800-4TB-DOCS (482-3627)

Office on Smoking and Health
National Centers for Chronic Disease Prevention and
    Health Promotion
Centers for Disease Control and Prevention
1600 Clifton Rd., N.E.
Atlanta, GA 30333
Phone: (404) 639-3311

Office of Disease Prevention and Health Promotion
P. O. Box 1133
Washington, DC 20013-1133
Phone: (202) 205-8611
http://mhic-nt.health.org

Part 3: Cardiovascular problems

American College of Cardiology
Heart and Healthlinks
http://www.acc.org

American Heart Association
7320 Greenville Ave.
Dallas, TX 75231
Phone: (214) 373-6300
http://www.amhet.org
http://www.americanheart.org

American Association of Critical Care Nurses
One Civic Plaza, Suite 330
Newport Beach, CA 92660
Phone: (714) 644-9310

American College of Cardiology
Heart House
9111 Old Georgetown Rd.
Bethesda, MD 20814-1699
Phone: 1-800-253-4636
Phone: (301) 897-5400
Fax: (301) 897-9745
http://www.acc.org

Coronary Club
9500 Euclid Ave.
Cleveland, OH 44106
Phone: (216) 444-3690

Heartlife
P. O. Box 54305
Atlanta, GA
Phone: (770) 952-1316

Heartmates
(An online resource for patients and loved ones to learn
    about cardiovascular care)
P.O. Box 16202
Minneapolis, MN 55416
Phone: 1-800-9HM-3331
Fax: (612) 929-6395
http://www.heartmates.com

High Blood Pressure Information Center
4733 Bethesda Ave., Suite 530
Bethesda, MD 20814
Phone: (301) 951-3260

Hypertension Network, Inc.
E-mail: info@bloodpressure.com

Midwest Heart Prevention Center
3825 Highland Ave., Tower #2, Suite 400
Downers Grove, IL 60515

National Heart, Lung, and Blood Institute
National Institutes of Health
9000 Rockville Pike
Building 31, Room 4A21
Bethesda, MD 20892
Phone: (301) 496-4236

Pulmonary Hypertension Association
P.O. Box 24733
Speedway, IN 46224-0733
Phone: 1-800-74-UPAPH

Renal-Electrolyte and Hypertension Division
University of Pennsylvania
700 Clinical Research Building
415 Curie Blvd.
Philadelphia, PA 19104-6144
Phone: (215) 662-3601
Fax: (215) 898-0189

Part 4: Metabolic function problems

Agency for Health Care Policy and Research, Public
    Health Service
Department of Health and Human Services
Acute Pain Management: Clinical Practice Guidelines
2101 East Jefferson St.
Rockville, MD 20852
Washington, DC, 1992

American Association of Diabetes Educators
444 N. Michigan Ave., Suite 1240
Chicago, IL 60611-3910
http://www.aadenet.org

American Diabetes Association
1660 Duke St.
Alexandria, VA 22314
Phone: 1-800-ADA-DISC or 232-3472

American Pain Society
4700 W. Lake Ave.
Glenview, IL 60025-1485
Phone: (847) 375-4715

American Society of Pain Management Nurses
2755 Bristol St., Suite 110
Costa Mesa, CA 92626
Phone: (714) 545-1305

Association for Professionals in Infection Control and
  Epidemiology
P. O. Box 79502
Baltimore, MD
Phone: (202) 296-2742
http://www.apic.org

Canadian Diabetes Association
15 Toronto St., Suite 1001
Toronto, Canada M5C2E3
Phone: (416) 363-3373
http://www.diabetes.ca

Diabetes Educational Research Center
Franklin Medical Building
829 Spruce St., Suite 302
Philadelphia, PA 19107
Phone: (215) 829-3426
http://www.liberty.net.org

Hospital Infections Program
National Center for Infectious Diseases
Centers for Disease Control and Prevention
1600 Clifton Rd. N.E.
Atlanta, GA 30333
Phone: (404) 639-3311
http://www.cdc.gov/ncidod/hip/hip.htm

National Diabetes Information Clearinghouse
Box NDIC
9000 Rockville Pike
Bethesda, MD 20892
Phone: (301) 468-2162

Oncology Nursing Society
501 Holiday Dr.
Pittsburgh, PA 15220-2749
Phone: (412) 921-7373

Pain Resources
http://www.pain.com

Part 5: Cancer

American Cancer Society
1599 Clifton Rd., N.E.
Atlanta, GA 30329-4251
Phone: (404) 329-7617
Phone: 1-800-ACS-2345
http://www.cancer.org
ACS Programs:
• Reach to Recovery
• Look Good, Feel Better
• I Can Cope

American Lung Association
1740 Broadway
New York, NY 10019
Phone: 1-800-LUNG-USA (1-800-586-4872)

American Society of Clinical Oncology
435 N. Michigan Ave., Suite 1717
Chicago, IL 60611-4067
Phone: (312) 644-0828
Fax: (312) 644-8557

Bone Marrow Transplant Family Support Network
P.O. Box 845
Avon, CT 06001
Phone: 1-800-826-9376
Phone: 1-800-Marrow2 (National Donor Line)

Cancer Care, Inc. and the National Care Center
  Foundation
1180 Ave. of the Americas
New York, NY 10036
Phone: (212) 302-2400
Phone: 1-800-813-HOPE
Fax: (212) 719-0263
E-mail: cancercare@aol.com

Leukemia Research Foundation
http://www.leukemiaresearch.org

Leukemia Society of America
Phone: 1-800-955-4LSA
http://www.leukemia.org

Make Today Count
Mid America Cancer Center
1235 East Cherokee
Springfield, MO 65804-2263
Phone: (417) 885-2273
Phone: 1-800-432-2273
Fax: (417) 888-7426

National Alliance of Breast Cancer Organizations
Phone: 1-800-719-9154
http://www.nabco.org

National Coalition for Cancer Survivorship
1010 Wayne Ave., 5th Floor
Silver Spring, MD 20910
Phone: (301) 650-8868
Fax: (301) 565-9670

National Hospice Organization
1901 North Moore St., Suite 901
Arlington, VA 22209
Phone: (703) 243-5900
Phone: 1-800-658-8898 (hospice helpline)
Fax: (703) 525-5762
E-mail: drsho@cais.com

Office of Cancer Communications
National Cancer Institute
National Institutes of Health
Bethesda, MD 20892
Phone: (301) 496-5583
Cancer Information Service: 1-800-4-CANCER

Oncology Nursing Society
501 Holiday Dr.
Pittsburgh, PA 15220-2749
Phone: (412) 921-7373
Fax: (412) 921-6565

Susan G. Komen Breast Cancer Foundation
Phone: 1-800-462-9273 (1-800-I'M AWARE)
http://www.komen.org

Y-ME National Breast Cancer Organization
Phone: 1-800-221-2141
http://www.y-me.org

Part 6: Renal disorders

Alliance for Aging Research (bladder training)
2021 K St., N.W., Suite 305
Washington, DC 20006

American Academy of Male Sexual Health
Norm Bowers, Executive Director
3101 Broadway, Suite 585
Kansas City, MO 64111
Phone: (816) 931-4455
Phone: 1-800-327-1885
Fax: (816) 561-7765
E-mail: robstan@robstan.com/aamsh/

American Association of Genitourinary Surgeons
Stuart Howards, MD, Secretary-Treasurer
University of Virginia Hospital
Box 422
Charlottesville, VA 22908
Phone: (804) 924-2224

American Association of Kidney Patients
100 South Ashley Dr., Suite 280
Tampa, FL 33602
Phone: (813) 223-7099
Phone: 1-800-749-2257
Fax: (813) 223-0001
http://cybermart.com/aakpaz/aakp.html

American Association of Kidney Patients
1 Davis Blvd., Suite LL1
Tampa, FL 33606
Phone: (813) 251-0725

American Foundation for Urologic Disease, Inc.
300 W. Pratt St., Suite 401
Baltimore, MD 21201

American Prostate Society
Claude Gerard, Chairman
1340-F Charwood Rd.
Hanover, MD 21076
Phone: (410) 859-3735

Continence Restored, Inc.
785 Park Ave.
New York, NY 10021

Family Focus Newsletter
National Kidney Foundation, Inc.
30 East 33rd St.
New York, NY 10016
Phone: 1-800-622-9010

For Patients Only Magazine
20335 Ventura Blvd., Suite 400
Woodland Hills, CA 91364
Phone: (818) 704-5555

Help for Incontinent People
P.O. Box 544
Union, SC 29379

Kidney Disease: A Guide for Patients and Their Families
American Kidney Fund
6110 Executive Blvd., Suite 1010
Rockville, MD 20852
Phone: 1-800-638-8299

National Kidney Foundation Patient Education Brochures
National Kidney Foundation, Inc.
30 E. 33rd St.
New York, NY 10016
Phone: 1-800-622-9010

National Kidney and Urologic Diseases Information
     Clearinghouse
Box KNUDIC
9000 Rockville Pike
Bethesda, MD 20892
Phone: (301) 654-4415

Renalife Magazine
American Association of Kidney Patients
Davis Blvd., Suite LL1
Tampa, FL 33606
Phone: (813) 251-0725

SIMON Foundation for Continence
P.O. Box 835
Wilmette, IL 60091

Understanding Kidney Transplantation
Edith T. Oberley, MA, and Neal R. Glass, MD, FACS
Charles C. Thomas Publishers, 1987
2600 S. First St.
Springfield, IL 62794-9265

*Your New Life With Dialysis — A Patient Guide for
Physical and Psychological Adjustment*
Edith T. Oberley, MA, and Terry D. Oberley, MD, PhD
Fourth Edition, 1991
Charles C. Thomas Publishers
2600 S. First St.
Springfield, IL 62794-9265

Part 7: Musculoskeletal problems

M & M Orthopedics
4115 Fairview Ave.
Downers Grove, IL 60515
Phone: (630) 968-1881
E-mail: moreinfo@mmortho.com

Roll-A-Bout Corporation
1124 Charles Dr.
Dover, DE 19904
Phone: (302) 736-6151

Dr. Thomas Schneider
Heinrich Heine University
Dept. of Orthopaedic Surgery
Moorenstr. 5
40225 Dusseldorf, Germany
E-mail: orthopae@uni-duesseldorf.de

United Amputee Services Association, Inc.
P.O. Box 4277
Winter Park, FL 32793
Phone: (407) 678-2920
Fax: (407) 678-2203

Part 8: Neurologic problems

American Heart Association — Stroke Connection
7272 Greenville Ave.
Dallas, TX 75231-4596
Phone: (214)373-6300
http://www.americanheart.org

The American Parkinson's Disease Association, Inc.
60 Bay St., Suite 401
Staten Island, NY 10301
Phone: 1-800-223-2732

Cushioning Solutions, Inc.
31093 Scappoose Highway
Scappoose, OR 97056
Phone: (503) 543-7679
Phone: 1-888-437-4535

Division of Neurosurgery
Allegheny General Hospital
320 E. North Ave.
Pittsburgh, PA 15212
Phone: (412) 359-6200
E-mail: bost@pgh.auhs.edu

Robert A. Fink, M.D., F.A.C.S.
2500 Milvia St., Suite 222
Berkeley, CA 94704-2636
Phone: (510) 849-2555
Fax: (510) 849-2557
E-mail: rafink@ibm.net

Mayo Foundation for Medical Education and Research
E-mail: mayo.ivi.com/mayo/library/htm/disease/htm

National Institute of Neurological Disorders and Stroke
National Institutes of Health
Bethesda, MD 20892
E-mail: ninds.nih.gov/orgznhp.htm

National Parkinson Foundation, Inc.
1501 NW 9th Ave., Bob Hope Rd.
Miami, FL 33136-1494
Phone: 1-800-433-7022

National Stroke Association
96 Inverness Dr. East, Suite I
Englewood, Colorado 80112-5112
Phone: (303) 649-9299
Fax: (303) 649-1328

Northstar Enterprises
3755 Avocado Blvd. #410
La Mesa, CA 91941
Phone: (619) 462-3738
Phone: 1-800-628-4997
Fax: (619) 462-4909
E-mail: twinflex@twinflex.com

Parkinson's Action Network
822 College Ave., Suite C
Santa Rosa, CA 95404
Phone: (707) 544-1994

Parkinson's Disease Foundation
650 W. 168th St.
New York, NY 10032
Phone: (212) 923-4700
Phone: 1-800-457-6676

United Parkinson's Foundation
833 W. Washington Blvd.
Chicago, IL 60607
Phone: (312) 733-1893

Part 9: Bowel elimination problems

American Cancer Society
1599 Clifton Rd., N.E.
Atlanta, GA 30329-4251
Phone: (404) 329-7617
Phone: 1-800-ACS-2345
http://www.cancer.org

Oncology Nursing Society
501 Holiday Dr.
Pittsburgh, PA 15220-2749
Phone: (412) 921-7373
Fax: (412) 921-6565
http://www.ons.org

United Ostomy Association
19772 MacArthur Blvd., Suite 200
Irvine, CA 92612
Phone: (714) 660-8624
Phone: 1-800-826-0826

Part 10: Pressure ulcers

American Academy of Wound Management
Kennedy Causeway, Suite 109
North Bay Village, FL 33141
Phone: (305) 866-9592
E-mail: Woundnet@aol.com

National Pressure Ulcer Advisory Panel
SUNY at Buffalo, Beck Hall
Main St.
Buffalo, NY 14214
Phone: (716) 662-8721
Fax: (716) 662-8804
http://www.npuap.org

U.S. Department of Health & Human Services
Public Health Service
Agency for Health Care Policy and Research
Executive Office Building, Suite 501
East Jefferson St.
Rockville, MD 20852

Wound, Ostomy and Continence Nurses Society
S. Coast Highway, Suite 201
Laguna Beach, CA 92651
Phone: 1-888-224-WOCN
http://www.wocn.org

Part 11: Psychiatric disorders

Alzheimer's Association
919 N. Michigan Ave., Suite 1000
Chicago IL 60611-1676
Phone: 1-800-272-3900

Alzheimer's Disease International
12 S. Michigan Ave.
Chicago, IL 60603
Phone: (312) 335-5777

American Association of Homes and Services for the
    Aging
901 E. St. N.W., Suite 500
Washington, DC 20004-2037
Phone: (202) 783-2242

American Society of Aging
833 Market St., Suite 512
San Francisco, CA 94103-1824
Phone: (415) 882-2910

Anxiety Disorders Association of America
6000 Executive Blvd.
Rockville, MD 20852
Phone: (301) 231-9350

Association for the Advancement of Behavior Therapy
305 7th Ave., Suite 16A
New York, NY 10001
Phone: (212) 647-1890

Center for the Study of Aging
706 Madison Ave.
Albany, NY 12208
Phone: (518) 465-6927

Children of Aging Parents
1609 Woodbourne Rd., Suite 302A
Levittown, PA 19057
Phone: 1-800-227-7294

Freedom From Fear
308 Seaview Ave.
Staten Island, NY 10305
Phone: (718) 351-1717

National Alliance for the Mentally Ill
200 N. Glebe Rd., Suite 1015
Arlington, VA 22203-3754
Phone: 1-800-950-6264

National Anxiety Foundation
3435 Custer Dr.
Lexington KY 40517
Phone: (606) 272-7166

National Depressive and Manic-Depressive Association
730 N. Franklin Square, Suite 501
Chicago, IL 60610
Phone: (312) 642-0049

National Foundation for Depressive Illness
P.O. Box 2257
New York, NY 10116
Phone: (212) 370-7190

National Institute of Mental Health
Information Resources and Inquiries Branch
5600 Fishers Lane, Room 7C-02
Rockville, MD 20857
Phone: (301) 443-4513
Phone: 1-800-421-4211 (depression awareness,
    recognition and treatment information)

National Institute of Mental Health
Panic Disorder Education Program
5600 Fishers Lane, Room 7C-02
Rockville, MD 20857
Phone: 1-800-64-PANIC

National Institute on Aging
Public Information Office
Federal Building, Room 5C27, Building 31
9000 Rockville Place
Bethesda, MD 20892
Phone: (301) 496-1752

The Psychiatric Institute of Washington
4228 Wisconsin Ave., N.W.
Washington, DC 20016
Phone: 1-800-369-2273

San Francisco Alzheimer's and Dementia Clinic
909 Hyde St., Suite 230
San Francisco, CA 94109
Phone: (415) 673-4600
Fax: (415) 673-9532
E-mail: SFHACLIN@aol.com

Suicide Prevention Center
184 Salem Ave.
Dayton, OH 45406
Phone: (513) 297-4777

Selected references

Arnold, E.N. "The Journey Clouded by Cognitive Disorders," in *Mental Health Nursing: The Nurse-Patient Journey.* Edited by Carson, V.B., and Arnold, E.N. Philadelphia: W.B. Saunders, 1996.

Baily, K.P. *Psychotropic Drug Facts.* Philadelphia: Lippincott-Raven Pubs., 1998.

Black, J. M., and Mattassarin-Jacobs, E. *Medical-Surgical Nursing,* 5th ed. Philadelphia: W.B. Saunders, 1997.

Carpenito, L. *Nursing Diagnosis: Application to Clinical Practice,* 7th ed. Philadelphia: Lippincott-Raven Pubs., 1997.

Farnsworth, B.J., and Biglow, A.S. "Psychiatric Case Management," in *Comprehensive Psychiatric Nursing,* 5th ed. Edited by Haber, J., et al. St. Louis: Mosby–Year Book, Inc., 1997.

Groenwald, S., et al. *Cancer Nursing: Principles and Practice,* 4th ed. Boston: Jones & Bartlett, 1997.

Guinane, C. *Clinical Care Pathways.* New York: McGraw-Hill, 1997.

Haber, J. "Mood Disorders," in *Comprehensive Psychiatric Nursing,* 5th ed. Edited by Haber, J., et al. St. Louis: Mosby–Year Book, Inc., 1997.

Haist, S.A., et al. *Internal Medicine on Call,* 2nd ed. Stamford, Conn.: Appleton & Lange, 1997.

Hess, C. *Nurse's Clinical Guide to Wound Care,* 2nd ed. Springhouse, Pa.: Springhouse Corporation, 1997.

Krainovich-Miller, K. "Anxiety Disorders," in *Comprehensive Psychiatric Nursing,* 5th ed. Edited by Haber, J., et al. St. Louis: Mosby–Year Book, Inc., 1997.

Lewis, S., et al. *Medical-Surgical Nursing: Assessment and Management of Clinical Problems,* 4th ed. St. Louis: Mosby–Year Book, Inc., 1996.

Makelbust, J., and Sieggreen, M. *Pressure Ulcers: Guidelines for Prevention and Nursing Management,* 2nd ed. Springhouse, Pa.: Springhouse Corporation, 1996.

Nursing Facts. Managed Care: Challenges and Opportunities for Nursing. Kansas City, Mo.: American Nurses Association, 1995.

Perry, A. and Potter, P. *Clinical Nursing Skills and Techniques,* 4th ed. St. Louis: Mosby–Year Book, Inc., 1998.

Resnick, W.M., and Carson, V.B. "The Journey Colored by Mood Disorders," in *Mental Health Nursing: The Nurse-Patient Journey.* Edited by Carson, V.B., and Arnold, E.N. Philadelphia: W.B. Saunders, 1996.

Richardson, K.W., and McMahon, A.L. "Delirium, Dementia and Amnesic and Other Cognitive Disorders," in *Comprehensive Psychiatric Nursing,* 5th ed. Edited by Haber, J., et al. St. Louis: Mosby–Year Book, Inc., 1997.

Robinson, L. "The Journey Threatened by Stress and Anxiety," in *Mental Health Nursing: The Nurse-Patient Journey.* Edited by Carson, V.B., and Arnold, E.N. Philadelphia: W.B. Saunders, 1996.

St. Anthony's DRG Guidebook 1997. Reston, Va.: St. Anthony Publishing, 1996.

Skidmore-Roth, L. *Mosby's Drug Guide for Nurses.* St. Louis: Mosby–Year Book, Inc., 1996.

Smeltzer, S., and Bare, B. *Brunner and Sudarth's Textbook of Medical-Surgical Nursing,* 8th ed. Philadelphia: Lippincott-Raven Pubs., 1996.

Standards of Clinical Nursing Practice. Kansas City, Mo.: American Nurses Association, 1993.

Thompson, J., et al. *Mosby's Clinical Nursing,* 4th ed. St. Louis: Mosby–Year Book, Inc., 1997.

Tucker, S.M., et al. *Patient Care Standards: Collaborative Practice Guides,* 6th ed. St. Louis: Mosby–Year Book, Inc., 1996.

Zander, K. "Evolving Mapping and Case Management for Capitation, Part III: Getting Control of Value," in *The New Definition,* vol. 11, 2. South Natick, Mass.: The Center for Case Management, Inc., 1996.

Index

t refers to a table.

t refers to a table.

t refers to a table.

t refers to a table.

t refers to a table.

t refers to a table.

W

White blood cells
  acute myelogenous leukemia and,
    90
  myocardial infarction and, 67
  respiratory problems and, 15, 29,
    39
Wound and skin consults, 138t
Wound cultures, 83, 145
Wound, ostomy, continence nurse,
    222t, 224t, 230t, 239t, 242t

X

X-rays
  chest. *See* Chest X-ray.
  colon, bowel surgery and, 197, 211
  for joint replacements, 153, 161
  skull, neurologic problems and,
    171, 189
  spine, for lumbar laminectomy,
    180

YZ

Y-ME, 98t

t refers to a table.